# Genetic Consultations in the Newborn

# Genetic Consultations in the Newborn

Robin D. Clark, MD and Cynthia J. Curry, MD

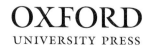

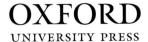

Oxford University Press is a department of the University of Oxford. It furthers
the University's objective of excellence in research, scholarship, and education
by publishing worldwide. Oxford is a registered trade mark of Oxford University
Press in the UK and certain other countries.

Published in the United States of America by Oxford University Press
198 Madison Avenue, New York, NY 10016, United States of America.

CIP data is on file at the Library of Congress
ISBN 978–0–19–999099–3

9 8 7 6 5 4 3 2 1

Printed by Sheridan Books, Inc., United States of America

# Contents

# Preface

In recent decades, stunning advances in neonatal medicine have dramatically reduced the morbidity and mortality of prematurity, sepsis, and respiratory distress. However, as the outcome for these conditions has improved, neonatal medicine has increasingly focused on addressing the needs of patients with congenital anomalies. Concurrently, astonishing progress in clinical genetics and genomics has facilitated diagnosis and delineation of both common and rare malformations and syndromes.

This book was written to assist clinicians who care for newborns with congenital abnormalities in their diagnosis, genomic testing, and management. Our goal was to make the evaluation of common neonatal anomalies and genetic syndromes accessible and understandable. In addition, we hoped that this book might serve as an initial guide for practitioners in areas where clinical genetic expertise is not readily available. As we wrote this book, the testing paradigm shifted to a genomic approach: Chromosome analysis gave way to microarrays, and single gene testing was largely replaced by gene panels and exome sequencing. This book, which was initially intended as a clinical primer, of necessity became a resource for gene-based information as well. Despite our frequent revisions, advances in genetic and genomic testing are certain to outpace the editing process.

We carefully considered how to simplify this complex subject matter to make it easier to use in a busy inpatient intensive care nursery. The 42 main chapters, written in a bulleted format, each focus on a different malformation or common clinical problem, such as hydrocephalus, hypotonia, or the growth-restricted infant, in which genetic diagnoses feature prominently in the differential diagnosis. Each chapter begins with a story—a brief case history illustrating a learning point. Malformations are defined and characterized as isolated or syndromic. Background information is followed by a differential diagnosis and a short guide to evaluation and management. Syndromic descriptions are brief, but the interested reader can obtain additional, updated information through links and references. For this purpose, we have included the unique MIM number that identifies each single gene disorder in the online database Mendelian Inheritance in Man. Most chapters contain "pearls" of practical information gleaned from our combined experience that have rarely been reported in the medical literature. The book concludes with short summaries of 19 conditions that are commonly diagnosed in neonates, focusing on features that make these syndromes recognizable as well as key points in their management. We used photographs of affected infants, whenever possible, to illustrate the phenotypes at this young age. We are grateful to the many colleagues and patient support organizations that contributed photographs to this effort.

Space constraints forced us to omit some and limit other topics. The differential diagnoses are broad but not encyclopedic. Some anomalies that might have filled a chapter of their own (e.g., duodenal atresia, tracheoesophageal fistula, vertebral anomalies and seizures) have been reviewed in an abbreviated form in a differential diagnosis or were left for possible inclusion in a future edition. Similarly, we could not include many biochemical and metabolic disorders, which could have filled their own book.

Six years after we began, we delivered this book to our patient publisher. The effort involved in writing this book far exceeded our projections, but it is clear to both of us that this joint effort, marked by mutual dedication and hard work, is a better book than either of us could have written alone. This book is not a substitute for a comprehensive genetic consultation by an experienced clinical geneticist or dysmorphologist, but it may provide the framework for initiating a complex workup in the nursery, neonatal intensive care unit, or office setting. We hope it offers timely assistance to you, your precious patients, and their deserving families.

Cynthia J. Curry, MD, and Robin D. Clark, MD
May 2018

# Acknowledgments

We thank our generous colleagues who provided expert opinions, guidance, and advice during the preparation of this book: John C. Carey, Dian Donnai, William Dobyns, Donna J. Eteson, Jamie Fisher, June-Anne Gold, Karen Gripp, Judith G. Hall, Julie Hoover-Fong, Louanne Hudgins, Kathreen Johnston, Kenneth L. Jones, Marilyn Jones, Jennifer Kalish, Deborah Krakow, Subhadra Ramanathan, Bianca Russell, Eric Villain, Andrew Wilkie, Elizabeth Woods, and any others we may have inadvertently omitted. We owe more than can be acknowledged here to our ever-inspiring mentors: Michael Baraitser, Bryan Hall, Charles Epstein,* David Rimoin,* and Robin Winter.* Our colleagues and genetic support groups who kindly provided photographs are acknowledged in each chapter.

We offer our thanks to the many neonatologists whose referrals and timely photos made this book possible, including David Aguilar, Douglas Deming, Stephen Elliott, Isabel Escalante, Angela Flores, Andrew Hopper, Alok Kumar, Shahriar Mokrian, Juanito Novales, Richard Peverini, William Phaklides, Anand Rajani, Krishna Rajani, Allan Wolpe.

Special thanks goes to Francis Fung, graphic designer at UCSF/Fresno, and Emily Kishibay for scanning countless slides and photographs.

We are grateful to the staff at Oxford University Press for their patience and flexibility, with particular thanks to our editors, Chad Zimmerman and Chloe Layman, for their unfailing encouragement, ready availability, and sound advice.

This book would not exist without our newborn patients. It has been and continues to be a privilege to work with deeply committed and caring families and their inspiring children during what is often the most difficult times of their lives. Through the decades, they have been our teachers as well as our patients. Our gratitude goes to them all.

Last here but first in our hearts, we thank our families: spouses Bjorn Nilson (CJC) and Terry Long (RDC) and our children and grandchildren. May they forgive us for many late dinners, lost evenings and weekends, and missed family events. Their love and support have made this long effort possible.

Robin D. Clark and Cynthia J. Curry
August 2018

*Deceased.

* Syndromes that appear with an asterisk (*) in the text are discussed more extensively in their own chapters. The authors ask that readers consult the table of contents for maximum clinical utility in these cases.

# Abbreviations

| | |
|---|---|
| 4p-, 5p-, 22q- | chromosome deletion syndromes for 4p, 5p, or 22q |
| AAP | American Academy of Pediatrics |
| ACE | angiotensin-converting enzyme |
| ADHD | attention deficit hyperactivity disorder |
| AED | antiepileptic drug |
| AFI | amniotic fluid index |
| AFP | α-fetoprotein |
| AIDS | acquired immune deficiency syndrome |
| aOR | adjusted odds ratio |
| AP | anteroposterior |
| ARM | anorectal malformation |
| ART | assisted reproductive technology |
| ASD | atrial septal defect |
| AV | atrioventricular |
| AVM | arteriovenous malformation |
| AVSD | atrioventricular septal defect |
| BAV | bicuspid aortic valve |
| BMI | body mass index |
| BP | breakpoint |
| BUN | blood urea nitrogen |
| BW | birth weight |
| $Ca^{2+}$ | serum calcium level |
| CBC | complete blood count |
| CDC | Centers for Disease Control and Prevention |
| CDH | congenital diaphragmatic hernia |
| CDP | chondrodysplasia punctata |
| cfDNA | cell-free DNA (test) |
| CHD | congenital heart disease or defects |
| Chr | chromosome |
| CI | confidence interval |
| CINCA | chronic infantile neurological cutaneous articular |
| CK | creatine kinase |
| CL | cleft lip |
| CLO | cleft lip only (without cleft palate) |
| CL/P | cleft lip with or without cleft palate |
| CLP | cleft lip with cleft palate |

| | | | | |
|---|---|---|---|---|
| CMV | cytomegalovirus | | ID | intellectual disability |
| CNS | central nervous system | | IDM | infant of a diabetic mother |
| CNV | copy number variant | | IgA | immunoglobulin A |
| CoA | coarctation of the aorta | | IGF | insulin-like growth factor |
| CoQ10 | coenzyme Q10 (ubiquinone) | | IgG | immunoglobulin G |
| CP | cleft palate | | IgM | immunoglobulin M |
| CPAP | continuous positive airway pressure | | IQ | intelligence quotient |
| CPK | creatine phosphokinase | | IUFD | intrauterine fetal demise |
| CPO | cleft palate only (without cleft lip) | | IUGR | intrauterine growth retardation |
| CSF | cerebrospinal fluid | | IVC | inferior vena cava |
| CT | computerized tomography | | LBW | low birth weight |
| CTD | conotruncal defect | | LCHAD | long-chain 3-hydroxyacyl-CoA dehydrogenase |
| CVS | chorionic villous sampling | | LCMV | lymphocytic choriomeningitis virus |
| CVSD | conoventricular septal defect | | LGA | large for gestational age |
| CSVT | cerebral sinus venous thrombosis | | LL | lower limb |
| DA/DC | diamniotic dichorionic (twins) | | LVOTO | left ventricular outflow tract obstruction |
| DD | developmental disability | | MAC | microphthalmia/anophthalmia/coloboma |
| DEB | diepoxybutane | | MC/DA | monochorionic diamniotic (twins) |
| DES | diethylstilbesterol | | MC/MA | monochorionic monoamniotic (twins) |
| DEXA | dual-energy X-ray absorptiometry | | MCV | mean corpuscular volume |
| DI | diabetes insipidus | | MIM | Mendelian Inheritance in Man (database) |
| DM | diabetes mellitus | | MLPA | multiplex ligation-dependent probe amplification (test for duplications/deletions) |
| DNA | deoxyribonucleic acid | | | |
| DORV | double-outlet right ventricle | | MMF | mycophenolate mofetil |
| DSD | disorder of sex development | | MMI | methimazole |
| dTGA | d-transposition of the great arteries | | MoM | multiple of the median |
| DVT | deep venous thrombosis | | mPKU | maternal phenylketonuria |
| DWM | Dandy–Walker malformation | | MRA | magnetic resonance angiography |
| DZ | dizygotic (twins) | | MRI | magnetic resonance imaging |
| ECG | electrocardiogram | | MSAFP | maternal serum α-fetoprotein |
| ECMO | extracorporeal membrane oxygenation | | mtDNA | mitochondrial DNA |
| EDTA | ethylenediaminetetraacetic acid (lavender-top blood collection tube) | | mTOR | mechanistic target of rapamycin (signaling pathway) |
| EEG | electroencephalogram | | MZ | monozygotic (twins) |
| ENT | otolaryngology (ear–nose–throat) | | NAI | nonaccidental injury |
| EXIT | ex utero intrapartum treatment | | NG | nasogastric |
| FDA | US Food and Drug Administration | | NIH | non-immune hydrops |
| FISH | fluorescence in situ hybridization | | NOMID | neonatal-onset multisystem inflammatory disorder |
| G tube | gastrostomy tube | | | |
| GA | gestational age | | NT | nuchal translucency |
| GERD | gastroesophageal reflux disease | | NTD | neural tube defect |
| GH | growth hormone | | OCA | oculocutaneous albinism |
| GI | gastrointestinal | | OCD | obsessive–compulsive disorder |
| GU | genitourinary | | OI | osteogenesis imperfecta |
| HCG | human chorionic gonadotropin | | OR | odds ratio |
| HCM | hypertrophic cardiomyopathy | | OTIS | Organization of Teratogen Information Services |
| HIE | hypoxic ischemic encephalopathy | | PAE | prenatal alcohol exposure |
| HLHS | hypoplastic left heart syndrome | | PAS | perinatal arterial stroke |
| HPE | holoprosencephaly | | PCD | primary ciliary dyskinesia |
| HSV | herpes simplex virus | | PCR | polymerase chain reaction |
| IAAa, IAAb | interrupted aortic arch, type a or b | | PDA | patent ductus arteriosus |
| IC | imprinting center | | PFO | patent foramen ovale |
| ICP | increased intracranial pressure | | Phe | phenylalanine |
| ICSI | intracytoplasmic sperm injection | | PKU | phenylketonuria |

| | | | |
|---|---|---|---|
| PPV | positive predictive value | TE | tracheoesophageal |
| PS | pulmonary stenosis | TGA | transposition of the great arteries |
| QT(c) | distance between Q wave and T wave on ECG; QTc is QT interval corrected for heart rate | TOF | tetralogy of Fallot |
| | | TPPA | treponema pallidum particle agglutination assay |
| RNA | ribonucleic acid | TS | Turner syndrome |
| RPR | rapid plasma reagin test (for syphilis) | TSHR-SAb | thyrotropin receptor-stimulating antibodies |
| RR | relative risk | TTTS | twin-to-twin transfusion syndrome |
| RSV | respiratory syncytial virus | uE3 | unconjugated estriol 3 |
| SA | situs ambiguus | UL | upper limb |
| SCID | severe combined immunodeficiency syndrome | UPD | uniparental disomy; maternal (matUPD) or paternal (patUPD) |
| SD | standard deviation | | |
| SGA | small for gestational age | US | ultrasound |
| SIDS | sudden infant death syndrome | VCUG | vesicourethrogram |
| SLE | systemic lupus erythematosus | VDRL | Venereal Disease Research Laboratory (test for syphilis) |
| SMA | spinal muscular atrophy | | |
| SMMCI | solitary median maxillary central incisor | VLCAD | very long-chain acyl-CoA dehydrogenase deficiency |
| SNHL | sensorineural hearing loss | | |
| SNP | single nucleotide polymorphism | VPA | valproic acid |
| SVT | supraventricular tachycardia | VSD | ventricular septal defect |
| T13, | trisomy 13 | VZIG | varicella zoster-specific immunoglobulin G |
| T18 | trisomy 18 | VZV | varicella zoster virus |
| T21 | trisomy 21, Down syndrome | WES | whole exome sequencing |
| TA | truncus arteriosus | WHO | World Health Organization |
| TAPVR | total anomalous pulmonary venous return | WHS | Wolf–Hirschhorn syndrome |

# Part I

## Common Issues in the Newborn

# 1

# Hypotonia

## Clinical Consult

A term infant with hypotonia and bilateral metatarsus adductus presented with relative pulmonary hypoplasia requiring full ventilatory support. The mother had mild polyhydramnios and reported decreased fetal activity. The physical exam was challenging due to multiple tubes and monitoring devices. His mouth was tented (Figure 1.1). He had hypoactive reflexes and minimal spontaneous movements of arms, legs, and fingers. The initial diagnosis was a disorder with Fetal Akinesia sequence, and exome sequencing was considered.

The family history was pertinent for three healthy children. Another child died 2 years previously with presumptive hypoxic ischemic encephalopathy. An autopsy did not reveal an underlying cause. The parents had been given a low recurrence risk. The mother reported no history of weakness or difficulty releasing a grasped object. She had subtle facial weakness. No grasp myotonia was elicited on initial examinations by genetics and neurology consultants, but careful reassessment revealed weak eyelids and suggestive grasp myotonia. Molecular testing for myotonic dystrophy in the infant revealed an expansion of 1,200 CTG repeats in *DMPK1*, consistent with **congenital myotonic dystrophy**.

Symptoms of myotonic dystrophy type 1 in affected mothers may be subtle and mild. Even experienced consultants can miss this diagnosis, which was the case when the first severely affected child was born to this mildly affected mother.

## Definition

- Hypotonia is low muscle tone for age, often caused by weakness or abnormalities of the central nervous system (CNS).
- 2–4% of term infants
- Male = Female
- Major types of hypotonia
  - Central hypotonia ~80%
    - Chromosome disorders (most frequent), CNS lesions, metabolic disorders
    - Clinical features: reflexes present, variable seizures and dysmorphic features
  - Peripheral hypotonia ~20%

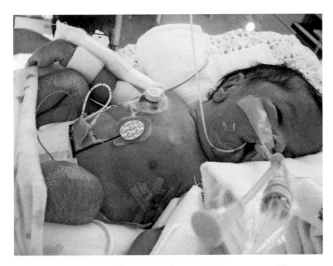

FIGURE 1.1 Congenital myotonic dystrophy in a neonate with pulmonary hypoplasia, tented mouth, facial edema, and hypotonic posture due to

- Congenital myopathies, spinal muscular atrophy, myotonic dystrophy
- Clinical features: reflexes hypoactive, lack of antigravity movements
- Prenatal findings often associated with hypotonia
  - Decreased fetal movements
  - Polyhydramnios
  - Breech presentation

## Differential Diagnosis

- We outline only a few of the hundreds of genetic conditions that can cause neonatal hypotonia. Many chromosomal and microarray abnormalities, single gene disorders, various metabolic diseases, and numerous complex syndromes cause congenital hypotonia. Multiple brain malformations are an important cause of neonatal hypotonia, but these are discussed in other chapters.
- The pace of new gene discoveries in infants with hypotonis is astonishing and as molecular pathways are elucidated, therapeutic targets are emerging.
- Using all tools available, a diagnosis can be achieved in ~90% of hypotonic infants. A detailed physical examination and thorough history remain essential for diagnosis, even in the genomic era.
  - More than 50% of patients can be diagnosed by exam and history alone.
  - In the remaining patients, a well-defined clinical phenotype facilitates choice of diagnostic tests and interpretation of molecular results.

- Chromosome disorders
  - **Down syndrome*** (MIM 190685)
    - Clinical features: characteristic facial findings, small ears < 3%, theatrical grimace (when crying), short broad hands with fifth finger clinodactyly, sandal gap, congenital heart defects in almost half
  - **Prader–Willi syndrome*** (MIM 176270)
    - Missing or inactive paternal contribution at chr 15q11.2
    - Clinical features: congenital generalized hypotonia a constant feature (Figure 1.2), poor feeding, absent or reduced suck, frog leg positioning, reflexes present, genital hypoplasia, clitoral hypoplasia (often overlooked in females—a helpful sign), cryptorchidism, decreased pigmentation for family background

*Pearl*: Unexplained poor feeding in a term infant without congenital anomalies warrants a brain MRI. If the MRI is normal, follow with DNA methylation study to rule out **Prader–Willi syndrome**.

  - **Smith–Magenis syndrome** (MIM 182290)
    - Deletion of 3.7-Mb interstitial deletion in chromosome 17p11.2
      - 10% caused by mutation in the *RAI1* gene at 17p11.2

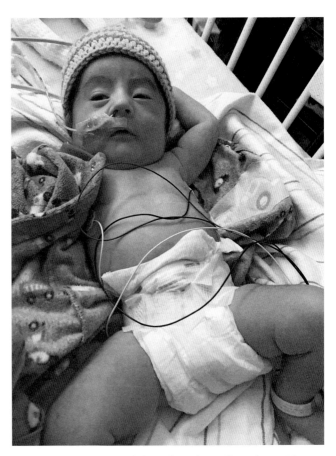

FIGURE 1.2 Hypotonia in baby with Prader–Willi syndrome. Note frog leg position of comfort and typical facial features.

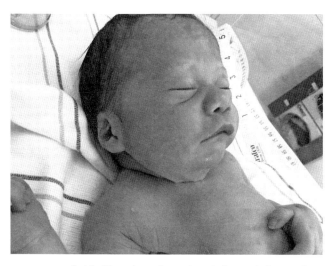

FIGURE 1.3 Smith–Magenis syndrome in an infant with dysmorphic features including small ears, downturned mouth corners, and lower canthal folds Note copious oral secretions reflecting decreased oral–motor tone.

- Clinical features: small ears, brachycephaly, midface hypoplasia, prognathism, hoarse cry, cardiac and other defects, seizures, intellectual disability (ID) (Figure 1.3)
  - Later: sleep problems and characteristic behaviors
  ○ **12p tetrasomy** (Pallister–Killian mosaicism, MIM 601803)
  - Mosaic marker chromosome consisting of two copies of short arm of chr 12; not present in all tissues
  - Clinical features: congenital diaphragmatic hernia, small ears, bitemporal alopecia, characteristic face and upper lip (see Figure 3.2), feeding problems, seizures, severe ID
  ○ **MECP2 duplication at Xq28** (MIM 300260)
  - Variable, mostly small <1-Mb duplications on chr Xq28, diagnosed on chromosome single nucleotide polymorphism (SNP) microarray; usually diagnosed in males
  - Clinical features: severe ID, hypotonia and spasticity, recurrent respiratory infections, neonatal renal calculi
- Dysmorphic single gene syndromes
  ○ **Kabuki syndrome** (MIM 147920)
  - Autosomal dominant disorder, caused by heterozygous variants in *MLL2* (*KMT2D*)
  - Clinical features: cleft palate, cardiac defects, genitourinary defects, mildly myopathic face with long palpebral fissures, blue sclerae, everted lateral third of lower eyelids, prominent fingertip pads, short fifth fingers (see Figure )
  ○ **Smith–Lemli–Opitz syndrome*** (MIM 270400)
  - Autosomal recessive disorder of cholesterol metabolism caused by variants in *DCHR7*
  - A multiple congenital anomaly syndrome with cleft palate, polydactyly, genital ambiguity, cardiac anomalies, and intrauterine growth restriction. Characteristic face with ptosis and anteverted nares.
  - Hypotonia a constant finding

  ○ **Rett syndrome variant** (MIM 613454)
  - Autosomal dominant, caused by de novo heterozygous variant in *FOXG1*
    • Occasionally, a parent has germline mosaicism.
  - Clinical features: progressive microcephaly, developmental delay, ID, stereotypic movements of hands
    • Hypoplasia of corpus callosum
  ○ **Bohring–Opitz syndrome** (MIM 605039)
  - Autosomal dominant, caused by de novo heterozygous variants in *AXL1*
  - Clinical findings: distinctive facial features, variable microcephaly, nevus flammeus, hypertrichosis, severe myopia, unusual posture of arms with flexion at elbows and wrists, hypotonia, severe feeding problems with vomiting, severe ID
    - Increased risk for Wilms tumor; ultrasound (US) surveillance indicated
  ○ **PURA associated hypotonia with neonatal respiratory distress** (MIM 616158)
  - Autosomal dominant , usually de novo variants in *PURA*
  - Gene responsible for much of phenotype seen in 5q31.3 deletion syndrome
  - Broad prominent forehead; myopathic face
  - May mimic HIE as neonatal apnea and seizures common; non-progressive but severe ID.
- Metabolic disorders
  ○ **Zellweger syndrome** (peroxisome biogenesis disorder 1A, MIM 214100)
  - Lethal autosomal recessive disorder, caused by homozygous or compound heterozygous variants in *PEX1* and other peroxisome biogenesis genes
  - Clinical features: characteristic face with high forehead, large fontanelles (Figure 1.4), severe progressive hypotonia, hepatomegaly, liver disease, poor feeding and seizures
  ○ **Congenital disorders of glycosylation** (CDG-1A, MIM 212605)
  - Expanding group of autosomal recessive disorders of protein glycosylation
    • CDG-1A is the most common type, caused by biallelic variants in *PMM2*.
  - Two main groups based on type of biochemical error: type I CDG and type II CDG
  - Clinical features: highly variable: liver disease, failure to thrive, microcephaly, developmental delay, dysmorphic features, abnormal fat distribution on buttocks and elsewhere
    • Brain MRI: cerebellar hypoplasia and other CNS lesions
  - Labs: carbohydrate-deficient transferrin electrophoresis and/or peroxisomal disorders sequencing panel
  ○ **Glycine encephalopathy** (nonketotic hyperglycinemia, MIM 605899)
  - Autosomal recessive disorder, caused by variants in *GLCD*, which encodes the P protein (MIM 238300) in

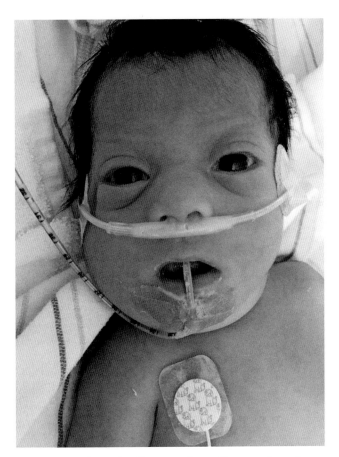

FIGURE 1.4 Infant with Zellweger syndrome. Note tented mouth, hypertelorism, and high forehead.

the mitochondrial glycine cleavage system. Other genes encode the T protein, GCST (MIM 238310); rarely others.
- The neonatal form of nonketotic hyperglycinemia is apparent in the first few days after birth.
- Clinical features: encephalopathy, failure to thrive, lethargy, severe illness, intractable seizures
  - Hiccups are a frequent and helpful clue.
  - Brain imaging: hydrocephalus, mega cisterna magna, white matter atrophy, corpus callosum hypoplasia
- Labs: Glycine accumulates in blood, urine, and cerebrospinal fluid.
  - It may not be detected by newborn screening programs.
  - Treat with sodium benzoate and dextromethorphan. Neonatal death is frequent, and survivors have severe ID.
- *FBXL4*-related encephalomyopathic mitochondrial DNA (mtDNA depletion syndrome, MIM 605471)
  - Autosomal recessive disorder, due to biallelic variants in *FBXL4*
  - Clinical features: congenital or early onset lactic acidosis, growth failure, feeding difficulty, hypotonia, global delay, seizures, movement disorders, ataxia, autonomic dysfunction, stroke-like episodes

- Hypertrophic cardiomyopathy, congenital heart malformations, arrhythmias
- Cataract, strabismus, nystagmus, optic atrophy
- Brain MRI: basal ganglia changes, periventricular cysts, cerebellar abnormalities, thin corpus callosum
  - Labs: elevated transaminases, lactic acidosis, neutropenia, hyperammonemia, mild creatine kinase (CK) elevations
  - Early death; median age at death, 2 years
- **Primary coenzyme $Q_{10}$** ($CoQ_{10}$ deficiency type I, MIM 607426)
  - Autosomal recessive disorder, caused by biallelic variants in nine genes involved in synthesis of CoQ
  - Clinical features: multisystem disease that may present as fatal neonatal encephalopathy with hypotonia
    - Steroid-resistant nephrotic syndrome may be initial manifestation. This occasionally may be an isolated finding.
    - Hypertrophic cardiomyopathy, retinopathy, optic atrophy, hearing loss
    - Later onset forms: slowly progressive multiple system disorder with parkinsonism, cerebellar ataxia, pyramidal dysfunction, dystonia, spasticity, seizures, ID
  - Labs: biochemical demonstration on frozen muscle homogenates of reduced levels of $CoQ_{10}$ (ubiquinone) in skeletal muscle or of complex I + III and II + III of the mitochondrial respiratory chain
  - Treat with oral high-dose $CoQ_{10}$
    - Neonatal death is frequent. There is occasional long survival with late-onset renal disease and neurologic and autonomic symptoms.

*Pearl*: Serum coenzyme Q levels reflect dietary intake. $CoQ_{10}$ levels in a tissue biopsy (preferably skeletal muscle) are needed to make the diagnosis of deficiency.

- Other metabolic disorders
  - Most are autosomal recessive and many are detected on newborn screening.
    - Rare inborn errors of metabolism are identified with exome sequencing or targeted panels.
  - Aminoacidurias
    - **Methylmalonic aciduria** (MIM 251000)
    - **Maple syrup urine disease** (MIM 248600)
    - **Propionic acidemia** (MIM 606054)
  - Lysosomal storage diseases
    - **Pompe disease** (glycogen storage disease type II, MIM 232300)
- Congenital lower motor neuron diseases
  - **Spinal muscular atrophy I** (Werdnig–Hoffman disease, SMA1, MIM 255300)
    - Autosomal recessive disorder: >95% of patients have a homozygous deletion in *SMN1* on chromosome 5q.

- Clinical features: alert infant, joint contractures, absent reflexes, variable tongue fasciculations
  - Relentless, progressive weakness due to lower motor neuron dysfunction, with eventual respiratory failure
- Treatment
  - Multiple clinical trials are in progress to ameliorate disease process; see https://clinicaltrials.gov.
  - Spinraza (Nusinersen) was approved by the U.S. Food and Drug Administration (FDA) in late 2016. Clinical trials suggest that motor milestones may be maintained when it is given to presymptomatic infants with later infancy onset forms of spinal muscular atrophy.
- **Spinal muscular atrophy with respiratory distress** (SMARD1, MIM 604320)
  - Autosomal recessive disorder, caused by biallelic variants in *IGHMBP2*
  - Clinical features: early weakness predominantly involving distal muscles, upper limb > lower limb, diaphragmatic eventration, respiratory infections, mild knee and foot contractures
    - Diaphragmatic palsy requires supportive ventilation.
    - Autonomic involvement: pain insensitivity, bowel and bladder problems, excessive sweating
  - Usually lethal during infancy
- Congenital muscular dystrophies and myopathies
  - Clinically and genetically heterogeneous group of disorders, with inconsistent and complex terminology and classification systems. Pathogenic variants in the same gene can produce variable phenotypes in both the myopathy and muscular dystrophy categories.
  - Collagen VI-related dystrophies
    - **Ullrich congenital muscular dystrophy** (MIM 254090)
      - Autosomal recessive trait, caused by biallelic mutations in one of three collagen VI genes: *COL6A1, COL6A2, COL6A3*
      - Clinical features: most severe end of spectrum has striking joint hypermobility of hands and feet, congenital hip dislocation, clubfeet, elbow and knee contractures, kyphoscoliosis, torticollis, progressive weakness
        - Respiratory insufficiency, especially at night
        - Normal IQ
    - **Bethlem myopathy** (MIM 158810)
      - Autosomal dominant trait, allelic to Ullrich congenital muscular dystrophy but milder, caused by heterozygous mutations in same three collagen VI genes

*Pearl*: A baby with both congenital hypotonia or joint laxity can present with contractures (e.g., SMA1, Marfan syndrome, Loeys–Dietz syndrome, and Ullrich muscular dystrophy).

- **Congenital myotonic dystrophy type 1** (MIM 160900) (see Clinical Consult)
  - Autosomal dominant disorder, caused by expanded number of trinucleotide (CTG) repeats in *DMPK* on chromosome 19p
    - Congenital presentation typically has >1,000 CTG repeats and is inherited from an affected mother, who may be mildly affected or asymptomatic.
  - Prenatal findings: polyhydramnios, decreased fetal activity, hydrops of upper body
  - Clinical features: variable severity, myopathic face, tented triangular mouth, high forehead, clubfeet; hypoactive reflexes, significant feeding and swallowing problems, oromotor weakness/dysfunction
    - Hypotonia and respiratory status usually improve gradually, but severe pulmonary hypoplasia may cause neonatal death.
    - There is global but variable developmental delay.
  - Maternal findings: subtle craniofacial weakness, mild bitemporal hair loss, grasp myotonia, learning disability, unconcerned affect ("la belle indifférence")
    - Affected mothers often deny symptoms. Ask about grasp myotonia in several ways: "Do you ever have difficulty letting go of a hairbrush or the steering wheel?" and "Do your hands ever get 'stuck' after picking up a heavy object?"

*Pearl*: The electromyogram (EMG), diagnostic of myotonic dystrophy in older children and adults, is usually not helpful in neonates.

- **Laminin alpha 2-related dystrophy** (LAMA2-RD, congenital merosin-deficient muscular dystrophy, MIM156225)
  - Autosomal recessive disorder, caused by biallelic variants in *LAMA2*
    - Complete *LAMA2* deficiency causes approximately half of congenital muscular dystrophy.
    - Partial deficiency has a more variable course.
  - Clinical features: hypotonia, weakness and occasional joint contractures; seizures 30%; several other presentations
    - Brain MRI: subcortical cysts, white matter changes, subcortical band heterotopia in 5%, variable cerebellar and pontine changes
    - Labs: CK elevated up to five times normal
- **Muscular dystrophy with eye and brain anomalies** (dystroglycanopathies, Walker–Warburg syndrome, muscle–eye–brain disease, MIM, 613150, 236670 and others)
  - Autosomal recessive disorders, caused by bialleic variants in *POMT1, POMT2, FKTN,* and others
    - A genetically heterogeneous group of disorders resulting from defective glycosylation of dystrophin-associated glycoprotein 1

- Clinical features: macrocephaly or microcephaly, cleft lip/palate, contractures
  - Eye: retinal malformations, microphthalmia, cataract, glaucoma, anterior chamber abnormalities
  - Brain MRI: a range from cobblestone (type II) lissencephaly to more focal polymicrogyria; cerebellar malformations, hypoplasia of midline brain structures, ventricular dilatation, Dandy–Walker malformation, posterior occipital encephalocele
  - Labs: strikingly elevated CK
  - Variable course from neonatal lethal to death in the first year, to less severe presentations
  - **RYR-related myopathies** (central core disease, minicore myopathy, MIM 180901)
    - Autosomal recessive disorder, caused by biallelic variants in *RYR1*, which encodes the sarcoplasmic reticulum calcium release channel
      - Recessive pathogenic variants usually result in a neonatal presentation.
    - Clinical features: facial weakness, early onset severe progressive scoliosis
      - Ophthalmoplegia in some forms of *RYR1* myopathy (central core and minicore myopathy) but may be absent in the congenital presentation
    - May require gastrostomy and nighttime ventilator support
- Nongenetic causes:
  - Most are not addressed here, including prematurity, congenital infection, botulism, hypothyroidism, cardiac failure, anemia, hypoxic and hemorrhagic brain lesions, hypothyroidism, and perinatal stroke. Hypoxic ischemic encephalophathy is discussed briefly.
  - **Hypoxic ischemic encephalopathy** (HIE)
    - HIE is caused by acute or chronic in utero or perinatal asphyxia.
    - Incidence 1–2/1,000 live births
    - Common clinical features: cord blood pH <7.0; base excess >12; Apgar score <3 for greater than 5 minutes; early onset moderate or severe encephalopathy; seizures within 12 hours of life, unresponsive to pyridoxine; multi-organ dysfunction: liver, kidney, lung
      - Magnetic resonance imaging (MRI)/computerized tomography (CT) show characteristic findings consistent with asphyxia; early brain MRI helps date injury
      - Other disease processes must be excluded.

*Pearl*: Low Apgar scores are neither necessary nor sufficient to make a diagnosis of HIE. Many other conditions cause low Apgar scores.

# Evaluation and Management

- Review pregnancy history: polyhydramnios, commonly due to reduced fetal swallowing, abnormal fetal lie, and decreased fetal activity.
  - Document fetal ultrasound abnormalities (e.g., clubfeet).
  - Note delivery complications, Apgar scores, resuscitation status at birth, and cord gases.
- Document the family history: consanguinity, infant death, weakness.
- Examine the parents for weakness and, especially in the mother, for slow grip release and other findings of myotonic dystrophy.
- Examine for distinctive features. Careful phenotyping will increase diagnostic yield.
  - Dysmorphic features: e.g. cleft palate, micrognathia, large fontanelles (e.g. **Zellweger syndrome**)
  - Eye exam for retinal dystrophy: e.g. in **muscular dystrophy with eye and brain anomalies (Walker–Warburg) syndrome**
  - Genitalia: e.g. small phallus, clitoral hypoplasia (e.g. **Prader–Willi syndrome***), cryptorchidism, genital ambiguity (e.g. **Smith–Lemli–Opitz syndrome***)
  - Neurological exam: Consult pediatric neurology to refine the neurologic phenotype.
    - Reflexes (absent in **spinal muscular atrophy**), extra ocular movements, seizures, head control, spontaneous movement of extremities, muscle bulk and so on.
- Imaging
  - Skeletal survey for epiphyseal stippling in suspected peroxisomal disorders
    - Order lateral view of the foot for heel stippling.
  - Abdominal US for organomegaly
  - Echocardiogram for cardiomegaly (**Pompe disease** MIM 232300)
  - Neuroimaging establishes the diagnosis in ~25%.
    - MRI gives best definition of anatomy.
    - Brain CT scan is useful for hemorrhagic events.
- Genetic testing
  - Chromosome analysis (for suspected trisomy 21); SNP microarray in all others. Excessive homozygosity may direct further testing.
  - DNA methylation for chr 15q11.2 for suspected **Prader–Willi syndrome***
  - Metabolic studies for hypotonia without an identified cause
    - Use an experienced reference laboratory.
    - Review newborn screening test results.
    - Initial baseline tests: quantitative urine organic acids, quantitative plasma amino acids, plasma and urine carnitine (total and esterified), plasma acylcarnitine profile, serum lactate, CK, ammonia, T4, thyroid-stimulating hormone

*Pearl*: Elevated CK narrows the differential diagnosis. Include it in initial round of tests.

○ For suspected congenital disorders of glycosylation
  ■ Serum carbohydrate-deficient transferrin analysis and plasma *N*-glycan profile
○ For suspected peroxisomal disorders, begin with biochemical testing.
  ■ Plasma very long-chain fatty acids (VLCFAs)
    • Elevated C26:0 and C26:1 and C24/C22 and C26/C22 ratios
      • When VLCFA is abnormal, consult with reference laboratory for further testing.
      • Consider peroxisomal disorders sequencing panel to expedite diagnosis
      • Patients with mild **Zellweger syndrome** may have (near) normal biochemical tests in plasma and urine, and further tests in fibroblasts or a gene panel may be needed.
○ Molecular genetic testing should be guided by clinical findings.
○ Single gene tests
  ■ **Spinal muscular atrophy**: exonic deletion in *SMN1*
  ■ **Congenital myotonic dystrophy**: increased CTG trinucleotide repeats in *DMPK*
○ Gene panels or exome sequencing trio testing (child and both parents if possible) for complex or unusual phenotypes
  ■ Consult genetic experts to interpret results and variants of unknown significance.

*Pearl*: Trinucleotide repeat disorders such as **congenital myotonic dystrophy** cannot be diagnosed with exome sequencing.

○ Locate genetic laboratories at
  ■ https://www.genetests.org
  ■ https://www.ncbi.nlm.nih.gov/gtr
○ Reserve invasive testing (EMG, nerve conduction, and muscle biopsy) for infrequent select cases.
  ■ Additional tests on muscle biopsy may include immunohistochemistry staining, electron microscopy, and respiratory chain enzyme analysis of mitochondrial DNA.
  ■ Include $CoQ_{10}$ levels in skeletal muscle homogenates.
  ■ Increasingly, molecular testing (panels, exomes) is replacing invasive testing.

## Further Reading

Bushby KM, Collins J, Hicks D. (2014) Collagen type VI myopathies. Adv Exp Med Biol. 802:185–99. PMID 24443028

Falsaperla R, Praticò AD, Ruggieri M, et al. (2016) Congenital muscular dystrophy: from muscle to brain. Ital J Pediatr. 42(1):78. PMID 27576556

Gonorazky HD, Bönnemann CG, Dowling JJ. (2018) The genetics of congenital myopathies. Handb Clin Neurol.148:549–564. PMID 29478600

Groen EJN, Talbot K, Gillingwater TH. (2018) Advances in therapy for spinal muscular atrophy: promises and challenges. Nat Rev Neurol. 14(4):214–24. PMID 29422644

Jungbluth H, Ochala J, Treves S, Gautel M. (2017) Current and future therapeutic approaches to the congenital myopathies. Semin Cell Dev Biol. 64:191–200. PMID 27515125

Salviati L, Trevisson E, Doimo M, Navas P. (2017) Primary coenzyme $Q_{10}$ deficiency. In: Pagon RA, Adam MP, Ardinger HH, et al., editors. GeneReviews [Internet]. Seattle, WA: University of Washington, Seattle; 1993–2017. PMID 28125198

Sparks SE, Krasnewich DM. (2017) Congenital disorders of N-linked glycosylation and multiple pathway overview. In: Pagon RA, Adam MP, Ardinger HH, et al., editors. GeneReviews [Internet]. Seattle, WA: University of Washington, Seattle; 1993–2017. PMID 20301507

Tanaka AJ, Bai R, Cho MT et al. (2015) De novo mutations in PURA are associated with hypotonia and developmental delay. Cold Spring Harb Mol Case Stud. E pub PMID 27148565

Tarailo-Graovac M, Wasserman WW, Van Karnebeek CD. (2017) Impact of next-generation sequencing on diagnosis and management of neurometabolic disorders: Current advances and future perspectives Expert Rev Mol Diagn. 17:307–9. PMID 28277145

# 2

# Intrauterine Growth Restriction

## Clinical Consult

An 800-g, 33-week gestation infant born to first cousin Palestinian parents had been in the neonatal intensive care unit (NICU) for 6 weeks. He had a benign course, but his growth was poor at less than the third percentile. Consultation revealed an extremely small baby with unusual craniofacial features: prominent eyes, a beaked nose, and microcephaly (Figure 2.1). As the infant's features became more noticeable and distinct over time, his mother researched her extensive family history and found a history of two other individuals with severe short stature and early death in her multiply consanguineous family. This history, consistent with autosomal recessive inheritance, plus this child's emerging facial characteristics over time allowed the diagnosis of **Majewski (microcephalic) osteodysplastic primordial dwarfism II (MOPD II)** (Figure 2.2). The diagnosis was later confirmed by demonstration of a mutation in the causative gene, *PCNT*, encoding pericentrin. He has had a very complicated course with severe short stature, delayed development, and multiple strokes due to Moyamoya malformation, a known complication of MOPD II.

## Definition

- Intrauterine growth restriction (IUGR) is the term used to describe infants who are below −2 SD of that expected for gestational age.
- May be genetic or environmental, including
  o Fetal/infant, placental, or maternal causes

## Differential Diagnosis

### Placental Factors

- Common etiology for IUGR
- **Placental lesions**
  o Structural abnormalities are usually associated with mild IUGR.
    ▪ Single umbilical artery

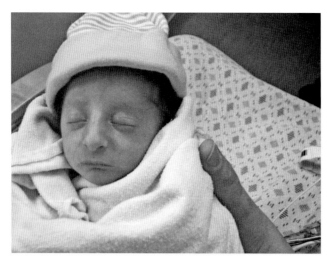

FIGURE 2.1 Infant with Majewski osteodysplastic dysplasia II as a newborn. Note prominent nose, prominent eyes, and small jaw.

- Short cord
- Velamentous or marginal cord insertion
- Circumvallate placenta
  - Anomalies that cause fetal underperfusion are more consequential.
    - Inflammatory lesions: infectious villitis, chronic villitis of unknown cause (most common)
    - Placental infarction, massive perivillous fibrin deposition (maternal floor infarction)
- Common comorbidities
  - Preterm delivery, stillbirth, oligohydramnios, placental abruption, preeclampsia
  - Hypospadias and other genital anomalies occur more often in IUGR males.

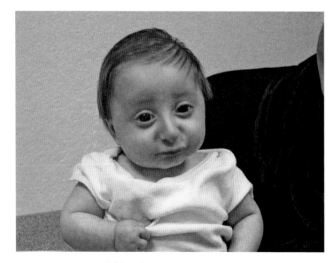

FIGURE 2.2 Same child as shown in Figure 2.1 at 8 months of age. Features are more recognizable over time.

## Maternal Factors

- **Maternal weight and nutrition**
  - Maternal and paternal size and weight; mother's small size more predictive of IUGR than father's size
  - Maternal weight gain; low birth weight common with famine
  - Mother's birth weight; mothers who were IUGR themselves have an increased risk for IUGR babies.
  - Prior bariatric surgery
- **Teratogens**
  - Chemotherapy, warfarin, anticonvulsants, alcohol, cigarettes
  - Caffeine probably not significantly associated with IUGR
  - Maternal hypertension and its treatment; preeclampsia
- Assisted reproductive technology (ART) increases the prevalence of low birth weight (LBW) and IUGR.
- Maternal thrombophilia: factor V Leiden heterozygosity (controversial)
- **Maternal disease**
  - Collagen vascular disease, renal insufficiency, malaria, diabetes, preeclampsia, severe anemia, congenital or acquired heart disease
- Multiple gestation: growth falls off particularly in third trimester.

## Fetal/Infant Factors

- **Chromosome abnormalities**
  - **Trisomies 18\*, 13\*, Turner syndrome\***, triploidy, mosaic trisomy 16
  - Confined placental mosaicism. A trisomic or abnormal cell line is confined to the placenta. Most pregnancy outcomes are normal but IUGR can result
  - Small deletions or duplications: 4p-\*, 5p-\*, 19q13.11, and many other copy number variants detected on microarray
  - Uniparental disomy (UPD) for chromosomes 6, 7, 11, 14, 16. Both involved chromosomes originate from one parent only.
    - Many cases are the result of trisomy or monosomy rescue that is more common with advanced maternal age.
    - Isodisomy, when both chromosomes are identical, can be detected on SNP microarray, but heterodisomy, when non-identical chromosomes are inherited from one parent, requires specific UPD testing.
- **Genomic imprinting errors**
  - **Russell–Silver syndrome** (Silver–Russell syndrome, RSS or SRS, MIM 180860)
    - Sporadic disorder caused by various complex epigenetic mechanisms
      - Hypomethylation of chromosome 11p15 imprinting center 1 (ICR1) ~60%
      - Maternal uniparental disomy 7 (matUPD7) ~18%

- Chromosome 11p15 rearrangements
- *CDKN1C* duplications or gain-of-function variants
- Heterozygous mutations in *HMGA2* and paternally inherited variants in *IGF2* account for rare familial cases of RSS.
■ Diagnosis based on compilation of features that can lead to both overdiagnosis and underdiagnosis
- Clinical features: prenatal growth restriction, height and weight <–2 SD, relative macrocephaly at birth, body asymmetry (frequent, not invariable) (Figure 2.3)
  - Fifth finger clinodactyly
  - Feeding difficulties: vomiting, gastroesophageal reflux disease (GERD), constipation
  - Later findings: postnatal growth restriction <–2 SD, protruding forehead at age 1–3 years, generally normal IQ
  - Occasional growth hormone deficiency
○ **IMAGe syndrome** (*i*ntrauterine growth restriction, *m*etaphyseal dysplasia, *a*drenal insufficiency, *ge*nital abnormalities, MIM 614732)
  ■ Caused by heterozygous gain-of-function mutation in *CDKN1C*. These mutations are more detrimental than those causing RSS.

■ Prenatal findings: severe IUGR, increased nuchal translucency (NT), abnormal serum screening, and, occasionally, short long bones
■ Clinical features: may present with life-threatening congenital adrenal insufficiency
- Increased pigmentation
- Subtle metaphyseal abnormalities
- Osteopenia and hypercalcemia
- Dysmorphic facial features: flat nasal bridge, short nose (Figure 2.4)
- Genital abnormalities in boys: micropenis, hypospadias
  - May be underdiagnosed
- Congenital anomalies/syndromes: 1–2% of **IUGR**
  ○ Suspect a chromosome abnormality/syndrome when IUGR occurs with anomalies and/or dysmorphic features. Many syndromes have IUGR
  ○ Some IUGR syndromes can be diagnosed prenatally by fetal US based on their patterns of congenital anomalies:
    ■ **Smith–Lemli–Opitz syndrome**\*: cardiac, genital ambiguity, polydactyly
    ■ **Cornelia de Lange syndrome**\*: limb anomalies, diaphragmatic hernia
- Congenital Infection: <5% of **IUGR**
  ○ Toxoplasmosis, cytomegalovirus, malaria, syphilis, Zika, and herpes are most common. Bacterial infections (e.g., tuberculosis and *Listeria*) are rare.
- Endocrine and metabolic: **rare**
  ○ **Laron dwarfism** (MIM 262500)
    ■ Autosomal recessive disorder due to pathogenic variants in growth hormone receptor gene
    ■ High serum growth hormone; low insulin-like growth factor 1 (IGF1) levels

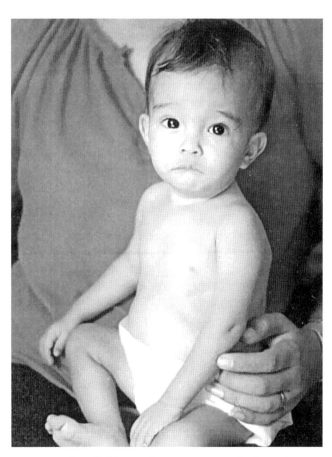

FIGURE 2.3 Russell–Silver syndrome. Note triangular face and downturned mouth corners.

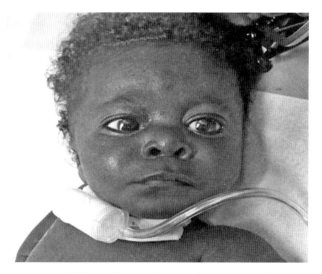

FIGURE 2.4 IMAGe syndrome. Infant is tracheotomy dependent. Note flat nasal bridge and mildly anteverted nares.
SOURCE: Courtesy of Julie Kaplan Parent MD, duPont Hospital for Children, Wilmington, DE.

- Suspect IGF1 deficiency with persistent hypoglycemia.
- **Mitochondrial disorders**, particularly respiratory chain defects, occasionally present with IUGR.
- **Primordial dwarfism**: In these syndromes, infants have low birth weights and in general remain small throughout life. Unlike the primary skeletal dysplasias, they are proportionate. Microcephaly accompanies several of these rare conditions.
  - **Microcephalic osteodysplastic dwarfism II** (MOPD, MIM 210720) (See Clinical Consult)
    - Autosomal recessive due to biallelic *PCNT* variants
    - Severe IUGR
    - Unusual facial features, including prominent eyes, beaked nose, a high squeaky voice; small and often dysplastic or missing teeth; usually mild ID but can be severe
  - **Seckel syndrome** (MIM 2106000)
    - Autosomal recessive disorder with significant clinical and molecular heterogeneity. Eight genes to date involving cell cycle regulation.
    - IUGR (not as severe as MOPD II), microcephaly, distinctive facial features; ID not as severe as predicted by head size
  - **Meier–Gorlin syndrome** (ear, patella, short stature syndrome, MIM 224690)
    - Autosomal recessive syndrome: multiple genes in the DNA pre-initiation complex including ORC1, ORC4, ORC6, and CDC45 and others
    - Clinically variable, with prenatal IUGR, microcephaly, and classic features of microtia, short stature, and hypoplasia/absence of patellae seen in ~80%. Intelligence can be normal or impaired (Figure 2.5)
- **Lipodystrophies and neonatal progeroid syndromes**
  - **Congenital lipodystrophy—SHORT syndrome** (MIM 269880)
    - Rare syndrome caused by de novo heterozygous variants in *PIK3R1*
    - Clinical features: IUGR, short stature, lack of subcutaneous fat, Rieger eye anomaly in some
      - Triangular face, thin alae nasi (Figure 2.6)
      - Hearing loss common

*Pearl*: Downregulation of genes in the PIK–AKT–mTOR pathway is the basis of SHORT syndrome and related overlapping phenotypes. This syndrome is a "mirror image" of the activating mutations in this pathway that cause macrocephaly/hemimegalencephaly/overgrowth syndromes.

- **Cutis Laxa IIA** (CLIIA, MIM 219200)
  - Autosomal recessive disorder with a defect in N- and O-glycosylation due to variants in *ATP6V0A2*. Other types do not have demonstrable metabolic error.

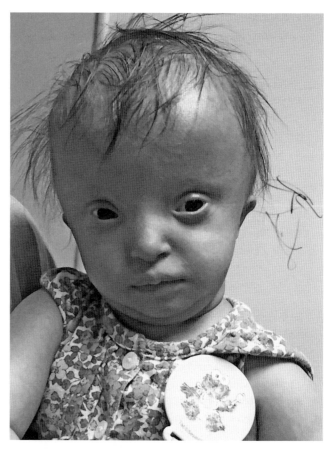

FIGURE 2.5 Meier–Gorlin syndrome. Note sparse scalp hair and eyebrows, and full lips. Ears were also very small.

- Clinical features: IUGR, failure to thrive, enlarged anterior fontanel, congenital hip dislocation, inguinal hernia, high myopia
  - Loose skin, joint hypermobility, long philtrum

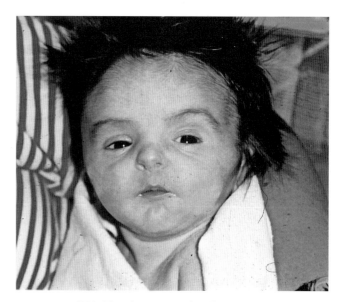

FIGURE 2.6 SHORT syndrome. Note thin alae nasi and small jaw and mouth.

- Cortical and cerebellar malformations (cobblestone lissencephaly) in most is associated with severe developmental delay, seizures, and neurologic regression.
- **Cutis laxa IIIA—DeBarsy syndrome** (MIM 219150)
  - Autosomal recessive, pathogenic variants in *ALDH18A1*
  - Clinical features: IUGR, failure to thrive, corneal clouding, cataracts
    - Progeroid appearance, pinched nose, small mouth, loose skin, hyperextensibility
    - ID, athetoid movements
- **Wiedemann–Rautenstrauch syndrome—neonatal progeroid syndrome** (MIM 264090)
  - Autosomal recessive disorder; recent report of biallelic variants in *POL3RA*
  - Clinical features: pseudohydrocephalic appearance with prominent forehead vessels
    - Late-onset IUGR in utero; failure to thrive; sparse hair, brows, and lashes; natal teeth
    - Variable ID and early death
- **Skeletal dysplasias**\*
  - Disproportionately short long bones and abnormal findings on skeletal X-rays can be subtle in newborns who present primarily with IUGR.
- **SHOX deficiency** (MIM 312865)
  - X-linked gene in the pseudoautosomal region of the short arm of the X chromosome at Xp22.3. Both males and females have functional SHOX genes so the inheritance is pseudoautosomal dominant. Variants cause non-specific short stature and IUGR. Loss of the SHOX gene is the probable cause of short stature in **Turner syndrome**.\*
  - **Leri–Weill dyschondrosteosis** (MIM 127300) is a mild skeletal dysplasia caused by heterozygous variants or deletion (80%) in *SHOX*
    - Clinical features: mesomelic short stature (short forearms), Madelung deformity of the wrist. More severe in females. Skeletal changes usually not seen in infancy
  - **Langer mesomelic dysplasia** (MIM 249700)
    - A more severe skeletal dysplasia with extreme mesomelic shortening caused by homozygous variants in *SHOX*

*Pearl*: SHOX deficiency, which causes 2–15% of idiopathic IUGR, has a prevalence of at least 1:1000 births.

  - Treatment with growth hormone is effective, so early diagnosis is important.
  - Check parents' stature and examine them for mesomelia and Madelung deformity, more severe in females.
- **Spondyloepiphyseal dysplasia congenita** (MIM 183900) and **Three M syndrome** (MIM 273750) are skeletal dysplasias that may present primarily with IUGR. The skeletal features may be subtle in newborns (see Skeletal Dysplasias-Viable\*).

# Evaluation and Testing

- Prenatal and family histories
  - Document known risk factors, parental heights, and birth weights.
- Physical examination
  - Measure skeletal proportions to detect disproportionate skeletal dysplasia that may present as IUGR (span, upper/lower segment ratio)
  - Examine for limb asymmetry, which is common in Russell–Silver syndrome.
  - Subcutaneous fat stores: Decreased fat may suggest malnutrition *in utero* or a lipodystrophy.
  - Note dysmorphic facial features and other anomalies, which may suggest chromosomal aneuploidy or syndrome.
- Genetic testing
  - Gross and histologic evaluation of placenta is indicated in all cases of IUGR.
  - Chromosomal microarray is indicated in IUGR, with or without dysmorphic features. Lack of striking dysmorphic features does not rule out a chromosomal cause (especially ring chromosomes or microdeletions).
  - Other tests depend on clinical findings and course.
  - Perform skeletal radiographs when short long bones are suspected.
  - Perform cranial imaging with IUGR and microcephaly (non-sedated MRI optimal).
  - When placenta is abnormal and thrombophilia is suspected, consider testing mother for antiphospholipid antibody syndrome, factor V Leiden, prothrombin mutation G20210A, protein C activity, and protein S activity levels (defer last test to 6 weeks postpartum because pregnancy lowers levels).
    - In neonates: factor V Leiden and prothrombin 20210 only
  - For suspected IMAGe syndrome, rapid assessment and treatment for adrenal insufficiency, *CDKN1C* sequencing and deletion/duplication analysis to confirm diagnosis.
  - For suspected Russell–Silver syndrome, start with 11p15 methylation studies and microarray; more studies may be indicated, especially if a parent is also affected (*HMGA2*, paternally inherited *IGF2*).
  - For suspected SHORT syndrome, consider clinical sequencing of *PIK3R1* or exome sequencing. Follow chronologically before testing.
  - For suspected *SHOX* deficiency, perform SNP microarray first and then, if negative, consider *SHOX* sequence analysis or gene panel testing.
  - For suspected *IGF1* spectrum disorders, order growth hormone levels and other endocrine investigations: IGF1 and IGF3.
  - Intrauterine growth restriction sequencing panels or microcephalic primordial dwarfism gene panels may be

appropriate. Exome sequencing may improve chances for a specific diagnosis in atypical cases.

## Further Reading

Alkuraya FS. (2015) Primordial dwarfism: an update. Curr Opin Endocrinol Diabetes Obes. 22(1):55–64. PMID 25490023

Avila M, Dyment DA, Sagen JV, et al. (2015) Clinical reappraisal of SHORT syndrome with PIK3R1 mutations: Towards recommendation for molecular testing and management. Clin Genet. 89:501–06. PMID 26497935

Azzi S, Salem J. (2015) A prospective study validating a clinical scoring system and demonstrating phenotypical–genotypical correlations in Silver–Russell syndrome. J Med Genet. 52:446–53. PMID 25951829

Binder G, Rappold GA. (2015) SHOX deficiency disorders. In: Pagon RA, Adam MP, Ardinger HH, et al. editors. GeneReviews®

[Internet]. Seattle, WA: University of Washington, Seattle; 1993–2017. PMID 20301394

Bober MB, Jackson A. (2017) Microcephalic Osteodysplastic Primordial Dwarfism, Type II: a clinical review. Curr Osteoporos Rep. 15(2):61–69. PMID 28409412

Cabrera-Salcedo C, Kumar P, Hwa V, et al. (2017) IMAGe and related undergrowth syndromes: The complex spectrum of gain-of-function CDKN1C mutations. Pediatr Endocrinol Rev. 14:289–97. PMID 28508599

de Munnik SA, Hoefsloot EH, Roukema J, et al. (2015) Meier-Gorlin syndrome. Orphanet J Rare Dis. 17(10):114. PMID 26381604

Hemsworth EM, O'Reilly AM, Allen VM, et al.; Knowledge Synthesis Group on Determinants of Preterm/LBW Births (2016) Association between factor V Leiden mutation, small for gestational age, and preterm birth: A systematic review and meta-analysis. J Obstet Gynaecol Can. 38:897–908. PMID 27720088

Wit JM, Oostdijk W, Losekoot M, et al. (2016) Mechanisms in endocrinology: Novel genetic causes of short stature. Eur J Endocrinol. 174:R145–73. PMID 26578640

# 3

# Overgrowth

## Clinical Consult

A genetic consultation was requested for a 36-week gestation female with feeding issues. Her birth weight and length were at the 97th percentile for gestational age and her head circumference was +3 SD. Examination revealed a mildly dysmorphic, slightly hypotonic infant (Figure 3.1A). She had a high forehead and down-slanting palpebral fissures. A clinical diagnosis was not apparent. When she returned at 3 months, her mother, a woman of low-average intelligence, was noted to have large hands and macrocephaly (Figure 3.1B). The baby continued to be large for her age, and her development was delayed. Chronologic follow-up revealed a gradual evolution of her facial features with a prominent pointed chin, ruddy cheeks, and high forehead consistent with a clinical diagnosis of **Sotos syndrome** (Figure 3.1C). An *NSD1* mutation was found in the child and subsequently in her affected mother.

The classic findings of Sotos syndrome may emerge over time, but the diagnosis can be made earlier, especially when a parent is affected. Affected adults often have high-normal stature and macrocephaly. The neurocognitive development of Sotos syndrome is variable: Some affected adults are employed and live independently. Such mildly affected individuals may escape ascertainment. The developmental outcome tends to be worse in infants with an *NSD1* deletion compared to those who have an *NSD1* gene mutation.

## Definition

- The large for gestational age (LGA) infant is defined as having a birth weight >90% for gestational age.
  - The American College of Obstetrics and Gynecology has adopted the standard of 97th percentile for gestational age or >4,500 g at term.
- Incidence: National Vital Statistics Report for US Births, in 2015
  - 7% of newborns had body weight (BW) >4,000 g.
  - 1% had BW >4,500 g.
    - Higher infant morbidity and mortality

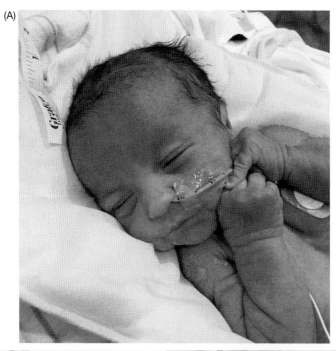

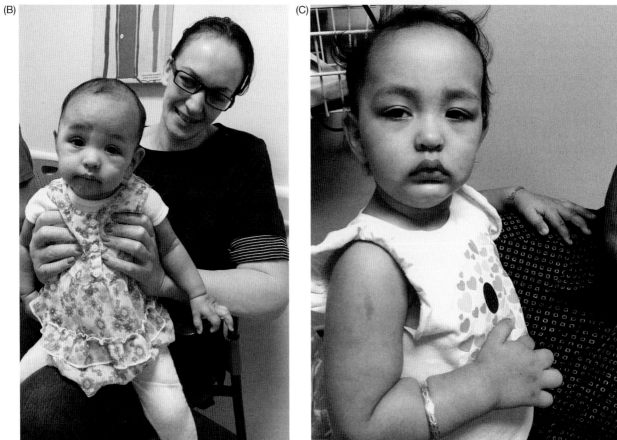

FIGURE 3.1A–C  Sotos syndrome. Same child as a newborn (A) and at several months of age (B) and as toddler (C). Note high forehead, long face and large hands in child and her mother.

- There are more NICU admissions (3× higher), shoulder dystocia (10× higher), and brachial plexus injury (20× higher) in this group compared to newborns with BW <4,000 g.
    - Mortality is greater for macrosomic infants of diabetic mothers than for other macrosomic infants.
  - 0.1% had BW >5,000 g.
- Risk factors
  - Male sex
    - Males weigh 100–200 g more than females, on average.
  - Advanced gestational age
  - High pre-pregnancy maternal body mass index (BMI)
    - Incidence of LGA infants has increased with the rising prevalence of maternal overweight, independent of maternal diabetes.
  - Maternal diabetes mellitus
  - Excess weight gain in pregnancy (>40 lbs)
  - Ethnicity is associated with LGA (even when controlling for diabetes): Hispanics, Caucasians, Native Americans, Samoans.

*Pearl*: Beware the macrosomic *pre*term infant "passing" as a term infant of normal BW. Large fetal size in the later months of pregnancy can lead to falsely "corrected" dates and to an unrecognized preterm delivery. Use early first-trimester US measurements to calculate gestational age.

## Differential Diagnosis

- Infant of diabetic mother (IDM)\*
  - By far, the most common etiology for LGA
  - Clinical features: increased risk for an array of birth defects
    - Poor feeding may persist for weeks without apparent cause.
    - Apparent dysmorphic features may be due to excessive facial fat.
    - The IDM with a large body and normal-sized head may appear relatively microcephalic.
- **Chromosomal anomalies**
  - Microarray abnormalities can cause abnormal dosage of growth-related genes.
    - Dup(4)(p16.3) includes *FGFR3*
    - Dup(15)(q26-qter) includes *IGF1R*
    - Dup(17)(p13.3)
    - Del(19)(p13.13) includes *NFIX*
    - Del(22)(q13)
  - **Pallister–Killian syndrome** (tetrasomy 12p mosaicism, MIM 601803)
    - A rare mosaic chromosome disorder with an additional chromosome, consisting of two copies of the short arm of chromosome 12

- It is occasionally mistaken for a derivative chromosome 21 and reported as a variant of **Down syndrome**.
- The extra chromosome disappears from blood over time. Neonatal microarray in blood detects the extra copies of 12p. Later, another tissue (buccal swab, skin biopsy) is needed for diagnosis.
  - Clinical features: high BW, bitemporal alopecia, unusual upper lip with the philtral skin extending into the middle of cupid's bow (Pallister lip) (Figure 3.2), epicanthal folds, full cheeks, diaphragmatic hernia, cardiac defects, hypotonia
    - Pigmentary streaks along lines of Blaschko
    - Facial features may suggest Down syndrome but overall phenotype is distinct.
    - Later: growth falls off with age; severe ID
- Syndromes with generalized overgrowth
  - **Beckwith–Wiedemann syndrome**\* (MIM 130650)
    - Relatively common autosomal dominant overgrowth disorder, caused by lack of a functioning paternal copy of a critical region on chromosome 11p15.5
    - Clinical features: large BW, macroglossia, posterior ear pits and creases, omphalocele, umbilical hernia, hypoglycemia

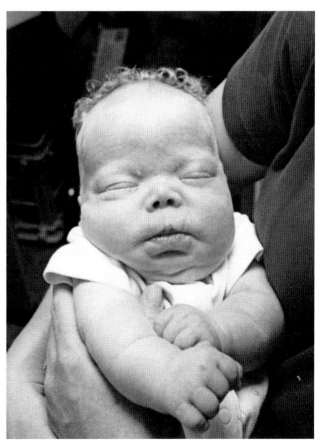

FIGURE 3.2 Pallister–Killian (12p tetrasomy). Note typical hair patterning, "Pallister" lip, and full cheeks.

- Surveillance guidelines for Wilms tumor and hepatoblastoma currently include serial AFP's until ~age 4, and abdominal US studies every three months through age 7.
  - **Sotos syndrome** (MIM 117550)
    - Autosomal dominant syndrome, caused by heterozygous variant or deletion of *NSD1* at chromosome 5q35; the most common syndromic cause of congenital macrosomia
      - *NSD1* variants are identified in 60–90%.
        - Variants in functionally related genes, *SETD2* and *DNMT3A*, cause a similar phenotype.
      - The family history may reveal an affected parent, although most cases are sporadic and de novo.
    - Clinical features: consistently increased birth length (98th %); hypotonia 75%, variable large hands and feet
      - Facial features may be subtle in the newborn: high prominent forehead, sparse frontoparietal hair, downslanting palpebral fissures, hypertelorism.
      - Joint laxity 20%, renal abnormalities 15%, cardiac anomalies 20%
      - Common neonatal problems: jaundice 65%, poor feeding 70%, and respiratory problems
        - Later findings: prognathism (not always apparent in newborns), increased risk (3%) for some cancers, scoliosis, seizures
          - Variable ID, usually mild
      - Brain imaging: ventriculomegaly, abnormalities of the corpus callosum and septum pellucidum
  - **Malan syndrome** (Sotos syndrome-2, MIM 614753)
    - Autosomal dominant disorder, due to a heterozygous (nonsense type) mutation or deletion causing haploinsufficiency for *NFIX*
    - Clinical features: postnatal overgrowth, macrocephaly, long face, high forehead, advanced bone age, hypotonia, strabismus, nystagmus, optic nerve pallor, feeding problems
      - Appearance similar to Sotos syndrome
      - Later: pectus excavatum, scoliosis, ID
        - Autism 25%, seizures 25%
  - **Costello syndrome** (MIM 218040)
    - Autosomal dominant disorder, caused by heterozygous pathogenic variant in *HRAS*
      - The rarest and most severe of the disorders in the **Noonan/CFC/LEOPARD/Costello RASopathy** spectrum*
    - Clinical features: large at birth; sparse curly hair; coarse facial features—thick full lips, wide mouth; redundant loose skin (cutis laxa); deep palmar creases (Figure 3.3A)
      - Later findings: failure to thrive, significant ID, increased tumor risk (Figure 3.3B)
  - **Marshall–Smith syndrome** (MIM 602535)
    - Rare autosomal dominant syndrome, due to heterozygous (frameshift, splice-site type) mutations in *NFIX*
      - Allelic to Malan syndrome

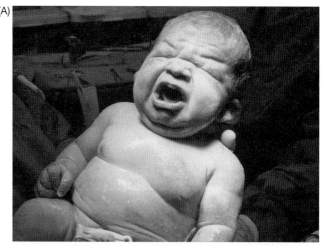

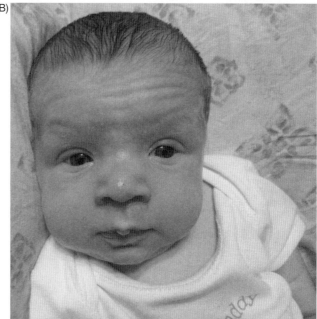

FIGURE 3.3 (A) Costello syndrome in a newborn. Note excessive skin folds, coarse features, and large size. (B) Same child in later infancy with failure to thrive. Wrinkled forehead persists.
SOURCE: Courtesy of Angelica Thomas and the Costello Syndrome Family Support Network.

- Clinical features: Severe failure to thrive and chronic respiratory distress can cause death in infancy.
  - Prominent forehead, bulging eyes, blue sclerae, large hands and feet
  - Later: osteopenia, accelerated bone age in the newborn, fractures; development very delayed
  - **Perlman syndrome** (MIM 267000)
    - Rare autosomal recessive syndrome, caused by biallelic variants in *DIS3L2*, which regulates cell proliferation and mitosis
    - Polyhydramnios common
    - Clinical features: characteristic face, inverted V-shaped upper lip, low-set ears, prominent forehead

- Cryptorchidism, interrupted aortic arch, marked enlargement of viscera: heart, liver, and kidneys
- Renal dysplasia with nephroblastomatosis
- Frequently lethal in infancy
- Later: poor growth, ID; high incidence of early onset Wilms tumor, often bilateral
  - **Simpson–Golabi–Behmel syndrome** (MIM 312870)
    - X-linked recessive condition, caused by hemizygous variants in *GPC3* or *GPC4*, which encode Glipican-3 and -4
      - Additional molecular heterogeneity likely
    - Clinical features: prenatal-onset overgrowth, BW ≤5.9 kg, macrocephaly, increased length
      - In severe neonatal form: diaphragmatic hernia, congenital heart disease, hypoglycemia. Early lethality is common.
      - Infants with milder presentation survive to adulthood.
      - There is an increased tumor risk, but no surveillance guidelines are published.
  - **Weaver syndrome** (MIM 277590)
    - Autosomal dominant disorder, caused by heterozygous variants in *EZH2*; a rare or underdiagnosed syndrome
      - Other genes recently identified
    - Clinical features: prenatal onset of overgrowth affecting weight > height, macrocephaly, down-slanting palpebral fissures, large ears, long philtrum, micrognathia; ventricular septal defect (VSD) and patent ductus arteriosus (PDA)
      - Limb anomalies: camptodactyly (joint contractures) of fingers, talipes, metatarsus adductus
      - Later: accelerated bone age, tall stature, variable ID
      - 5% risk for tumors; no recommended surveillance protocol. Evaluate based on symptoms.
- Segmental overgrowth syndromes
  - Somatic variants in the phosphatidylinositol/AKT/mTOR pathway cause segmental overgrowth disorders.
  - **Klippel–Trenaunay syndrome** (KTW, MIM 149000)
    - *AGGF1* and *PIK3CA* variants have been found in a few patients' affected tissues.

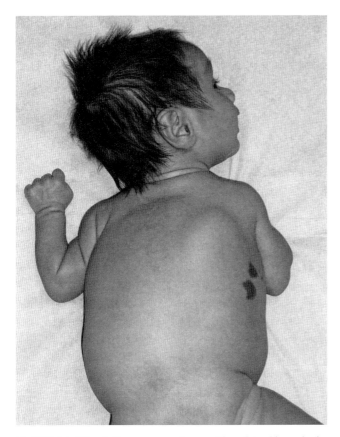

FIGURE 3.4 Klippel–Trenaunay syndrome with unilateral lower limb overgrowth with diffuse hemangiomatous skin findings.

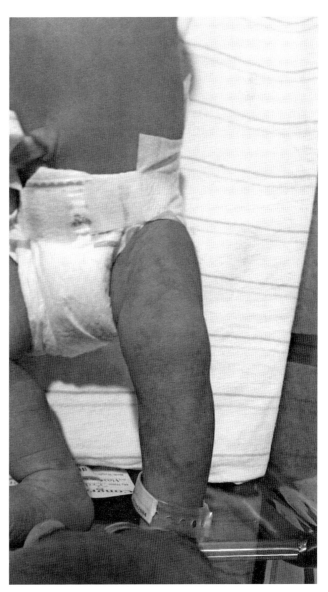

FIGURE 3.5 CLOVES syndrome. Note lipomatous mass over the back and hemangiomas.

- Usually sporadic, rarely reported with positive family history or recurrence
- Clinical features: hemangiomas and soft tissue and/or skeletal (usually lower limb) overgrowth, venous varicosities (Figure 3.4)
  - Thrombophlebitis and thromboembolism risks can be significant.
  - Kasabach–Merritt syndrome (thrombocytopenia) in approximately half
  - Vaginal and rectal bleeding; hematuria in ~15%
- Noninvasive techniques and local compression are preferred. Surgery rarely results in improvement; frequent recurrence of varicosities.
  - *PIK3CA-related overgrowth syndromes* (PROS, MIM 171834)
    - A diverse group of sporadic segmental overgrowth disorders
    - Somatic mosaicism for activating heterozygous variants in *PIK3CA* usually limited to affected tissues
    - Phenotypes vary based on which tissues are primarily affected.
      - Not all affected children are large at birth.
  - **Congenital *l*ipomatous *o*vergrowth, *v*ascular malformations, *e*pidermal nevi, *s*coliosis/skeletal and spinal syndrome** (CLOVES, MIM 612918)

- Clinical features: progressive and disproportionate segmental overgrowth syndrome involving subcutaneous, muscular, vascular, and adipose tissue with skeletal overgrowth (Figure 3.5)
  - ***M*egalencephaly *ca*pillary malformation *p*olymicrogyria syndrome** (MCAP, MIM 602501)
    - Clinical features: prenatal overgrowth, megalencephaly, perisylvian pachygyria, brain and body asymmetry, cutis marmorata, mosaic skin changes and cutaneous vascular malformations (Figure 3.6), digital anomalies—syndactyly, postaxial polydactyly
    - More limited phenotypes can be expressed as macrodactyly, hemihypertrophy, isolated macrocephaly, or hemimegalencephaly with relatively good outcomes.
  - **Proteus syndrome** (MIM 176920)
    - Somatic heterozygous activating variant in *AKT3*
    - Clinical features: severe, variable asymmetric overgrowth, usually of postnatal onset, epidermal nevi, cerebriform connective tissue nevi, usually on the sole, vascular malformations, exostoses

*Pearl*: In the overgrown newborn, build the differential diagnosis around the rarest feature: ear pits/creases in Beckwith–Wiedemann syndrome, camptodactyly in Weaver, and unusual lip in 12p tetrasomy.

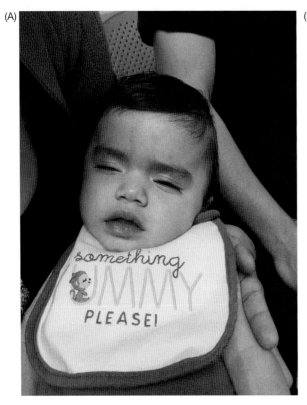
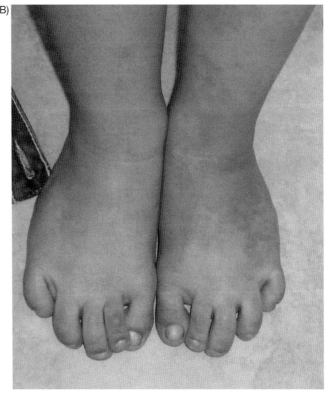

FIGURE 3.6  (A) Macrocephaly in MCAP (megalencephaly, capillary malformation, polymicrogyria syndrome). (B) Different MCAP patient with unusual flat wide feet with hemangiomatous skin changes on one foot.

## Evaluation and Management

- Document prenatal history: maternal obesity, excess weight gain, maternal diabetes.
- Review family history: ethnicity, consanguinity, learning disabilities, parental height and BW.
- Evaluate for segmental versus generalized overgrowth, and document associated abnormalities and dysmorphic features.
  - Ear pits/creases, camptodactyly
  - Echocardiogram
  - Brain imaging
- Genetic testing
  - Chromosomal microarray when generalized overgrowth is unexplained or there are other anomalies
  - Other genetic tests according to the clinical features
    - Methylation studies of 11p15 for suspected Beckwith–Wiedemann syndrome
    - RASopathy gene panel for suspected Costello or other RASopathy
    - Obtain skin or other tissue in segmental overgrowth or tissue-specific mosaic conditions: 12p tetrasomy, MCAP and CLOVES syndromes.
  - Consider exome sequencing for undiagnosed syndromic overgrowth; yield is 50% in recent study (Tatton-Brown et al, 2017).
- Anticipate common complications: hypoglycemia, poor feeding.
- Follow surveillance guidelines (abdominal US q 3mo) for tumor risk in Beckwith–Wiedemann syndrome. Many other overgrowth syndromes have cancer predisposition without a specific tumor being implicated. Base monitoring on careful observation for symptoms.
- Consider enrolling patients in clinical trials for medical therapy (mTOR-inhibiting drugs) rather than surgical intervention in PROS. Recent clinical trial data suggests that a drug inhibiting PIK3CA may be effective in stabilizing and reversing symptoms in PROS related disorders.

## Further Reading

Edmondson AC, Kalish JM. (2015) Overgrowth syndromes. J Pediatr Genet. 4:136–43. PMID 27617124

Keppler-Noreuil KM, Parker VE, Darling TN, Martinez-Agosto JA. (2016) Somatic overgrowth disorders of the PI3K/AKT/mTOR pathway and therapeutic strategies. Am J Med Genet C Semin Med Genet. 172:402–21. PMID 27860216

Malan V, Chevallier S, Soler G, et al. (2010) Array-based comparative genomic hybridization identifies a high frequency of copy number variations in patients with syndromic overgrowth. Eur J Hum Genet. 18:227–32. PMID 19844265

Martinez-Lopez A, Blasco-Morente G, Perez-Lopez I, et al. (2017) CLOVES syndrome: Review of a PIK3CA-related overgrowth spectrum (PROS). Clin Genet. 91:14–21. PMID 27426476

Neylon OM, Werther GA, Sabin MA. (2012) Overgrowth syndromes. Curr Opin Pediatr. 24:505–11. PMID 22705997

Tatton-Brown K, Loveday C, Yost S, et al. (2017) Mutations in epigenetic regulation genes are a major cause of overgrowth with intellectual disability. Am J Hum Genet. 100:725–36. PMID 28475857

Venot Q, Blanc T, Rabia SH, et al. (2018) Targeted therapy in patients with PIK3CA-related overgrowth syndrome. Nature. 558(7711):540–46. PMID 29899452

# 4

## Twins

### Clinical Consult

A 36-year-old G3 woman presented at 14 weeks' gestation for an initial fetal US. Monochorionic, diamniotic twins (monozygotic–MZ) with suspected congenital heart defects were identified. At 19 weeks, fetal echocardiograms suggested tetralogy of Fallot (TOF) in both twins. The family declined invasive testing. At 26 weeks' gestation, mild discrepancies in amniotic fluid volumes between the twins suggested **early twin-to-twin transfusion syndrome (TTTS)**. Serial US revealed progression of TTTS. At 31 weeks, Doppler studies showed reversed diastolic flow in both twins. The decision was made to deliver by C-section. Apgar scores were 7/8[1] and 6/8[5]. The twins were non-dysmorphic, with mild pulmonary hypertension complicating their tetralogy. Microarray in one twin was normal. Clinically, they did well and underwent uncomplicated repair of TOF at 6 and 11 months of age.

This case illustrates the increased frequency of birth defects in monozygotic twins, especially congenital heart defects, which may be present in one or both twins. Heart defects in MZ twins can have an early embryonic etiology but, in addition, early TTTS can give rise to right ventricular outflow abnormalities such as pulmonary atresia. Given the poor prognosis for untreated TTTS, the decision to deliver preterm was timely.

### Definition

- Twins account for 3% of live births and 96% of multiple births.
  - Dizygotic (DZ) twins are more common than monozygotic (MZ): 70:30.
    - The rate of DZ twins varies by population.
    - The rate of MZ twins is uniform worldwide at 3–5/1,000 births.
- "Vanishing twin" phenomenon is common. A significant percentage of twin pregnancies, especially those conceived after assisted reproductive technology (ART), later become singleton pregnancies.

*Pearl*: Many birth defects in apparent singletons may be related to the twinning process, with subsequent loss of the co-twin.

- Factors affecting twin prevalence
  - Assisted reproductive technology (ART) is the main cause of increased twinning
    - The frequency of twins has risen 20% in the United States, 15% in South Korea, and 29% in Denmark.

*Pearl*: ART increases the frequency of both DZ twins and MZ twins.

  - Maternal age: increased maternal age is a factor in approximately one-third of spontaneous DZ twins
  - Ethnicity: Africans have highest DZ twinning rates and Asians the lowest.
  - Increased parity is associated with increased twinning.
  - Family history: Positive maternal family history of DZ twins increases the chance of twins.
    - A paternal family history of twins does not affect the risk for twins, but father's daughters may have more twins in their offspring.
  - Obese and tall women have increased twin rates.
- **Chorionicity determined by timing of cleavage in MZ twins**
  - All DZ twins and MZ twins that divide within the first 3 days post fertilization have two placentas, two chorions (dichorionic, DC), and two amnions (diamniotic, DA).
    - 20–30% of MZ twins are DC/DA
    - Some DZ twins have fused placentas and shared circulation.

*Pearl*: Because MZ twins can occur with any type of chorionicity, having two separate amnions and chorions does not rule out MZ twinning.

  - MZ twins that divide 4–8 days post fertilization have one placenta, one chorion (monochorionic, MC), and two amnions.
    - 70% of MZ twins are MC/DA.
  - MZ twins that divide 8–12 days post fertilization have one placenta, one chorion, and one amnion:
    - <1% of MZ twins are MC/MA.
  - MZ twins that divide after 12 days post fertilization are MC/MA conjoined twins.
  - Mirror-image MZ twins have mild asymmetries in hair patterning and hair whorls and hand creases. They are thought to separate late, after body axis determination, but early enough to avoid conjoined twinning.
- **Conjoined twins**
  - Abnormally late cleavage causes conjoined twinning; joined ventrally 87% or dorsally 13%
  - Ventrally joined twins: cephalopagus 11%, thoracopagus 19%, omphalopagus 18%, ischiopagus 11%, parapagus (pelvis and trunk) 28%
  - Dorsally joined twins: craniopagus 5%, rachiopagus (vertebral column) 2%, pygopagus (sacrum) 6%
- **Morbidity and mortality are higher in twins than in singletons.**

  - Preterm birth
  - Low birth weight, growth restriction
  - Congenital anomalies, especially in MZ twins
  - Fetal and neonatal death
    - Prematurity and TTTS are the leading causes of neonatal mortality in twins.
    - Neonatal sudden infant death syndrome (SIDS) is more common in same-sex twins than in opposite-sex twins, suggesting that monozygosity is a risk factor for SIDS.

# Diagnosis

- Fetal US allows early diagnosis and determination of chorionicity.
  - Fetal US at ~7 weeks' gestation is the most accurate time to determine placentation.
- Twins may have variable but similar phenotypes or mirror-image features.
  - A twin presumed to be unaffected may have a milder expression compared to a more severely affected co-twin, making them concordant for the disorder.

# Differential Diagnosis

- Discordant phenotypes
  - Single gene disorders, teratogenic effects (e.g., dilantin embryopathy), brain abnormalities, chromosome abnormalities, epigenetic abnormalities, autism, and isolated congenital anomalies (e.g., cleft lip/palate) can be discordant in MZ twins, as in the MZ twins shown in Figure 4.1, one with hemifacial microsomia.
  - Etiology
    - DZ twins have different genetic backgrounds and minor differences in embryonic timing.
    - MZ twins can have variable mosaicism due to somatic mutations and placental and epigenetic changes.
      - Discordance for late-onset illnesses, such as migraine, diabetes, and cancer, increases over a lifetime.

*Pearl*: MZ twins often show significant phenotypic discordance. Although genetically "identical," MZ twins can express their genes differently due to epigenetic changes. The term "identical twins" can be misleading and should be avoided.

- Congenital anomalies
  - Congenital anomalies are two or three times more common in MZ twins compared to DZ twins or singletons. DZ twins also have more birth defects compared to singletons.

(A)
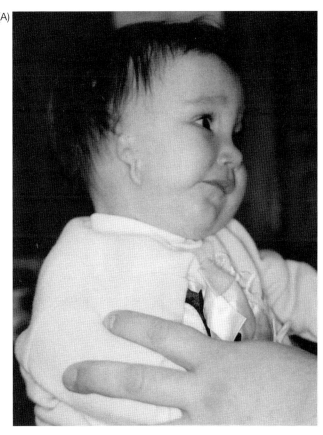

(B)
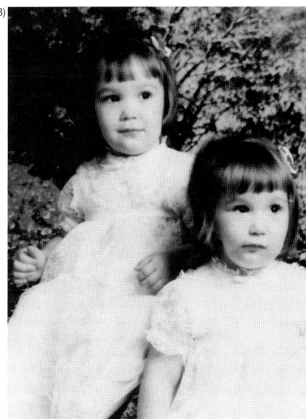

FIGURE 4.1  Hemifacial macrosomia (OAVS) with microtia and asymmetric mandibular hypoplasia in one of MZ twins at birth and at age 4.

○ Birth defect risks in twins may be increased by use of fertility treatment.
○ Congenital anomalies with increased frequency in MZ and DZ twins
  ▪ Congenital heart disease
    • ~5% of MC twins have congenital heart disease (CHD), most commonly VSD.
  ▪ Arthrogryposis, specifically amyoplasia, often discordant in MZ twins
  ▪ CNS: anencephaly, holoprosencephaly
  ▪ Gastrointestinal (GI): omphalocele, especially after ART
  ▪ Genitourinary (GU): hypospadias, obstructive uropathy, exstrophy of the cloaca
  ▪ VATER/VACTERL association, hemifacial microsomia, sacrococcygeal teratoma, sirenomelia
• **Beckwith-Wiedemann syndrome\*** (MIM 130650) slightly more common after ART. Twins can be DZ or MZ and concordant or discordant.
  ○ Deformations are more common in twins.
    ▪ Intrauterine constraint disproportionately affects the infant with the lower position in utero.
    ▪ Cranial asymmetry: plagiocephaly, torticollis, micrognathia
    ▪ Clubfoot, positional foot abnormalities

*Pearl·* Twinning is not a risk factor for developmental hip dysplasia.

• Specific problems in MC/DA twins
  ○ **Twin to Twin Transfusion Syndrome** (TTTS)
    ▪ 10–15% of MC twins
    ▪ Clinical features: Amniotic fluid volume discrepancy is early cardinal sign; differences in hemoglobin (Hgb), hematocrit (Hct), and fetal weight later.
      • Right ventricular outflow tract abnormalities occur in ~9% of recipient twins with TTTS: pulmonary atresia, pulmonic stenosis, and tricuspid insufficiency.
        • After successful laser ablation, ~30% of recipient twins have persistent cardiac lesions.
    ▪ TTTS <26 weeks' gestation should be monitored at a specialized center with laser ablation capability.
    ▪ Up to 60% improve or stabilize over time.
    ▪ TTTS is progressive in 40%.
      • May have a lethal outcome in second trimester
      • Abnormal neurologic outcome primarily associated with prematurity and its complications
  ○ **Twin anemia/polycythemia syndrome** (TAPS)
    ▪ Clinical features: a milder form of TTTS that is not accompanied by changes in amniotic fluid volume

- Follows laser ablation for TTTS in one-third or more of cases
  - May occur in the absence of overt TTTS; may be slow and chronic, avoiding TTTS symptoms
  - Discrepancies occur in weight as well as Hgb and Hct.
- Detected by serial monitoring of peak systolic Doppler measurements of fetal middle cerebral arteries
○ **Twin reversed arterial perfusion (TRAP) sequence**
- Rare complication in MC twins, 1%
- Pump twin has normal fetal circulation, but a portion of its cardiac output goes through arterial–arterial anastomoses in the placenta to umbilical artery and to systemic circulation of recipient co-twin.
  - Risks to pump twin: congestive heart failure, hydrops, death
- Recipient twin is acardiac, nonviable.
  - Circulation in recipient is "reversed": Blood is pumped from normal twin to acardiac twin without passing through a capillary bed.
  - Deoxygenated blood is supplied to lower body through iliac arteries with poor perfusion and resorption of upper body.
    - Heart is absent. Severe craniofacial and limb anomalies. Florid edema and excessive fat are common.
- Prenatal diagnosis possible as early as 11 weeks. Assessment of vasculature helps determine TRAP diagnosis.
  - Diagnostic confusion in US can occur when there is a deceased co-twin or co-twin with anomalies.
- Intervention increases survival to ~85% in pump twin.
○ **Vanishing twin and death of a co-twin**
- "Vanishing" twin is the early loss of one MC twin, <10 weeks. Rates vary; may be more common after ART.
- Most "vanishing" twins are MZ, lost due to vascular disruption, cord entanglement, severe malformations, or spontaneous mutations incompatible with life.
- Death of a MC twin usually occurs after ~12 weeks.
- Damage to survivor has rarely been reported when death of co-twin occurs as early as 9 weeks' gestation. Most documented cases of damaged surviving twins are in the second and third trimesters.
  - Death of co-twin causes release of thromboplastin and disseminated intravascular coagulation; thromboemboli travel through shared vascular connections and cause hemorrhage, ischemia, and disruptive birth defects in survivor.
- Surviving fetus has increased risk for the following:
  - IUGR, very low BW, prematurity, low Apgar scores, perinatal mortality, severe hypotension, anemia due to massive blood volume loss from surviving twin into deceased twin (vascular sink)
  - Renal failure due to acute tubular necrosis
  - CNS insults, porencephaly, schizencephaly, microcephaly, hydranencephaly, cerebral palsy in the survivor (Figure 4.2)

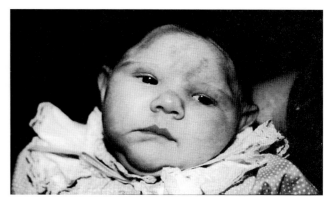

FIGURE 4.2 Severe microcephaly with extensive encephalomalacia after death of a MZ co-twin at 24 weeks' gestation.

  - Gastroschisis, intestinal atresia, limb amputation, aplasia cutis congenita of the trunk and elsewhere (Figure 4.3)

- **MC/MA twins**
  ○ Incidence 1–3% of all MZ twins

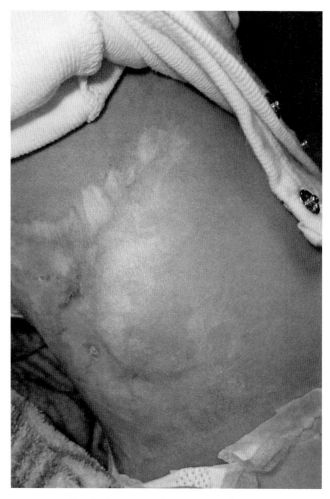

FIGURE 4.3 Death of a MZ co-twin at ~16 weeks' gestation. Extensive healed cutis aplasia of trunk that required skin grafts.

- ○ Survival is poor.
  - ■ Only approximately half of MC/MA twins are alive at 16 weeks' gestation.
  - ■ Of those alive at 16 weeks, only 50% survive to 24 weeks; 25% are lost due to elective termination (secondary to anomalies) and 25% to spontaneous miscarriage.
  - ■ Of those alive at 24 weeks, 4.5% are not viable at term.
- ○ Fetal death primarily due to cord entanglement
- ○ Increased risk of birth defects 26%
  - ■ Increased risk of cerebral injury to the survivor following twin death from cord entanglement

- • To improve outcome, hospitalization of mother after 24 weeks with continuous monitoring and early elective delivery
- • Evaluate twins for concordant or discordant expression of syndromes and birth defects.
  - ○ For known MC twins, genetic testing (microarray, molecular) can be done in just one twin.
  - ○ Evaluate the apparently unaffected twin for anomalies seen in the affected twin (e.g., echocardiogram, renal US) because penetrance for the abnormality may be reduced and the unaffected twin may have minor manifestations.

## Evaluation and Management

- • Determine zygosity
  - ○ Fetal US: Examination of membranes may not determine zygosity because DZ twins can occasionally have fused placentas and shared vascular connections.
  - ○ The most accurate way to determine zygosity after birth is with DNA analysis.
  - ○ Microchimerism can occur in ~8% of DZ twins, making them immune tolerant and a good source for organ transplant.
  - ○ Zygosity may be important in understanding a birth defect present in one or both twins.
- • **Fetal management**
  - ○ After death of a co-twin, monitor surviving fetus.
    - ■ Serial US for head circumference and anomalies
    - ■ Fetal MRI best predictor of CNS damage
      - • When cerebral damage is evident <24 weeks, counsel about neurodevelopmental disability and available pregnancy management options.
  - ○ Treatment options *in utero*.
    - ■ TTTS: laser ablation of vascular connections may produce better outcome (improved survival and normal neurologic exam) than amnio reduction.
    - ■ TRAP: laser ablation of the acardiac twin's umbilical cord at 16–26 weeks
    - ■ For MC/MA twins

## Further Reading

Bartels E, Schulz AC, Mora NW, et al. (2012) VATER/VACTERL association: identification of seven new twin pairs, a systematic review of the literature, and a classical twin analysis. Clin Dysmorphol. 21:191–5. PMID 22895008

Conte G, Righini A, Griffiths PD, et al. (2018) Brain-injured survivors of monochorionic twin pregnancies complicated by single intrauterine death: MR findings in a multicenter study. Radiology. 288:582–90. PMID 29688161

Dawson AL, Tinker SC, Jamieson DJ, et al. (2016) Twinning and major birth defects, National Birth Defects Prevention Study, 1997–2007. J Epidemiol Community Health. 70:1114–21. PMID 27325867

Evron E, Sheiner E, Friger M, et al. (2015) Vanishing twin syndrome: Is it associated with adverse perinatal outcome? Fertil Steril. 103:1209–14. PMID 25772775

Prefumo F, Fichera A, Pagani G, et al. (2015) The natural history of monoamniotic twin pregnancies: A case series and systematic review of the literature. Prenat Diagn. 35:274–80. PMID 25399524

Ruiz-Cordero R, Birusingh RJ, Pelaez L, et al. (2016) Twin reversed arterial perfusion sequence (traps): an illustrative series of 13 cases. Fetal Pediatr Pathol. 35:63–80. PMID 26847661

Quintero RA, Kontopoulos E, Chmait RH. (2016) Laser treatment of twin-to-twin transfusion syndrome. Twin Res Hum Genet. 19:197–206. PMID 27203606

Springer S, Mlczoch E, Krampl-Bettelheim E, et al. (2014) Congenital heart disease in monochorionic twins with and without twin-to-twin transfusion syndrome. Prenat Diagn. 34:994–9. PMID 24827120

# 5

# Non-Immune Hydrops

## Clinical Consult

A 35-year-old G3P2 teacher presented for fetal ultrasound at 18 weeks' gestation. She reported a rash lasting 2 or 3 days at 15 weeks' gestation. Female monochorionic diamniotic twins were identified, and one twin had mild abdominal ascites. Middle cerebral artery peak systolic flow velocity was normal in both twins. Fetal echocardiogram was normal. STAT maternal immunoglobulin G (IgG) and IgA levels ruled out TORCH infections, but parvovirus B19 titers were positive with high IgM titers and slightly elevated IgG titers. Amniotic fluid polymerase chain reaction (PCR) for parvovirus B19 was positive. At 22 weeks' gestation, the weekly fetal ultrasound showed increased ascites and mild generalized hydrops with early pleural effusion. Referral to a major fetal treatment center was expedited. A few days later, when the peak systolic flow velocity in the middle cerebral artery was >1.5 multiple of the median (MoM), an *in utero* transfusion of maternal red cells was undertaken in the affected twin. After two transfusions, the hydrops and ascites slowly resolved, and serial monitoring revealed continued improvement. The twins delivered at term. With the exception of redundant abdominal skin folds, the affected infant appeared well at 6 months (Figure 5.1). At age 14 months, the affected twin was developmentally approximately 6 weeks behind her co-twin.

**Parvovirus infection** causes a generally benign illness, but it may result in a severe fetal aplastic anemia. The peak systolic flow velocity in the middle cerebral artery is a sensitive gauge of fetal anemia and the need for *in utero* treatment. Data on long-term neurologic outcome are limited though generally encouraging. Anecdotal reports, such as this, suggest the need for developmental follow-up in surviving children.

## Definition

Hydrops fetalis refers to excessive fluid accumulation in at least two serous cavities (pleural, abdominal, pericardial) and/or the presence of diffuse body wall edema. Cystic hygroma may or not be present.

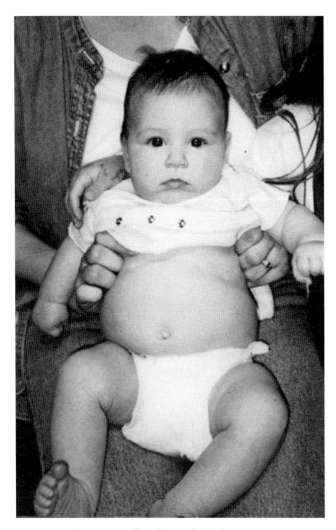

FIGURE 5.1 Parvovirus-affected twin who had severe ascites prior to in utero transfusions. At several months of age she had redundant abdominal skin but was otherwise well.

- Non-immune hydrops (NIH), responsible for >90% of cases of hydrops, occurs in 1/1,700–1/3,000 pregnancies.
  - In the past, Rh isoimmunization was the primary cause.
- NIH is the end stage of a large number of disorders with varying pathophysiology: congenital lymphatic dysplasia, congestive heart failure, fetal anemia, hypoproteinemia, and obstruction to venous return.
  - The primary cause can be obscured by end-stage disease, and more than one mechanism may be operative terminally.
- Usually recognized by ultrasound in the first or second trimester. Polyhydramnios can precede other findings. Oligohydramnios is a late finding usually preceding demise.
  - Approximately 10% of patients with hydrops are not diagnosed before birth.
- NIH is associated with high infant morbidity and mortality. Only ~20% amenable to treatment.
  - Approximately 45% survive the perinatal period.

- Early diagnosis before 22 weeks' gestation has lower survival versus diagnosis after 30 weeks' gestation.
  - Long-term disabilities and neurologic sequelae are frequent with severe disease.
  - The prognosis depends on the underlying cause.
    - Best prognosis: isolated chylothorax, chylous ascites, isolated pleural effusion, meconium peritonitis, cardiac arrhythmia
    - Poor prognosis: presence of congenital anomalies, low birth weight or chromosome abnormality
      - Many die in utero, especially those with aneuploidy. Families with early diagnosis of severe hydrops may elect to discontinue the pregnancy.

## Differential Diagnosis

- Cardiovascular abnormalities ~22%
  - Arrhythmias including supraventricular tachycardia (SVT), heart block due to SSA, SSB antibodies, Wolf–Parkinson–White syndrome, flutter
  - Structural cardiac disease: Ebstein anomaly, tetralogy of Fallot, hypoplastic left heart, truncus arteriosus, transposition of the great vessels, aortic atresia, premature closure of ductus arteriosus
  - Cardiomyopathy, endocardial fibroelastosis, cardiac rhabdomyomas
- Chromosomal abnormalities ~14%
  - **Turner syndrome\*** is the most common aneuploidy with hydrops. Cystic hygroma and dramatic swelling of hands and feet may predominate. Most 45,X fetuses are miscarried (Figure 5.2A) due to extreme hydrops. In survivors, swelling of the hands and feet or redundant neck skin may be the only residua of fetal hydrops (Figure 5.2B).
  - **Trisomy 21\*** (T21) and **Trisomy 18\*** (T18) are common causes.
    - The following prenatal findings suggest T21: short long bones, absent nasal bone, fifth finger clinodactyly, and sandal gap between toes. Overlapping, clenched fingers may assist in diagnosing T18. Cystic hygroma is occasionally seen.
    - Many other chromosome disorders present with NIH (e.g., deletion 13q).

*Pearl*: In an affected fetus with NIH, cell-free DNA (cfDNA) can establish some diagnoses (e.g., T21 and T18).

- Congenital infection ~7%
  - Most common are parvovirus, syphilis, and cytomegalovirus. Less common are toxoplasmosis, Coxsackie viruses, varicella, respiratory syncytial virus (RSV), Lyme disease, and HIV.

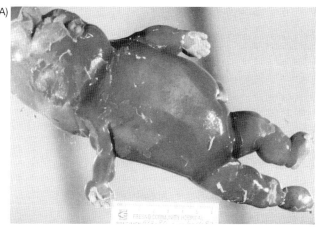

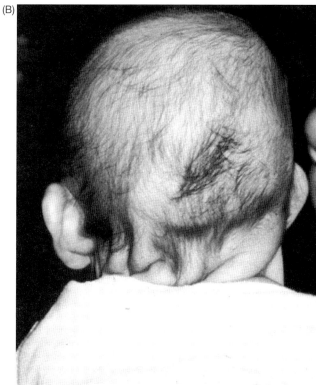

FIGURE 5.2  (A) Severe hydrops in 45,X leading to fetal demise in 18-week fetus. (B) Webbing and redundant neck skin following resolution of cystic hygroma in 45,X.

- o **Parvovirus B19**
  - ■ Incidence of acute parvovirus B19 infection in pregnancy is ~3.5%.
    - • 40–60% of pregnant women are not immune.
  - ■ Risk of NIH is ~4% in an infected pregnant woman.
    - • It presents 3–13 weeks after maternal infection.
  - ■ Diagnosis: Elevated IgM indicates current infection.
    - • Elevated IgG without IgM elevation indicates past infection.
  - ■ Approximately 30% of hydrops cases resolve; other cases progress and may lead to death due to fetal anemia.
    - • The risk of fetal loss after infection is ~11% before 20 weeks and ~1% after 20 weeks.

- • In utero transfusion may be life-saving.
- • It is probably *not* teratogenic but long-term developmental concerns remain.
- o **Syphilis**
  - ■ **Rising** incidence in several U.S. states, doubled in past 5 years
    - • Fetal transmission 70–100% in primary syphilis
    - • May occur anytime during pregnancy
  - ■ Prenatal features: ascites, pleural effusion, hydrops, IUGR
  - ■ Clinical findings: hydrops, thrombocytopenia, hepatosplenomegaly, metaphyseal bone changes (Figure 5.3A)
    - • Red, peeling hands and feet (other areas also) are characteristic (Figure 5.3B).
  - ■ Treatment: penicillin *only*

*Pearl*: Congenital syphilis is on the rise. Order rapid test on all mothers at delivery. Red peeling hands and feet are a distinctive clue. Peeling areas are very infectious.

- o **Cytomegalovirus (CMV)**
  - ■ Incidence of congenital CMV infection is 0.5–2%.
    - • Only 10–15% of infants with congenital CMV are symptomatic.
  - ■ Prenatal findings: echogenic bowel, IUGR, hepatosplenomegaly, pleural and pericardial effusion, intracranial calcifications at the borders of lateral ventricles, microcephaly and ventriculomegaly (late)
  - ■ Clinical features in neonate: thrombocytopenia, "blueberry muffin rash," chorioretinitis
    - • Sensorineural hearing loss is the most common sequela.
- • Skeletal dysplasias and NIH
  - o Many lethal skeletal dysplasias can present with NIH, including the following:
    - ■ **Achondrogenesis** (MIM 200600): severely shortened long bones, small chest, cystic hygroma
    - ■ **Atelosteogenesis I** (MIM 108720) is dominant; Type II is recessive (MIM 256050): cleft palate, clubfeet
- • Metabolic disorders >5%
  - o These disorders often go undiagnosed because of lack of specific staining for lysosomal storage. Autopsy is critical. Molecular testing can confirm a suspected diagnosis using newborn screening blood spots

*Pearl*: Consider metabolic causes, especially when a previous infant in the family has also had NIH.

- ■ Most metabolic causes are lysosomal storage disorders: most commonly **mucopolysaccharidoses VII** (MIM 253220), **perinatal lethal Gaucher** (MIM 608013), and **GM1 gangliosidosis** (MIM 230500). Rare

(A)

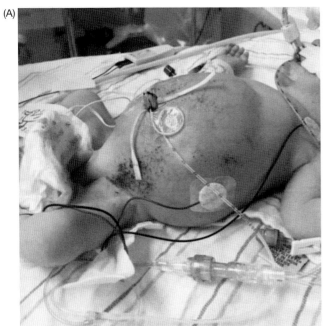

(B)

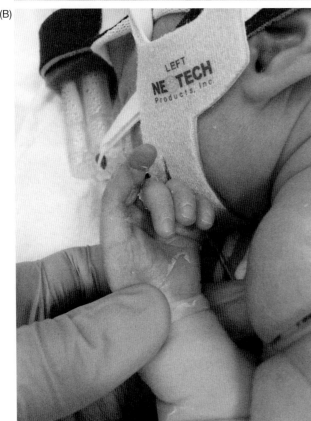

FIGURE 5.3   (A) Congenital syphilis with hepatosplenomegaly, ascites, and petechiae. (B) Peeling skin is a helpful diagnostic clue in congenital syphilis.

metabolic causes of NIH are **Hurler syndrome MPS I** (MIM 60701), **sialidosis (neuraminidase deficiency)** (MIM 256550), **infantile sialic acid storage disease** (MIM 269920), **galactosialidosis** (MIM 256540),

**Niemann–Pick type C** (MIM 257220), **Neiman–Pick type A** (MIM 257200), **mucolipidosis II** (MIM 252500)

○ Congenital disorders of glycosylation, diagnosed with abnormal transferrin electrophoresis followed by confirmatory molecular testing

- Syndromic **NIH**
  ○ **Noonan\*** (MIM 163950), **cardiofaciocutaneous** (CFC, MIM 115150), **Costello** (MIM 218040), and rarely **neurofibromatosis type 1** (MIM 162200)
    ▪ Fetal lymphatic abnormalities occur in 43%.
      • Increased nuchal translucency, increased nuchal fold, cystic hygroma, fetal edema, excess amniotic fluid (AFI >25 cm)
    ▪ At birth, 57% have lymphatic abnormalities.
  ○ **Neu–Laxova syndrome** (MIM 256520)
    ▪ Autosomal recessive disorder of the L-serine biosynthesis pathway, caused by biallelic variants in *PHGDH* or *PSAT1*
    ▪ Clinical features: lethal disorder with severe edema of hands and feet, microcephaly, cataracts, ectropion, ichthyosis (Figure 5.4)
  ○ **Hennekam syndrome** (MIM 235510)
    ▪ Autosomal recessive disorder: Biallelic variants in *CCBE1* are detected in ~25%.
    ▪ Clinical findings: lymphedema of all four limbs, lymphangiectasia of the intestines and/or lungs
      • Variable learning difficulties
      • Characteristic face: flat face, flat and broad nasal bridge, hypertelorism
  ○ **Microcephaly–chorioretinal dysplasia–lymphedema–mental retardation** (MCLMR, MIM 152950).

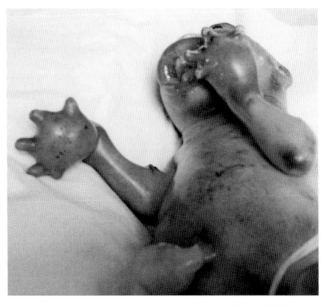

FIGURE 5.4   Neu–Laxova syndrome. Dramatic swelling of the hands and feet is a frequent finding.

- Autosomal dominant disorder: Most have a de novo heterozygous variant in *KIF11*.
- Clinical features: Microcephaly (–2 to –7 SD) is consistent, but other features are variable: chorioretinopathy, retinal folds, microphthalmia, lower limb lymphedema, which can be confined to the dorsa of the feet.
  - This phenotype overlaps with that of congenital infection.
  - Moderate intellectual disability
- **Fetal Akinesia Deformation Sequence** (FADS MIM 208150) Syndromes with markedly decreased fetal activity often result in FADS. Many present with hydrops:
  - **Lethal multiple pterygia syndrome** (MIM 253290)
    - Hypoplastic lungs, contractures with pterygia, cystic hygroma
    - Autosomal recessive variants in gene CHRNG
  - **Escobar syndrome** (MIM 265000)
    - Non-lethal syndrome also caused by variants in CHRNG
- **Congenital myotonic dystrophy** (MIM 160900)
  - Edema often only of upper body

- **LYMPHATIC DYSPLASIA ~15%**
  - Genes that function in early lymphatic development are implicated in autosomal dominant and recessive types of fetal hydrops.
  - **Milroy disease** (hereditary lymphedema IA, MIM 153100)
    - Autosomal dominant disorder; 85% penetrant
      - 70% have a heterozygous variant in *FLT4*.
    - Onset is usually at birth but may occur later.
    - Clinical features: typically presents with congenital edema of both legs, may affect hands; hydrocele, pleural effusion, chylous ascites less common
  - **Lymphedema–distichiasis syndrome** (MIM 153400)
    - Autosomal dominant with incomplete penetrance due to heterozygous variant in *FOXC2*
    - Clinical features: distichiasis in 95% (double row of eyelashes), lymphedema of the extremities usually presents in childhood, cleft palate; can present with NIH
  - **Lymphedema III** (MIM 616843)
    - Autosomal recessive disorder caused by biallelic variants in *PIEZO1*
    - Clinical features: recurrent facial swelling with secondary cellulitis, recurrent chylothorax; four limb lymphedema in childhood and adulthood
  - **Hypotrichosis–lymphedema–telangiectasia syndrome** (MIM 137940)
    - Both autosomal dominant (with renal defect, proteinuria) and autosomal recessive disorders are caused by variants in *SOX18*.
    - Clinical features: alopecia, swelling of eyelids, hydroceles, edema of scrotum. NIH can be the presenting sign.
      - Survivors may have late-onset lymphedema and recurrent fluid accumulation.

- **SINGLE SYSTEM ABNORMALITIES**
  - Lung: cystic pulmonary airway malformation, pulmonary sequestration, diaphragmatic hernia, congenital pulmonary lymphangiectasia
  - Gastrointestinal: meconium peritonitis, volvulus
  - Liver: hepatic fibrosis, biliary atresia
  - Renal: polycystic kidneys
  - Other: sacrococcygeal teratoma, other tumors
- **PLACENTAL AND CORD ABNORMALITIES**
  - Fetal–maternal hemorrhage
  - Chorioangioma of the placenta
  - **Neonatal hemochromatosis** (MIM 231100)
    - Long thought to be genetic but now known to be an alloimmune phenomenon with nearly 100% recurrence risk
      - Unrelated to adult-onset hemochromatosis
      - Prenatal treatment with IVIG may ameliorate or prevent iron accumulation in tissues.
  - Torsion or true knot in cord

- **TWIN INTERACTIONS**
  - Twin-to-twin transfusion in monochorionic, diamniotic twins; rare in monochorionic, monoamniotic twins (see Twins*)
- **MATERNAL DISEASE**
  - Severe maternal anemia
  - **α-Thalassemia** (MIM 141800)
    - Both parents must be carriers of the α-thalassemia trait. Suspect when both maternal and paternal mean corpuscular volumes (MCVs) are low.
  - Diabetes (rare)
- **IDIOPATHIC**
  - Overall, ~20% of all cases of NIH elude diagnosis.
  - Document features thoroughly and save cord blood or tissue for molecular studies or exome sequencing.

# Evaluation and Management

- **Maternal evaluation *during pregnancy***
  - Refer to a tertiary perinatal center for thorough pre- and postnatal evaluation to increase diagnostic yield, which may be critical for the few conditions in which intervention may be life-saving.
    - Seek early genetics consultation.
  - Document family history, including consanguinity, previous fetal losses, history of lymphedema, and other anomalies (cardiac anomalies, distichiasis).
  - IgG and IgM for TORCH infections including syphilis and parvovirus (STAT), varicella, Lyme disease, RSV, and AIDS
    - Hydrops associated with parvovirus B19 infection may be cured with fetal transfusion. Timing is critical.

- o Perform Betke–Kleihauer test to rule out fetal–maternal hemorrhage.
- o When MCV is low, without evidence of iron deficiency, investigate further:
  - ▪ Quantitative hemoglobin electrophoresis, especially in ethnic groups at risk for β-thalassemia
  - ▪ Molecular testing for α-thalassemia carrier status when hemoglobin electrophoresis is normal, especially if mother is Asian.

- **Fetal evaluation**
  - o Detailed ultrasound including arterial and venous Doppler
    - ▪ Middle cerebral artery peak systolic velocity in all after 16 weeks for fetal anemia
  - o Fetal echocardiogram—for arrhythmia and structure
  - o Amniocentesis with fluorescence in situ hybridization (FISH) for common trisomies followed by microarray if negative
    - ▪ Consider saving cells for other specific testing.
    - ▪ Offer cfDNA for aneuploidy screening if amniocentesis is declined.

- **Neonatal evaluation**
  - o Obtain family history as previously discussed.
  - o Recommend tests outlined above *for mother*.
  - o Examine placenta for lysosomal storage, excessive iron, evidence of infection, and lymphatic dysplasia.
  - o Take photographs for documentation and evaluation of dysmorphic features.
  - o Radiographs for skeletal findings, calcified meconium, etc.
  - o Order laboratory studies in the infant:
    - ▪ Complete blood count (CBC) with red blood cell (RBC) indices STAT
      - • If abnormal: Order parental MCV to rule out parental carrier status for α-thalassemia.
      - • Follow with quantitative hemoglobin electrophoresis and DNA for α-globin gene sequencing and enumeration.
    - ▪ Blood type and antibody screen

- ▪ Chromosome analysis (Na heparin green top tube), microarray (lavender top tube)
- ▪ Test for viral infectious diseases, as previously discussed.
- ▪ Consider testing for lysosomal storage disorders when other evaluations are negative.
- ▪ Bank DNA for future use (EDTA lavender top tube). Freeze tissue in the event of infant's demise.
- ▪ Several genetic testing laboratories offer NIH sequencing panels. Consider exome sequencing when no diagnosis has been made.
  - o Echocardiogram
  - o Genetic consultation
  - o Autopsy is essential when fetal/neonatal death occurs without a known cause.

# Further Reading

Bascietto F, Liberati M, Murgano D, et al. (2018) Outcomes associated with fetal Parvovirus B19 infection: a systematic review and meta-analysis. Ultrasound Obstet Gynecol. [Epub ahead of print]. PMID 29785793

Bellini C, Donarini G, Paladini D, et al. (2015) Etiology of non-immune hydrops fetalis: An update. Am J Med Genet A. 167A:1082–88. PMID 25712632

Desilets V, Audibert F, and Society of Obstetricians and Gynecologists of Canada. (2013) Investigation and management of non-immune hydrops. J Obstet Gynecol Can. 35:923–38. PMID 24165062

Gimovsky AC, Luzi P, Berghella V. (2015) Lysosomal storage disease as an etiology of nonimmune hydrops. Am J Obstet Gynecol. 212:281–90. PMID 25305402

Myers A, Bernstein JA, Brennan ML, et al. (2014) Perinatal features of the RASopathies: Noonan syndrome, cardiofaciocutaneous syndrome and Costello syndrome. Am J Med Genet A. 164A:2814–21. PMID 25250515

Ota S, Sahara J, Mabuchi A, et al. (2016) Perinatal and one-year outcomes of non-immune hydrops fetalis by etiology and age at diagnosis. J Obstet Gynaecol Res. 42:385–91. PMID 26712114

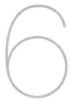

# Teratogenic Agents

## Clinical Consult

A term female infant had lack of facial movement and a left clubfoot. She was delivered to a 26-year-old mother with poor prenatal care, who reported marijuana use until pregnancy was confirmed at 5 months' gestation. All growth parameters were at the 4th–10th percentile. She was transferred to a regional NICU for apnea while breast-feeding. A geneticist interviewed the mother there at the baby's bedside in the NICU. The genetics exam was pertinent for absent lateral eye movements, left esotropia, disconjugate gaze, laterally built-up nasal bridge, micrognathia, hypoplastic nails, low-volume cry, exaggerated startle response, and hypertonia. Bilateral palsies of the sixth and seventh cranial nerves established the diagnosis of **Moebius sequence** (Figure 6.1). The baby went home on oral feedings at 3 weeks of age.

When her baby returned for a follow-up visit at 2 months, the mother met with a genetic counselor in a private setting and reported that she had requested a pregnancy termination at 8 weeks' gestation. Her physician gave her five pills that she took as directed. After passing tissue vaginally, she assumed that she had miscarried and failed to keep her scheduled follow-up appointment. At 5 months' gestation, she realized she was pregnant and started prenatal care. Medical records were not available to confirm her medication exposure, but one of the medications she took was probably misoprostol (Cytotec). This drug in combination with methotrexate is frequently used for early pregnancy termination. In 5% of cases, pregnancy termination is unsuccessful. Infants born after misoprostol/methotrexate exposure have an increased risk for Moebius sequence, transverse limb anomalies, and/or the teratogenic effects of methotrexate. The likely diagnosis is **misoprostol embryopathy**. This case illustrates the importance of speaking privately with the mother to elicit an accurate history of teratogen exposures.

## Definition

- Teratogens, extrinsic agents that interrupt normal morphogenesis, cause 5–6% of congenital anomalies.

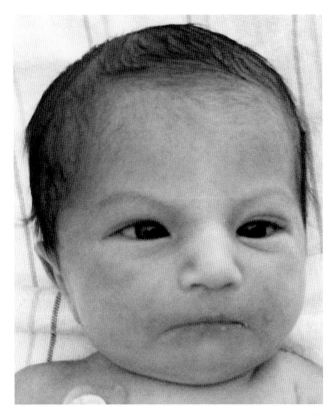

FIGURE 6.1  Moebius sequence in a newborn exposed to misoprostol in an unsuccessful attempt to induce an abortion. Note expressionless face, lack of lateral gaze, and esotropia.

○ Common teratogens, including infectious agents, are reviewed here. Fetal alcohol spectrum disorders* are reviewed in a separate chapter.
- Prescription drug use is common in pregnancy. Alcohol and tobacco use is even more prevalent.
  ○ In the United States, approximately half of pregnant women take at least one medication in the first trimester, and 90% take at least one medication while pregnant.
  ○ Drugs known to be teratogenic are prescribed commonly to women of childbearing age: once in every 13 ambulatory visits, in one study.
    ■ Among women who take potentially teratogenic drugs, >6% become pregnant.

## Congenital Infections

- TORCH (*T*oxoplasma, *r*ubella, *c*ytomegalovirus, *h*erpes, including syphilis)

*Pearl*: TORCH infections account for 5–15% of IUGR.*

  ○ **Congenital toxoplasmosis infection** is the most common parasitic infection in the United States

○ Caused by a parasite, *Toxoplasma gondii*, found in undercooked meat and cat feces
  ■ Incidence 0.1–1/1,000 live births, affects 400–4,000 infants/year in the United States
    • ~85% of women of childbearing age in the United States are susceptible to *Toxoplasma* infection.
  ■ Infection occurs by ingestion of oocysts from fecal material in contaminated soil, cat litter, garden vegetables or water, or ingestion of pseudocysts in undercooked meat.
  ■ Domestic cats are the primary host.
    • In the United States, 12% of cats have *T. gondii* in feces. Rates vary in other countries.
    • Kittens are more likely than adult cats to excrete oocytes in feces.
  ■ Most infected women are asymptomatic; 15% have flu-like symptoms with lymphadenopathy.
  ■ Fetal infection
    • More severe in the first trimester
    • Less likely when infection occurs early in pregnancy: <2% in the first 10 weeks; 80% near term
  ■ Clinical features
    • Asymptomatic 70–90%
      • Up to 80% develop learning and vision problems later.
      • Preterm infants often develop CNS manifestations by 3 months of life.
    • Symptomatic 10–30%
      • Term infants may have milder symptoms: hepatosplenomegaly and lymphadenopathy.
      • Systemic presentation: maculopapular rash, lymphadenopathy, thrombocytopenia, jaundice
      • Predominantly CNS presentation: hydrocephalus, intracranial calcifications, microcephaly, seizures, meningoencephalitis, chorioretinitis, deafness
      • Can be fatal
  ■ Diagnosis
    • Follow up positive maternal IgM titers with *T. gondii* serology testing in a specialty reference laboratory (http://www.pamf.org/serology).
    • PCR in amniotic fluid to diagnose fetal infection
    • Prenatal maternal serology may miss neonatal cases when transmission occurs later in pregnancy.
  ■ Treat pregnant mothers with spiramycin or, after 18 weeks gestational age (GA), pyrimethamine–sulfadiazine and folinic acid; hepatotoxicity and bone marrow suppression can develop with the latter.
○ **Congenital rubella embryopathy**
  ■ Incidence unknown
    • Rare disease in developed countries; lack of vaccination causes outbreaks.
    • Incidence is higher in the developing world; fewer women of reproductive age are immune.

- Infection before 12 weeks' gestation causes miscarriage or fetal death in ~30%.
- Clinical features after first-trimester infection
  - IUGR 34%, microcephaly 78%, microphthalmia, cataracts 37%, pigmentary retinopathy, cardiac defects 34% (especially septal defects, pulmonary artery stenosis), hepatosplenomegaly, thrombocytopenia, "blueberry muffin syndrome"
  - Brain anomalies 12.5%: Dandy–Walker malformation, ventriculomegaly, periventricular calcifications
  - Deafness 15%; ID is common.
- Diagnose with viral isolation (preferred), serology for IgM (may not be detectable), PCR, rubella antigen detection, placental biopsy.
  - o Diagnose with serology (IgM, IgG, IgG avidity) and real-time quantitative PCR (more sensitive) in urine, blood, saliva.
  - o Only 25% of symptomatic children are diagnosed.
  - o Treatment with antiviral agents (IV ganciclovir and the oral prodrug, vanganciclovir) is more effective in the first few weeks of life.
- o **Congenital cytomegalovirus infection** (CMV)—the most common congenital infection
  - Congenital CMV infection occurs in 0.3–0.7% of newborns worldwide; 1% or 2% in high-risk, low socioeconomic groups.
    - Affects >25,000 infants/year in the United States
  - ~40% of pregnant women in the United States are at risk for primary CMV infection.
  - 1% of pregnant women seroconvert during pregnancy.
  - Vertical transmission from mother to fetus occurs in 30% of primary CMV infections and in 1.4% of reactivated past infections.
    - Premature babies can acquire CMV infection from infected breast milk or blood transfusions.
  - Clinical features
    - Symptomatic patients: 10–12% of infected infants
      - Hepatomegaly, splenomegaly, hydrops, jaundice, sepsis-like syndrome, petechiae, hemolytic anemia, microcephaly, IUGR, pneumonia, hydrops, seizures
      - Less common: microphthalmia, chorioretinitis, cataracts, myocarditis
      - MRI/CT findings: intracranial calcifications, periventricular cysts, cerebellar hypoplasia, migration disorders, cerebellar vermis hypoplasia, ventriculomegaly, absent corpus callosum
      - Later: developmental delay/intellectual disability 40–58%, cerebral palsy, visual impairment, seizures, autism
    - Hearing loss 40–50%
    - Asymptomatic infants: 88–90% of infected infants
      - 10–20% have neurologic sequelae.

*Pearl*: Among children with autism, 3–7% have evidence of congenital CMV infection on newborn dried blood spots.

- Sensorineural hearing loss (SNHL), in 7–15%, is increased 20 times compared to the general population of infants.
- SNHL median onset: 27 months
- Among children with unexplained SNHL, 23% test positive for CMV DNA on newborn dried blood spots.

*Pearl*: Up to 10% of infants who failed newborn hearing screen had congenital CMV infection in Australia.

- o Treatment with antiviral agents (IV ganciclovir and the oral prodrug, vanganciclovir) is more effective in the first few weeks of life.
- o Diagnose with serology (IgM, IgG, IgG avidity) and real-time quantitative PCR (more sensitive) in urine, blood, and saliva.
- o Only 25% of symptomatic children are diagnosed.
- o **Congenital herpes simplex infection** (HSV-1, HSV-2)
  - Incidence 1/3,200 live births
    - In United States, ~1,500 cases/year
  - 20–30% of pregnant women are infected with HSV-2.
    - 2% of at-risk women seroconvert for HSV-1 or HSV-2 during pregnancy.
      - Most are unaware of their infection.
      - Only ~35% have symptoms.
    - With a past history of genital herpes: 1% shed virus at delivery.
  - Risk to the fetus is greatest when mothers seroconvert in the third trimester near delivery.
    - Seroconversion occurs after primary maternal infection in 50%; after recurrent infection: <3%
  - Timing of fetal infection
    - Intrauterine HSV infection: ≤5% of all congenital HSV infection
      - Increased miscarriage, stillbirth, congenital anomalies
    - Infection at delivery 85–90%; early postnatal life 5–10%
      - Morbidity and mortality for HSV-2 are 50%; those for HSV-1 are 70%.
  - Clinical features
    - Perinatal HSV infection
      - Localized vesicles on skin, eyes, or mouth within 1–3 weeks of birth
      - Untreated disseminated disease in 70%: coagulopathy, pneumonitis, liver failure, meningitis, encephalitis
    - Up to 40% with disseminated disease do not develop skin lesions.

- Intrauterine HSV infection
  - ~50% have disseminated disease.
  - Scarring, active skin lesions, microphthalmia, cataract, retinal dysplasia, microcephaly, hydranencephaly, intracranial calcifications, IUGR
  - Developmental delay and seizures occur with both intrauterine and perinatal infection.
  - Perinatal mortality >80% without therapy.
  - Treat infants with high-dose acyclovir.
- **Congenital syphilis infection**
  - Incidence 11.6/100,000 live births (United States, 2014), highest rate since 2001
    - Incidence is rising in the United States in all regions and all racial groups.
    - Lack of prenatal care is a risk factor.
  - It is caused by the spirochete, *Treponema pallidum*.
  - Transplacental transmission, the most common route of fetal infection, occurs from 14 weeks GA.
    - Risk of fetal infection increases with gestational age.
    - Infant can be infected by genital lesions at delivery.
    - Within the first 4 years of maternal infection, an untreated pregnant woman has a 70% chance of transmitting the infection to her fetus.
  - Maternal treatment with benzathine penicillin G is 98% effective in preventing congenital syphilis.
    - Initiate ≥30 days before delivery. Penicillin dose must be appropriate for stage of infection (primary, secondary, latent).
  - Clinical features
    - Among untreated infected women, 50–80% have an adverse pregnancy outcome.
      - Miscarriage, late stillbirth, low birth weight, preterm delivery, early infant death, congenital syphilis in the offspring
    - Asymptomatic infants: ~60% of infected live-born infants
      - Low birth weight can be the only symptom of congenital syphilis.
    - Symptomatic infants: hydrops, ascites (Figure 5.3), jaundice, anemia, hepatosplenomegaly 50–90%, thrombocytopenia 30%, fever, petechiae, desquamation (especially of hands and feet), maculopapular rash (1 or 2 weeks of life to 3 months), rhinitis, symmetric long bone lesions 50–95% (6 weeks–6 months), lymphadenopathy (4–8 weeks), chorioretinitis, meningitis 40–60%, calcification of vessels at basal ganglia

*Pearl*: Consider congenital syphilis in a hydropic infant with hemolytic anemia and a negative Coombs test.

  - Neonatal evaluation includes lumbar puncture, eye exam, long bone films, CBC.
  - Diagnosis
    - All mothers should be screened in all three trimesters.

- Screening at birth with IgG treponemal rapid antigen is fast: Further screening is indicated in those testing positive with the *Treponema pallidum* particle agglutination assay (TPPA) and then the rapid plasma reagin test (RPR),
- The organism cannot be cultured.
- Dark field microscopy of placenta for spirochetes can be diagnostic.
  - Treat with penicillin IV or IM for 10 days.
    - Refer to American Academy of Pediatrics guidelines in *Red Book: 2015 Report on the Committee on Infectious Diseases.*

- **Lymphocytic choriomeningitis virus (LCMV) infection**
  - LCMV is a rodent-borne virus.
  - Congenital LCMV infection is underascertained; incidence is unknown.
  - Prenatal findings: IUGR, hydrops, ascites, microcephaly, ventriculomegaly, hydrocephalus, polyhydramnios
  - Clinical features: microcephaly, neuronal migration anomalies, pachygyria, periventricular calcification, porencephalic cysts, intracranial hemorrhage, ventriculomegaly, hydrocephaly, seizures, chorioretinitis, bilateral optic nerve atrophy or dysplasia

*Pearl*: LCMV serology should be included whenever TORCH studies are done, especially when brain and eye findings are present.

- **Congenital parvovirus B19 virus infection**
  - Affects 1–5% of pregnant women; causes fifth disease ("slapped cheek disease") in children
    - Maternal infection is asymptomatic or associated with erythema infectiosum (rash, fever, polyarthralgia), postinfectious arthropathy, or anemia. Most have a normal pregnancy outcome.
  - Fetal transmission occurs in 39% of maternal infections.
    - Among infected newborns, ~40% of mothers had symptomatic infection.
    - Parvovirus is cytotoxic to erythroid precursor cells; inhibits erythropoiesis; and causes fetal anemia, ascites, pleural effusion, and fetal death/stillbirth.
    - Fetal death 10% overall
      - Highest risk for death when infection occurs in ≤20 weeks of gestation
      - Higher risk with ascites/hydrops (Figure 5.1), survival drops to 70%
        - *In utero* fetal transfusion for severe hydrops increases survival to 86%.
        - Passive immunization with gammaglobulin injection into the peritoneal cavity in utero may be beneficial.
  - Clinical features in newborns: anemia, hydrops, high-output cardiac failure, myocarditis, corneal opacities, meconium peritonitis, hepatic calcifications

- Isolated ascites or pleural effusion may occur in the absence of anemia.
  ○ Diagnose with IgM antibodies and DNA detection with PCR (combination gives highest sensitivity) in maternal and infant sera.
    - Evaluate for parvovirus B19 whenever there is non-immune hydrops, ascites, or unexplained fetal death.
    - Fetal ascites should prompt STAT maternal parvovirus titers as treatment may be life-saving.
- **Congenital varicella zoster virus syndrome** (VZV)
  ○ Incidence 1–7/10,000 pregnancies
    - It affects 1% or 2% of fetuses exposed to maternal chickenpox in the first 20 weeks of pregnancy, globally.
    - Among infected fetuses, 12% have congenital anomalies.
  ○ Fetal transmission
    - Primary maternal varicella infection in the first 20 weeks of gestation is the main cause.
      • Reactivation of latent herpes zoster in the mother is a theoretical risk.
    - Intrauterine infection has not been reported with primary maternal infection after 28 weeks.
    - The highest risk for fetal transmission is when primary maternal infection occurs 5 days before to 2 days following delivery.
      • Mortality is ~20% in neonatal varicella acquired by peripartum infection.
        • The greatest risk of death is when the infant's rash develops at 5–10 days of age.
    - Prophylaxis with varicella zoster-specific IgG (VZIG) is recommended for exposed infants whose mothers have negative IgG and IgM titers.
      • Prenatal findings: hydrops, IUGR, CNS and limb anomalies, fetal death
  ○ Clinical features: CNS lesions 48–62%, microcephaly, hydrocephaly, cortical atrophy, ventriculomegaly, seizures, eye disorders 44–52% (chorioretinitis, microphthalmia, cataract), limb and digit hypoplasia 46–72%, skin lesions 70% (dermatomal distribution, denuded skin, scarring)
    - Mortality ~30%
    - Long-term learning and developmental problems in some
  ○ Diagnose with both VZV DNA PCR analysis and IgG and IgM specific for VZV, in mother and infant.
  ○ Treat active neonatal infection: VZIG treatment and antiviral drugs.
    - Treat pregnant non-immune women exposed to infection with VZIG.
- **Congenital Zika virus infection**
  ○ Zika, an RNA flavivirus, is endemic in more than 50 countries.
  ○ In 2015, Zika virus infection was associated with 20-fold annual increase in microcephaly in northeast Brazil, for a prevalence of 99.7/100,000 live births.

  ○ Risk is greatest in countries with mosquito-borne transmission: Mexico, Central and South America, Caribbean and Pacific Islands, Cape Verde, Africa.
  ○ Modes of infection
    - *Aedes* mosquito is the primary vector.
    - Infection can occur through sexual contact with an infected partner who traveled to an endemic area.
    - Laboratory transmission has been reported.
    - Zika virus has been found in breast milk, and evidence of mother-to-infant transmission via breast feeding has been reported.
  ○ 80% of infected individuals are asymptomatic.
    - In symptomatic adults, illness is usually mild; fever, rash, joint pain, conjunctivitis.
    - Guillain–Barre syndrome can occur.
  ○ Infected pregnant women, symptomatic or asymptomatic, may transmit the virus to their fetus.
    - Congenital infection results from transplacental transmission.
    - Peripartum infection also occurs.
  ○ Infection in all three trimesters is associated with risk for congenital microcephaly and other adverse developmental outcomes. Infected infants with normal head circumference at birth can develop microcephaly by 6 months. Microcephaly may be most obvious but not the most common adverse outcome.
    - Recent estimates from combined studies for adverse outcome after Zika infection range from 29% to 40%.
    - Specific information on the range of effects, the critical period for teratogenicity, and the mechanism of pathogenesis (brain disruption) is emerging.
  ○ Prenatal findings
    - Gradual fall off in head circumference to microcephalic range (<3 percentile for GA) in the mid to late second trimester
    - Abnormal CNS findings on fetal US: ventriculomegaly, vermis hypoplasia, may help make diagnosis
  ○ Clinical features: fetal loss, IUGR, severe microcephaly, redundant scalp folds/rugae, prominent occipital shelf, seizures, spasticity, pigmented maculopathy (~30%) (Figure 14.4A, B)
    - Joint contractures ~11%
    - CNS imaging: dramatic volume loss (fetal brain disruption), poor gyral formation, ventriculomegaly, enlarged cisterna magna, small cerebellum, widespread intracranial calcifications (not periventricular)
      • Calcifications in the brain stem are associated with arthrogryposis.
  ○ Follow Centers for Disease Control and Prevention (CDC) and World Health Organization (WHO) guidelines for diagnosis and reporting: https://www.cdc.gov/zika/index.html.
    - PCR for viral antibodies in symptomatic and exposed patients. Repeat in 2–12 weeks if negative.

- Test mother's partner or others with travel history, 2–12 weeks after possible exposure with Zika-specific IgM antibodies.
- Test exposed women and those with travel history in all three trimesters.
- In the United States, Zika virus infection is reportable to public health departments.
- Recommendations for prenatal testing are evolving.
  - When Zika infection is documented in pregnancy (positive virus, RNA or serology testing), amniocentesis can be considered at 15 weeks, for molecular detection of the Zika virus.
  - After fetal loss in a Zika-exposed pregnancy, collect multiple tissue specimens: cord blood, placenta, cerebrospinal fluid (CSF).
- Newborn and maternal testing
  - Test infants with microcephaly, CNS calcifications, and mother with positive or inconclusive Zika test.
    - If she has not been tested, consider testing mother first.

## Prescription Medications

- **Angiotensin-converting enzyme inhibitors and angiotensin II receptor antagonists** (ACE inhibitors)
  - These drugs (Lisinopril, Captopril, Enelopril, Fosinopril) interfere with the renin–angiotensin system.
    - They are associated with toxic effects on the fetal kidney in the second and third trimesters.
    - Pregnant women should change to another antihypertensive medication by 8–10 weeks' gestation.
  - Clinical features: hypotension, renal failure, renal dysplasia, oliguria, oligohydramnios, IUGR, pulmonary hypoplasia, PDA, incomplete ossification of the skull, scalp defects
  - No confirmed major teratogenic effects with first trimester use
    - Comorbidities, such as maternal diabetes and obesity, can also cause congenital anomalies.
- **Antiepileptic drugs** (AEDs)—General
  - AEDs are commonly prescribed teratogenic medications.
  - AEDs are used to treat neuropathic pain, migraine headaches, psychiatric disorders, and epilepsy.
  - AED exposure roughly doubles the risk for congenital anomalies.
    - 6.1% versus 2.8% among untreated epileptic women
    - Risk varies with the AED.
    - Most data show a dose-dependent risk relationship and higher risk in polytherapy versus monotherapy.
  - **Phenobarbital**: congenital malformations ~5.5%, especially nail hypoplasia, distal phalangeal hypoplasia, primarily of fifth fingers

  - **Hydantoin** (Phenytoin, Dilantin): congenital malformations 3–7%
    - Clinical features: midface hypoplasia, upturned nose, long philtrum, thin upper lip, nail hypoplasia, distal phalangeal hypoplasia, primarily of fingers; oral clefts, cardiac, genitourinary anomalies, growth deficiency, microcephaly, developmental delay
  - **Carbamazepine** (Tegretol): Malformation rate is low; congenital malformations ~2.9%, but risks for spina bifida are increased; odds ratio (OR) 2.6.
  - **Topiramate** (Topamax): congenital malformations 4.2–4.6%, especially small for gestational age, microcephaly, facial clefts, hypospadias
  - Newer AEDs: Lamotrigine (Lamictal), levetiracetam (Keppra), and gabapentin (Neurontin) are likely less teratogenic, but clinical data are limited.
- AEDs: **Valproic acid (VPA) embryopathy** (Depakote, Depakene)
  - VPA is the most teratogenic of all AEDs.
    - *In utero* exposure to VPA poses a two- to sevenfold increased risk of major congenital malformations compared to other common AED exposures.
  - Used to treat epilepsy, depression, bipolar disorder, migraine headache prophylaxis
  - Congenital malformations: 6–18% of children exposed to VPA in the first trimester of pregnancy
    - Higher risk with higher doses: ≥1,000 mg/day
    - Higher risk with polytherapy versus monotherapy
    - Congenital anomaly in a previous child exposed to VPA strongly increases the chance of anomalies in VPA-exposed siblings
  - Clinical features
    - First-trimester exposure associated with a 1% or 2% risk for lumbar meningomyelocele (adjusted odds ratio (aOR) 9.7).
      - Although folic acid supplementation is recommended, it does not reduce the risk for neural tube defects due to VPA.
    - Microcephaly 11%
    - Metopic craniosynostosis
    - Typical facial features: small nose, depressed nasal bridge, long flat philtrum, thin upper lip; oral clefts (aOR 4.4)
    - Cardiac lesions (aOR 2.0), especially septal defects
    - Limb defects, especially radial aplasia and thumb hypoplasia (Figure 6.2), clubfeet
    - Hypospadias (aOR 2.4)
    - IQ less than 70 in 10%, autism 4–9%
    - Delayed development relative risk (RR) 3.38
  - Neonatal fibrin depletion, thrombocytopenia, and fatal hemorrhage have been reported in a few cases.
- **Isotretinoin embryopathy**
  - Isotretinoin or 13-*cis*-retinoid acid (Accutane) is a vitamin A derivative.

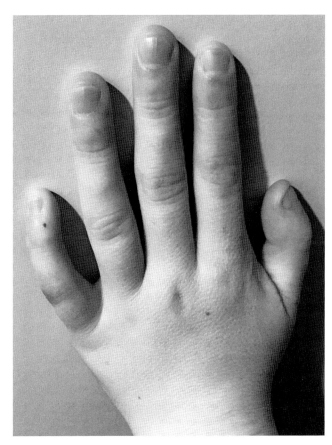

FIGURE 6.2 Thumb hypoplasia is a form of radial ray defect caused by valproic acid embryopathy.

- When taken orally, it is a potent human teratogen.
- Topical preparations (Isotrex, RetinA) are not teratogenic.
○ It is approved for severe recalcitrant cystic acne but often used off-label for milder acne.
  - Other uses: rosacea, generalized lichen planus, psoriasis, cutaneous systemic lupus erythematosus (SLE)
○ Adverse outcomes of pregnancy
  - Miscarriage 40%, for fetuses exposed in the first trimester
  - Premature birth 16%
  - Congenital anomalies 20–35%
○ Clinical features: craniofacial anomalies, anotia/microtia (Figure 9.1), cleft palate, micrognathia, facial and oculomotor nerve palsies (typically asymmetric), conotruncal and aortic arch heart defects, retinal or optic nerve anomalies, hydrocephalus cerebellar or vermis hypoplasia, abnormal pons and medulla
  - Neurocognitive impairment 30–60%
    • Affects those with and without congenital anomalies
    • Borderline to low IQ: 47% by 5 years
- **Methimazole embryopathy**
○ Methimazole (MMI, Tapazole) interferes with synthesis of thyroid hormones.

- For thyrotoxicosis of Graves disease in pregnancy
- Considered by some the drug of choice for hyperthyroidism in pregnancy
○ Clinical features: aplasia cutis congenita of scalp, underlying skull defects, supernumerary, hypoplastic or absent nipples (athelia), syndactyly, dystrophic nails, choanal atresia, tracheoesophageal fistula, esophageal atresia, imperforate anus
  - Large population-based surveys have not reported increased birth defects, but minor features may not be ascertained.
- **Methotrexate and aminopterin embryopathy**
○ Folic acid antagonists block synthesis of thymidine and inhibit DNA synthesis.
○ Used for cancer; autoimmune, dermatologic, and rheumatologic disorders; ectopic pregnancy; early interruption of pregnancy
○ Higher doses, 50 mg/m$^2$, for cancer, ectopic pregnancy, pose greater risk for congenital anomalies. Lower dose, >10/mg/week, for psoriasis, SLE, rheumatoid arthritis, also teratogenic
○ Most sensitive period is 6–8 weeks' gestation
  - Preconceptional use may cause inadvertent first-trimester fetal exposure due to variable maternal methotrexate metabolism.
○ Adverse outcomes of pregnancy
  - Miscarriage: 25–40%
  - Major congenital anomalies: 6% or 7% (aOR 3.1) among infants born to exposed rheumatologic patients
○ Clinical features: microcephaly, upswept frontal hair pattern, shallow supraorbital ridges, hypoplasia of the skull bones, wide fontanels, short palpebral fissures, cleft palate, microtia (Figure 6.3), hypospadias, diaphragmatic hernia, cardiac anomalies ~70%, pulmonary atresia
  - Skeletal anomalies: coronal or lambdoid craniosynostosis, short limbs, clubfeet, oligodactyly, syndactyly
  - Developmental delay, ID
- **Misoprostol embryopathy**: See Clinical Consult.
○ Misoprostol (Cytotec) is a synthetic prostaglandin E1 analog.
  - Approved to treat peptic ulcer disease; commonly used off-label to induce labor
  - In combination with methotrexate or mifepristone, used to induce early abortion, 80–95% effective
    • Increases uterine artery resistance and reduces uteroplacental perfusion
○ Clinical features in survivors: unilateral or bilateral Moebius syndrome (facial and abducens nerve palsies), brain stem ischemia, hydrocephalus, posterior encephalocele, cleft palate, micrognathia, Pierre–Robin sequence, limb defects, Poland sequence (hypoplasia of the pectoralis major muscle, syndactyly of fingers, hypoplasia of the forearm), clubfoot, joint contractures, autism

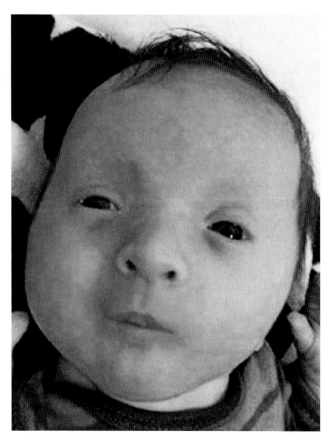

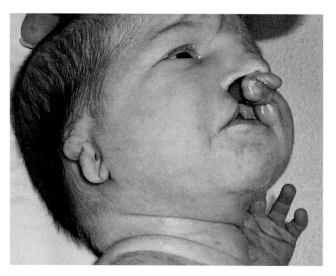

FIGURE 6.4 This infant with Mycophenylate embryopathy has microtia and bilateral cleft lip and palate.
SOURCE: Courtesy of Antonio Pérez Aytés, MD, Hospital Universitario y Politecnico La Fe, Valencia, Spain.

FIGURE 6.3 This infant with methotrexate embryopathy has short palpebral fissures, hypoplastic supraorbital ridges, and a small mouth.
SOURCE: Courtesy of Karen Gripp, MD, Nemours Children's Hospital, Wilmington, DE.

o Misoprostol is available without a prescription in Brazil. There, first-trimester exposure was documented in half of all infants with Moebius syndrome.
  ▪ Most had been exposed to the drug for only one day.
  ▪ Misoprostol exposure increases the risk of Moebius syndrome from 1/50,000–1/500,000 to ~1/1,000 (OR 38.8).

*Pearl*: Whenever Moebius syndrome, unilateral or bilateral, is diagnosed, seek a history of misoprostol exposure.

- **Mycophenolate embryopathy**
  o Mycophenolate mofetil (MMF, CellCept) and other mycophenolic acid preparations are immunosuppressants that inhibit *de novo* purine synthesis.
  o It prevents organ rejection after renal, hepatic, and cardiac transplantation.
    ▪ Often used off-label in bone marrow, stem cell transplants, and for inflammatory and autoimmune disorders (rheumatoid arthritis, SLE)
  o Miscarriage: 45% after first trimester exposure
  o Clinical features: major malformations 26%, especially orofacial clefts, hearing loss, and microtia/

anotia with external auditory canal atresia (Figure 6.4); hypertelorism; coloboma; micrognathia; hypoplastic fingers, fingernails, and toenails; congenital heart defects; tracheoesophageal fistula; myelomeningocele; diaphragmatic hernia

- **Thalidomide embryopathy**
  o From 1957 to 1962, thalidomide caused an epidemic of congenital anomalies affecting more than 10,000 children worldwide.
  o It is prescribed (Immunoprin) under controlled circumstances for leprosy, multiple myeloma, and other chronic disorders.
    ▪ Originally used as a sedative, then for nausea in pregnancy
  o Exposed pregnancies are uncommon where prescribing safeguards are strictly followed.
    ▪ Most cases have been reported in South America; several involved sharing the drug among relatives of patients with leprosy.
  o Critical period for exposure is 21–49 days.
    ▪ A single dose taken within the critical period can cause birth defects.
  o Clinical features: bilateral amelia, phocomelia, other limb, cardiac, CNS, ear and eye anomalies
    ▪ Major anomalies 35–40%
    ▪ Miscarriage 25%
    ▪ Autism and ID
- **Warfarin embryopathy**
  o Anticoagulant (Coumadin) used for deep vein thrombosis, cardiac valve replacement
  o Adverse pregnancy outcome ~25%

- Spontaneous abortion, stillbirth, recognizable embryopathy
  - ○ Critical period: 6–12 weeks' gestation
    - Embryopathy associated with >5 mg/day
  - ○ Clinical features: low birth weight, growth retardation, skeletal anomalies, hypoplastic nasal bone (most common feature), stippled epiphyses (proximal femurs, calcanei), chondrodysplasia punctate, brachydactyly, optic atrophy, microphthalmia, laryngomalacia, CNS anomalies, fetal hemorrhage, encephalocele and congenital heart defects (atrial septal defect (ASD), PDA)

*Pearl*: A hypoplastic nose should prompt a skeletal survey (including a lateral view of the heel) to identify stippled epiphyses or extraosseous calcifications.

## Maternal Disorders

- **Chronic hypertension**
  - ○ Incidence is 1–5% of the pregnant population.
    - Rising with rates of obesity, advanced maternal age, diabetes
  - ○ Adverse perinatal outcomes correlate with duration and severity of hypertension.
    - Maternal complications: preeclampsia 25%, placental abruption, cesarean delivery, postpartum hemorrhage, death
    - Fetal complications: prematurity, IUGR, small for gestational age, perinatal mortality
    - Many outcomes are unaffected by treatment with antihypertensive medications during pregnancy.
  - ○ Congenital malformations of all types are more prevalent in the offspring of chronically hypertensive women, regardless of treatment.
    - With treatment: OR 1.7; without treatment: OR 1.5
    - Cardiac anomalies are equally prevalent in the offspring of treated hypertensive mothers (OR 1.6) and untreated hypertensive mothers (OR 1.5).
- **Maternal hyperthyroidism**
  - ○ Fetal effects occur in 1% or 2%, regardless of treatment in mothers with hyperthyroidism.
    - The risk of fetal and neonatal hyperthyroidism correlates with maternal antibody levels.
  - ○ Thyrotropin receptor-stimulating antibodies (TSHR-SAb) cross the placenta, causing an overactive fetal thyroid.
  - ○ Clinical features: goiter, prominent staring eyes, exophthalmos, hepatosplenomegaly, congestive heart failure, fever, tachycardia, sweating, vomiting, diarrhea, jaundice
    - Mortality ≤25%, significant morbidity
  - ○ Short-term anti-thyroid therapy (usually methimazole and propranolol) is indicated.
- **Maternal phenylketonuria** (mPKU)
  - ○ Incidence 1/10,000 (Europe)
    - With newborn screening, PKU (MIM 261600) has been successfully treated with an early protein-restricted diet, resulting in normal intellectual function in adulthood.
    - Strict dietary control of phenylalanine (Phe) is recommended throughout life in PKU, but control is often suboptimal in the adult years.
  - ○ Elevated maternal Phe levels in maternal serum are teratogenic and fetotoxic.
    - Cause congenital anomalies, miscarriage, intrauterine fetal demise (IUFD), preterm delivery
    - Maternal Phe levels during pregnancy correlate with neonatal sequelae.
      - Neonatal outcome is worse for women with untreated classic mPKU (serum Phe >1,200 μmol/L) during pregnancy.
      - Milder hyperphenylalaninemia (Phe <600 μmol/L), also causes microcephaly and other sequelae
    - Clinical features: IUGR 20–40%, congenital cardiac anomalies 6–12%, tetralogy of Fallot, VSD, microcephaly 50–70%, esophageal atresia, bladder exstrophy, bifid thumbs, vertebral and renal anomalies
      - Facial features: flat nasal bridge, anteverted nares, micrognathia, ptosis, brachydactyly
      - Later: ID 47–92%, seizures
  - ○ Diagnose with *maternal* phenylalanine level.

*Pearl*: Whenever a new diagnosis of PKU is made in a newborn, check the mother for undiagnosed mPKU.

## Differential Diagnosis

- For fetal anuria that is suspected to be due to third trimester use of ACE inhibitors, also consider **renal tubular dysgenesis** (MIM 267430), an autosomal recessive disorder that causes fetal anuria, oligohydramnios, pulmonary hypotension, and perinatal death.
- For suspected isotretinoin embryopathy, consider **CHARGE syndrome\*** (MIM 214800) and **22q11.2 deletion.\***
- For suspected methimazole embryopathy, also consider **Adams–Oliver syndrome** (MIM 100300), autosomal dominant disorder of aplasia cutis congenita of the scalp and limb defects.
- When suspecting mycophenolate embryopathy, also consider **Fryns syndrome** (MIM 229850) and **Treacher–Collins syndrome** (MIM 154500).
- When TORCH infection is suspected, also consider
  - ○ **CINCA syndrome** (MIM 607114), an autosomal dominant multisystem autoinflammatory disorder that causes intracranial calcifications, hydrocephalus, hepatosplenomegaly, and rash. See Clinical Consult in Chapter 18.

- ○ *COL4A1, COL4A2* (MIM 175780, 614483) heterozygous pathogenic variants cause autosomal dominant vascular disruption of the CNS with IUGR, schizencephaly, microcephaly, periventricular calcifications, hydrocephalus, porencephaly, intraventricular hemorrhage, and cataract.
- When thalidomide embryopathy is suspected, consider **Okihiro syndrome** (MIM 607323), an autosomal dominant trait caused by a heterozygous pathogenic variant in *SALL4*, characterized by Duane anomaly with radial ray abnormalities.
- When Warfarin embryopathy is in the differential diagnosis, consider maternal autoimmune diseases such as SLE, scleroderma, and mixed connective tissue disease, which may disrupt fetal vitamin K metabolism, causing a clinical picture similar to that of chondrodysplasia punctata. Hyperemesis gravidarum and gastric bypass surgery can also cause maternal vitamin K deficiency, mimicking warfarin embryopathy or maternal Vitamin A deficiency and fetal anophthalmia.
- When suspecting Zika virus embryopathy, also consider other causes of microcephaly* due to fetal brain disruption sequence.

## Evaluation and Management

- Ask about the mother's health status and habits: history of gastric bypass surgery, travel history, habits (eating raw meat or cheese), occupational exposures to solvents, pesticides, contact with animals, cat litter, acute or chronic infections, sick contacts, rashes, fevers, hyperemesis, hypertension, thyroid disease, special diets, diabetes, cancer, and autoimmune disorders.
- Document teratogen exposure: recreational drug use, prescription, nonprescription or shared medications, medication use prior to positive pregnancy test and in the early months of pregnancy, suspected ectopic pregnancy, and vaginal bleeding after taking a medication.
  - ○ In private, ask about any medication exposure for pregnancy interruption.
- Consult online sources for up-to-date information.
  - ○ The Organization of Teratogen Information Services (OTIS) produces fact sheets in English and Spanish for medications and maternal medical conditions: https://www.mothertobaby.org/fact-sheets-parent.
- Fetal intervention/therapy when appropriate (e.g., *in utero* transfusion, VZIG)
- Offer referral for counseling for prevention of recurrence.

## Further Reading

Anderson JL, Levy PT, Leonard KB, et al. (2014) Congenital lymphocytic choriomeningitis virus: When to consider the diagnosis. J Child Neurol. 29:837–42. PMID 23666045

Araujo AQ, Silva MT, Araujo AP. (2016) Zika virus-associated neurological disorders: A review. Brain. 139:2122–30. PMID 27357348

Bateman BT, Huybrechts KF, Fischer MA, et al. (2015) Chronic hypertension in pregnancy and the risk of congenital malformations: A cohort study. Am J Obstet Gynecol. 212:337.e1–e14. PMID 25265405

Chitayat D, Keating S, Zand DJ, et al. (2008) Chondrodysplasia punctata associated with maternal autoimmune diseases: Expanding the spectrum from systemic lupus erythematosus (SLE) to mixed connective tissue disease (MCTD) and scleroderma report of eight cases. Am J Med Genet A. 146A:3038–53. PMID 19006208

Hoeltzenbein M, Elefant E, Vial T, et al. (2012) Teratogenicity of mycophenolate confirmed in a prospective study of the European Network of Teratology Information Services. Am J Med Genet A. 158A:588–96. PMID 22319001

Lammer EJ, Chen DT, Hoar RM, et al. (1985) Retinoic acid embryopathy. N Engl J Med. 313:837–41. PMID 3162101

Lamont RF, Sobel JD, Carrington D, et al. (2011) Varicella-zoster virus (chickenpox) infection in pregnancy. BJOG. 118:1155–62. PMID 21585641

Naing ZW, Scott GM, Shand A, et al. (2016) Congenital cytomegalovirus infection in pregnancy: A review of prevalence, clinical features, diagnosis and prevention. Aust N Z J Obstet Gynaecol. 56:9–18. PMID 26391432

Neu N, Duchon J, Zachariah P. (2015) TORCH infections. Clin Perinatol. 42:77–103. PMID 25677998

Običan S, Scialli AR. (2011) Teratogenic exposures. Am J Med Genet C Semin Med Genet. 157:150–69. PMID 21766437

Orbach H, Matok I, Gorodischer R, et al. (2013) Hypertension and antihypertensive drugs in pregnancy and perinatal outcomes. Am J Obstet Gynecol. 208:301.e1–e6. PMID 23159698

Prick BW, Hop WC. (2012) Maternal phenylketonuria and hyperphenylalaninemia in pregnancy: Pregnancy complications and neonatal sequelae in untreated and treated pregnancies. Am J Clin Nutr 95:374–82. PMID 22205310

Rodríguez-García C, González-Hernández S, Hernández-Martín A, et al. (2011) Aplasia cutis congenita and other anomalies associated with methimazole exposure during pregnancy. Pediatr Dermatol. 28:743–5. PMID 21995270

Smigiel R, Cabala M, Jakubiak A et al. (2016) Novel COL4A1 mutation in an infant with severe dysmorphic syndrome with schizencephaly, periventricular calcifications, and cataract resembling congenital infection. Birth Defects Res A Clin Mol Teratol. 106:304–7. PMID 26879631

Tanoshima M, Kobayashi T, Tanoshima R, et al. (2015) Risks of congenital malformations in offspring exposed to valproic acid in utero: A systematic review and cumulative meta-analysis. Clin Pharmacol Ther. 98:417–41. PMID 26044279

Tian C, Ali SA, Weitkamp J-H. (2010) Congenital infections, Part I: Cytomegalovirus, toxoplasma, rubella, and herpes simplex. NeoReviews. 11:e436.

Tomson T, Dina Battino D. (2012) Teratogenic effects of antiepileptic drugs. Lancet Neurol. 11:803–13. PMID 22805351

Weber-Schoendorfer C, Chambers C, Wacker E, et al. (2014) Pregnancy outcome after methotrexate treatment for rheumatic disease prior to or during early pregnancy: A prospective multicenter cohort study. Arthritis Rheumatol. 66:1101–10. PMID 24470106

# Part II

## Cardiovascular System

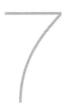

# Cardiac Defects

## Clinical Consult

A genetic consult was requested for a non-obstructing intracardiac mass, likely to be a rhabdomyoma, in a term newborn. The mother had taken an anticonvulsant medication throughout the pregnancy for a long-standing seizure disorder. The mother had angiofibromas on her nose and malar areas, raised leathery patches of skin (Shagreen patch) on her forehead (Figure 7.1), hypopigmented macules, and a learning disorder.

The baby did not have hypopigmented macules, but a brain MRI revealed subependymal glial nodules, confirming the clinical suspicion of **tuberous sclerosis complex** (TSC). As expected, the rhabdomyoma resolved spontaneously by 9 months. The infant had delayed development consistent with the diagnosis.

TSC is a variable multisystem autosomal dominant condition caused by heterozygous pathogenic variant in *TSC1* or *TSC2*. TSC is rarely diagnosed in the newborn period in the absence of an intracardiac tumor.

## Definition

- Various isolated structural cardiac anomalies and some syndromes that include congenital heart defects (CHD) are considered here. Heterotaxy* and some syndromes that include cardiac anomalies are reviewed elsewhere.
- CHD are the most common type of congenital anomaly.
  - o Incidence 10.8/1,000 live births
    - ■ One-third are severe
  - o 3 M:2 F
    - ■ M > F: aortic stenosis, coarctation of the aorta (CoA), hypoplastic left heart syndrome (HLHS), d-transposition of the great arteries (dTGA)
    - ■ F > M: atrial septal defect (ASD), pulmonic stenosis
- Family history
  - o Most CHD are sporadic.
  - o Only 2.2% of patients with CHD have an affected first-degree relative.
- Risk factors
  - o Assisted reproductive technology (ART)
  - o Folic acid insufficiency

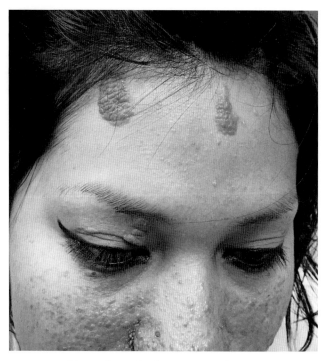

FIGURE 7.1 This mother with tuberous sclerosis has shagreen patches on her forehead and multiple angiofibromata on her nose and cheeks.

- o Increased nuchal translucency in first trimester
- o Maternal diabetes or obesity
- o Maternal hypertension, maternal antihypertensive medication use (beta blocker, renin–angiotensin blocker)
- o Maternal opioid use
- o Maternal smoking
- o Twins*: Monochorionic (MC) twins have the highest risk: 6–10× the risk for cardiac anomalies in singletons.
- o MC/DA twins with twin–twin transfusion syndrome: the risk is further increased at 15–23×.
- Recurrence risk
  - o Isolated nonsyndromic CHD: 4%, 2–4× the general population risk
  - o Higher risk for relatives of female probands
  - o Risk varies with the type of cardiac lesion in the proband.
    - ▪ Highest risk: HLHS 10–15%, tetralogy of Fallot (TOF)
    - ▪ Lowest risk: dTGA
    - ▪ Affected siblings have concordant lesions in 69%.
- Etiology of CHD
  - o Unknown in >50%
  - o Genes are known to contribute to ~45%, both isolated and syndromic CHD
    - ▪ MZ twins have concordant CHD in 94%, DZ twins 33%
    - ▪ Exome sequencing (ES) data from the Congenital Heart Disease Genetics Network Study
      - • De novo point mutations in several hundred genes collectively contribute to ~10% of severe CHD.
      - • Familial CHD (three generations): 30% have pathogenic variants.

- • Genes responsible for monogenic familial CHD may also cause isolated sporadic CHD.
  - • TOF: *JAG1, GDF1, NKX2.5, ZFPM2, GATA4, NOTCH1, MYH6*
- Associated comorbidities
  - o Extracardiac anomalies ~25%
  - o Developmental disability (DD)
    - ▪ DD affects 10% of all CHD, 50% in severe
      - • Microcephaly at age 2 is the most predictive sign of DD.
    - ▪ Attention deficit hyperactivity disorder (ADHD) 3–4× greater than the general population

## Differential Diagnosis

- Specific types of CHD
  - o Septal defects: most common CHD
    - ▪ ASD
      - • Two types: ASDI (ostium primum, type I); ASDII (ostium secundum, type II) ~10% of CHD
      - • 6 M:10 F
      - • Isolated ASD ~80%
      - • Usually sporadic but occasionally familial
        - • Autosomal dominant ASD (MIM 108800) can be caused by heterozygous pathogenic variant in *GATA4* (MIM 607941), *NKX2-5* (MIM 180900), and other genes, including two sarcomeric genes: *MYH6, ACTC1.*
        - • It can be associated with autosomal dominant hypertrophic and noncompaction cardiomyopathy or with arrhythmia and prolonged PR interval.
    - ▪ Ventricular septal defect (VSD) the most common CHD, approximately one-third of all CHD
      - • Affects up to 0.5% of the population
      - • Most are hemodynamically insignificant and close spontaneously without treatment
      - • Risk for CHD among first-degree relatives of a proband with VSD: 3%
    - ▪ Atrial ventricular septal defect (AVSD) 4-5% of CHD
      - • Incidence 0.3–0.4/1,000 live births
      - • Unknown genetic cause in 40%
      - • Pathogenic variants in single genes (*NR2F2*) have been identified in nonsyndromic AVSD.
      - • Syndromic AVSD
        - • **Heterotaxy***
        - • **Down syndrome*** (T21)
        - • AVSD accounts for 39% of CHD in T21.
        - • Incidence of AVSD varies with race in Down syndrome.
        - • Higher in Blacks

- Lower in Hispanics, compared to non-Hispanic Caucasians
- **Patent ductus arteriosus** (PDA) 5–7% of CHD
  - Incidence 1/2,000 1/5,000 among full-term infants
  - Caused by disruption of the prostaglandin E4 receptor
  - Isolated PDA can be autosomal recessive or dominant.
- **Conotruncal defects** (CTD)
  - Abnormal outflow vessels of the heart
  - Genetic causes not defect specific
  - Six types
    - Double-outlet right ventricle (DORV)
    - TOF
    - Interrupted aortic arch types a and b (IAAa, IAAb)
    - TGA
    - Truncus arteriosus (TA)
    - Conoventricular septal defect (CVSD)
- **Left ventricular outflow tract obstruction** (LVOTO)
  - CoA 5% of CHD
    - Prenatal diagnosis is difficult.
    - More common in males
    - Clinical features: often occurs with other CHD, cyanosis, diminished femoral pulses, tachypnea and cardiogenic shock, blood pressure may be different in four extremities
    - Treat empirically with prostaglandin E1 infusion until CoA is ruled out by echocardiogram.
    - Associated with **Turner syndrome**\* and **Kabuki syndrome** (MIM 147920)
  - HLHS: most severe LVOTO, 1–3% of CHD
    - Incidence 2 3/10,000 live births in the United States

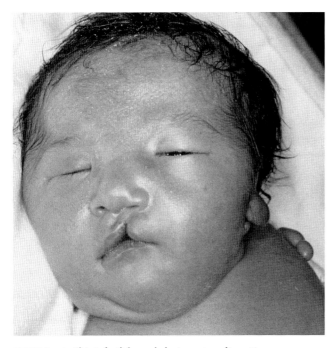

FIGURE 7.2 This infant's has subclavian artery disruption sequence due to hypoplastic left heart syndrome, which caused many left-sided anomalies—cleft lip, microtia, facial palsy, pulmonary agenesis, vertebral anomalies, and amelia of the upper extremity.

- 1.5 M:1 F
- Recurrence risk
  - After one affected child: 2–4%, up to 15% for some types of left ventricular outflow tract anomalies
  - After two affected children: 25%
  - First-degree relatives often have milder, undiagnosed left-sided cardiac lesions on echocardiogram aortic stenosis, CoA, hypoplastic aorta, bicuspid aortic valve.
  - Isolated HLHS: Most are sporadic and multifactorial, but autosomal recessive inheritance occurs.
  - Syndromic HLHS: extracardiac anomalies in 15–28%
  - Maternal diabetes accounts for 6–8% of HLHS.
  - Aneuploidy: **trisomies 13\* and 18,\* Turner syndrome\***
  - De novo microarray abnormalities 12%
  - **HLHS with subclavian artery disruption sequence.** Hypoperfusion in that vascular distribution can cause left-sided anomalies: cleft lip, microtia, pulmonary agenesis, amelia of the left upper extremity (Figure 7.2).
  - Single gene disorders
    - **Noonan syndrome\*** (MIM 163950)
    - **Holt–Oram syndrome** (MIM 142900)
    - **Smith–Lemli–Opitz syndrome\*** (MIM 270400)
- Chromosome anomalies cause 9–18% of all CHD; almost all have extracardiac anomalies.
  - Aneuploidy accounts for 5–8% of all CHD.
    - CHD occur in ~30% of children with chromosome anomalies.
    - These have high rates of CHD:
      - **Down syndrome\*** 35–50%
      - **Trisomy 13\*** 60–80%
      - **Trisomy 18\*** 90–100%
      - **Turner syndrome\*** 33%
  - Microarray abnormalities are common causes of CHD.
    - Similar copy number variants (CNVs) are found among patients with different cardiac defects, indicating phenotypic heterogeneity.
      - Gene pathways that lead to particular types of cardiac defects are not distinct.
      - De novo microarray abnormalities, excluding deletion 22q11.2, occur in 8–14% of isolated CHD versus 2–4% of controls.
        - Single ventricle 13.9%
        - Conotruncal defect 8%
        - Nonsyndromic TOF 10%
        - HLHS 12.7%
    - Syndromic CHD (extracardiac anomalies and/or dysmorphic features): 15–20% have a CNV.
  - **Chromosome 22q11.2 deletion\***—75% have CHD
    - The most common deletion in patients with CHD
      - TOF: 10% have 22q deletion.

- Tricuspid atresia 35%
- IAAb 50%
  - **Williams syndrome***—50–85% have CHD
  - Recurrent microarray abnormalities: ~25% of the CNVs found in CHD are recurrent.
    - Deletions: 2q23.1, 8p23 including *GATA4*, 15q11.2–13
    - Duplications: 1q21.1 including *GJA5*, 15q11.2–13, 16p13.11, 22q11.2
  - CNV phenotypes are highly variable with reduced penetrance.
    - Unaffected parents may have the CNV.
- Teratogens*
  - **Rubella embryopathy**: rare among immunized populations
  - Maternal prepregnancy diabetes mellitus* aRR 4 for CHD
    - Elevated first-trimester HgbA1c level increases the risk for various CHD.
    - Cardiac anomalies
      - ~50% are conotruncal defects: TGA, TA, visceral heterotaxy, single ventricle.
      - HLHS, TOF
    - Gestational and pregestational diabetes mellitus are associated with hypertrophy of the septum and cardiomyopathy, especially, but not exclusively, in LGA babies.
  - **Maternal phenylketonuria** (mPKU)
    - Incidence 1/10,000–1/15,000

*Pearl*: In the United States, the number of babies born to mPKU mothers is now equal to the number of babies born with PKU.

- mPKU is underdiagnosed.
  - Women with mPKU are often unaware of their diagnosis or that they were treated with a protein-restricted diet in childhood.
- Pregnant women with mPKU should maintain a carefully monitored phenylalanine (Phe)-restricted diet *prior* to conception and throughout gestation.
  - Elevated maternal serum Phe is extremely teratogenic.
  - ~50% of Phe-restricted pregnancies achieve optimal Phe levels.
  - In poorly controlled mPKU pregnancies, ≥95% of fetuses are affected.
    - The risk of CHD increases with the maternal Phe level in the first 8 weeks of gestation.
    - The risk of CHD is also increased, ~2%, among offspring of mothers without classical PKU who have mild hyperphenylaninemia.
- Clinical features
  - Growth restriction, microcephaly, dysmorphic features, intellectual disability
  - Cardiac anomalies 7–15%
    - Typically, CoA, TOF, VSD, HLHS

- ART
  - Increases risk of CHD by 40–50% (aOD 1.4–1.5)
    - Similar to the increase seen for all anomalies after ART
    - The degree to which this increased risk is attributable to the procedure of ART versus the underlying cause of the infertility has not been determined.
  - In one study, ART was significantly more common among infants with TOF, but not other types of CHD, compared to controls (6.6% vs. 3.5%, *p* = 0.002).
    - Intracytoplasmic sperm injection (ICSI) further increased risk for TOF (aOR 3.0, 95% confidence interval (CI) 1.0–8.9)
  - Other teratogenic agents*
    - Lithium
      - Ebstein anomaly: low risk after first trimester exposure, 0.05–0.1%
  - **Fetal alcohol spectrum disorder***
    - In classical fetal alcohol syndrome, 30–100% have CHD (OR 18.0).
      - Typically, ASD, VSD, TOF
    - Folic acid antagonists
      - Anticonvulsants
      - Methotrexate, trimethoprim
    - Retinoic acid and vitamin A derivatives
      - Excessive vitamin A intake or isotretinoin (Accutane) exposure in the first trimester affects cardiac neural crest cells.
        - Typically, conotruncal, aortic arch abnormalities
- Single gene disorders with cardiac defects
  - **Alagille syndrome** (MIM 118450)
    - Autosomal dominant trait, caused by heterozygous pathogenic variant in *JAG1* (94%) or *NOTCH2*
    - Clinical features: pulmonary artery stenosis, peripheral pulmonary stenosis (PS), TOF, ASD, broad forehead, deep-set eyes, long pointed chin, cholestatic jaundice, paucity of bile ducts (90%), neonatal hepatitis, posterior embryotoxon, butterfly vertebrae (Figure 7.3)
  - **Char syndrome** (MIM 169100)
    - Autosomal dominant disorder, caused by heterozygous pathogenic variant in *TFAP2B*
    - Clinical features: characteristic face, high forehead, flat profile, hypertelorism, short nose with flat tip, thick lips; clinodactyly with missing middle phalanx of little fingers; PDA almost universal; CoA, bicuspid aortic valve
  - **Holt–Oram syndrome** (MIM 142900)
    - Autosomal dominant trait, caused by heterozygous pathogenic variant in *TBX5*
    - Clinical features: variable CHD, typically secundum ASD or VSD; conduction defects; can be severe: HLHS, TAPVR, TA; thumbs hypoplastic (may be subtle),

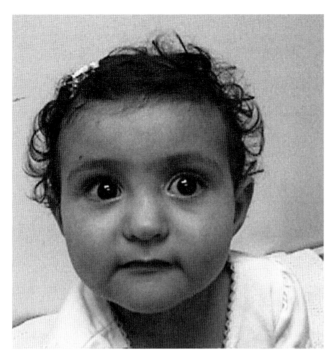

FIGURE 7.3 This toddler with Alagille syndrome has the characteristic broad forehead, deep-set eyes, and slightly pointed chin. SOURCE: Courtesy of Ian Krantz, MD, Children's Hospital of Philadelphia, PA.

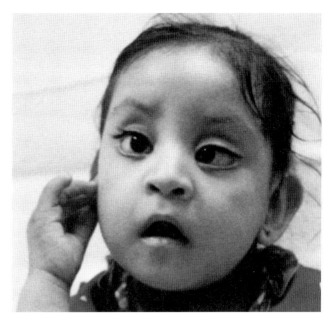

FIGURE 7.4 This child with Kabuki syndrome has long palpebral fissures, eversion of lower eyelids, and eyebrows that look interrupted due to segmental hypoplasia. Note the open mouth, myopathic facial appearance, and large ears.

triphalangeal, or absent; thenar, carpal, or radial bony anomalies

- Upper limb and shoulder anomalies are bilateral and often asymmetric, can be severe.
- Phocomelia can simulate thalidomide embryopathy.

○ **Kabuki syndrome** (MIM 147920)

■ Autosomal dominant trait, caused by heterozygous pathogenic variant in *KMT2D, KDM6A*

■ Clinical features: coarctation of the aorta, bicuspid aortic valve, VSD, mitral stenosis, TOF, single ventricle, DORV, TGA, prenatal growth deficiency, long palpebral fissures (Figure 7.4), eversion of lower lids, deficient lateral eyebrows, large prominent ears, cleft palate, prominent fetal pads on the fingertips, hypotonia, poor feeding

○ **Rubinstein–Taybi syndrome** (MIM 180849)

■ Autosomal dominant trait, caused by heterozygous pathogenic variant in *CREBBP* (50–70%) or *EP300*

■ Clinical features: ASD, VSD, PDA, CoA, PS, bicuspid aortic valve, polyhydramnios, microcephaly, arched eyebrows, down-slanting palpebral fissures, beaked nose, broad thumbs and great toes (Figure 7.5), feeding and respiratory problems

○ These syndromes with CHD are reviewed elsewhere:

■ **CHARGE syndrome**,* **Cornelia de Lange syndrome**,* **Cri-du-Chat syndrome/5p minus**,* deletion of chromosome 22q11.2,* Down syndrome,*

**Heterotaxy**,* Noonan syndrome,* **Smith–Lemli–Opitz syndrome**,* trisomy 13,* trisomy 18,* Turner syndrome,* **VATER/VACTERL association**,* Williams syndrome,* **Wolf–Hirschhorn syndrome/4p minus***

- Syndromes that cause aortic dilation

○ **Loeys–Dietz syndrome** (MIM 609192)

■ Autosomal dominant trait, caused by heterozygous pathogenic variant in *TBFBR1, TGFBR2, SMAD3, TGFB2*

■ Clinical features: widespread arterial ectasia and tortuosity, aggressive early aortic and other arterial dilation and aneurysms, dissection of smaller arteries than in Marfan syndrome, craniosynostosis, hypertelorism, bifid uvula or cleft palate, club feet, pes planus, translucent skin

■ Monitor with frequent imaging (MRA or CT angio) and treatment with beta blockers

○ **Marfan syndrome** (MIM 154700)

■ Autosomal dominant trait, caused by heterozygous pathogenic variant in *FBN1*

■ Clinical features in the severe neonatal presentation: dilated aortic root, mitral valve prolapse, arachnodactyly, early severe scoliosis, pectus deformities, lens dislocation, myopia

■ Treat with beta blockers

- Arrhythmias and long QT syndromes

○ **Jervell and Lange–Nielsen syndrome** (MIM 220400)

■ Autosomal recessive disorder, caused by biallelic pathogenic variants in *KCNQ1* or *KCNE1*

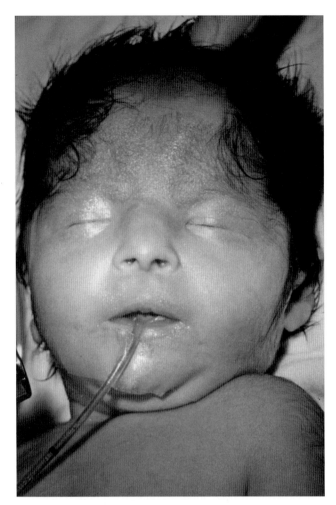

FIGURE 7.5 This newborn with Rubinstein–Taybi syndrome has down-slanting palpebral fissures, a prominent nose, and a columella that extends below the alae nasi. A prominent nevus flammeus is present on the forehead.

■ Clinical features: long QT, bilateral congenital profound sensorineural hearing loss, syncopal episodes during stress

*Pearl*: To detect Jervell and Lange–Nielsen syndrome, check electrocardiogram (ECG) for long QT in babies who fail the newborn hearing screen *prior to* hospital discharge. Early diagnosis saves lives. More than half die by age 15 years.

- ○ **Timothy syndrome** (MIM 601005)
  - ■ Autosomal dominant disorder, caused by heterozygous pathogenic variant in *CACNA1*c; often de novo
    - • Parental gonadal mosaicism can occur.
  - ■ Clinical features: Structural cardiac defects (PDA, patent foramen ovale, TOF, VSD, hypertrophic cardiomyopathy) occur with conduction defects (AV block or bradycardia in the fetus, severe QT prolongation, severe ventricular tachyarrhythmia, torsade de pointes).
    - • Facies: characteristic features 85%
      - • Thin upper lip, depressed nasal bridge, round face
    - • Variable syndactyly of the fingers (not the thumb) and toes 2 and 3 (Figure 33.5)

- • Hypoglycemia, fetal hydrops
- • Later findings: seizures, developmental delay, autism
- ■ Presents in the first few days of life
  - • Early diagnosis is key.
  - • Implantable cardioverter defibrillator should be considered in every patient.
    - • Without therapy, often lethal by age 3 years
- ○ Various channelopathies can cause arrhythmia and SIDS.
  - ■ **Oculodentodigital syndrome** (MIM 164200)
    - • Autosomal dominant disorder, caused by a heterozygous pathogenic variant in *GJA1*, that encodes connexin 43, a gap junction protein
      - • Widely distributed in the cardiac conduction system
    - • Clinical features: pinched nose, microphthalmia (Figure 33.1), syndactyly of ring and little fingers, arrhythmia can cause sudden death, SIDS
- ○ Autoimmune congenital heart block
  - ■ **Neonatal lupus syndrome** occurs with various maternal autoimmune disorders (SLE, Sjogren) with transplacental passage of cross-reacting antibodies.
    - • Anti-SSA/SSB
  - ■ Clinical features: congenital complete atrioventricular heart block, dilated cardiomyopathy, hydrops, prematurity, rash, growth retardation
- • Syndromes associated with cardiac tumors
  - ○ **Basal cell nevus syndrome** (Gorlin syndrome, MIM 109400)
    - ■ Autosomal dominant disorder, caused by heterozygous pathogenic variant or microdeletion involving *PTCH1*, *PTCH2*, or *SUFU*
      - • De novo pathogenic variant in 40%
    - ■ Clinical features: macrocephaly, hydrocephalus, calcified falx cerebri, hypertelorism, cleft palate, bifid ribs, scoliosis, cardiac fibroma 3%, polydactyly of the feet
      - • Later findings: basal cell carcinoma before age 40 years, palmar and plantar pits, jaw cysts, ovarian cysts; medulloblastoma usually >5 years
        - • Avoid ionizing radiation, especially radiation therapy.

*Pearl*: Suspect Gorlin syndrome in an infant with a cardiac fibroma. Examine the parents for small dermal pits in their palms, which can be enhanced by rubbing pencil lead on the palms and wiping off the excess with a paper towel.

- ○ **Tuberous sclerosis complex** (TSC, MIM 19110, 191092): See Clinical Consult.
  - ■ Autosomal dominant condition, caused by heterozygous pathogenic variant in *TSC1* or *TSC2*
  - ■ Clinical features: TSC causes hamartomas in multiple organ systems.
    - • Congenital cardiac rhabdomyoma ~20%
      - • 80–90% of congenital cardiac rhabdomyomas are due to TSC.

- Often detected by fetal US
- Tends to regress
  - Kidney: angiomyolipomas
    - Enlarged cystic kidneys can be confused with poly-cystic kidneys.
  - Skin: Hypomelanotic "ash-leaf" spots are usually evident at birth; other skin findings develop before puberty.
  - CNS: Intracranial calcifications may be evident by CT scan in neonates.
  - Later findings: developmental disabilities ~50%, variable intellectual disability, autism, learning disabilities, infantile spasms
  - Childhood brain tumors, especially subependymal giant cell astrocytoma, 5–14%
    - Treatment with mTOR inhibitors (rapamycin, sirolimus) may improve outcome.
- Cardiomyopathy
  - **Infants of diabetic mothers**\* or babies with hyperinsulinism can present with myocardial, usually septal, hypertrophy.
  - Syndromes with cardiomyopathy
    - Noonan syndrome\* and especially in **Costello syndrome**
    - **Beckwith–Wiedemann syndrome**\*—cardiomyopathy is occasional.
  - Viral myocarditis produces dilated cardiomyopathy.
  - More than 40 inborn errors of metabolism cause ~5% of neonatal cardiomyopathy.
    - 27% of hypertrophic neonatal cardiomyopathy
    - Common mechanisms are accumulation of storage material or deficiency of a cellular organelle.
    - **Mitochondrial oxidative phosphorylation dysfunction** causes hypertrophic cardiomyopathy with profound lactic acidosis, hydrops, arrhythmia.
    - Other metabolic causes of cardiomyopathy:
      - Fatty acid oxidation defects: commonly very long-chain acyl-CoA dehydrogenase deficiency (VLCAD), long-chain 3-hydroxyacyl-CoA dehydrogenase (LCHAD)
      - Peroxisomal disorders
      - Lysosomal storage disorders
      - Organic acidemias
      - Aminoacidemias
      - Glycogen storage diseases
      - Congenital disorders of glycosylation
- **Barth syndrome** (MIM 302060)
  - X-linked cardiomyopathy, caused by a pathogenic variant in *TAZ*
    - Reduces remodeling of cardiolipin, a phospholipid in the inner mitochondrial membrane
  - ~3–5% of boys with cardiomyopathy have Barth syndrome.
    - Clinical features: left ventricular noncompaction, dilated or (rarely) hypertrophic cardiomyopathy, endocardial fibroelastosis, ventricular arrhythmia, neutropenia, growth retardation, skeletal myopathy. Can cause fetal hydrops\*, fetal death, or stillbirth in males.

  - Diagnosis: Increased urine 3-methylglutaconic acid should lead to *TAZ* gene sequencing.

## Evaluation and Management

- Document pregnancy history: teratogen exposure, twins, maternal PKU or dietary restriction in childhood, maternal diabetes, twin gestation, infertility, or ART.
- Take a detailed family history: consanguinity, affected relatives, other types of CHD.

*Pearl*: Suspect mPKU when all the children in a family are affected with poor growth, intellectual disability, microcephaly, and/or CHD.

- Examine the parents: dysmorphic features, extracardiac anomalies (e.g., palmar pits, thumb anomalies, hypopigmented macules).
  - Recommend parental echocardiograms when their child has HLHS or any LVOTO defect.
  - Consider checking maternal phenylalanine level.
- Examine for extracardiac anomalies: head imaging, ophthalmologic exam, abdominal ultrasound, skeletal radiographs.
- Check for arrhythmias, especially in deaf infants.
  - When the infant has a cardiomyopathy, a metabolic genetics consultation can be helpful.
- Genetic testing
  - Start with microarray analysis, unless a specific chromosome aneuploidy is suspected.
    - When microarray is abnormal, test parents for the CNV identified in their child.
  - Start with chromosome analysis, when aneuploidy, such as Down syndrome, is suspected.
  - Test for single gene disorders when the physical findings and history suggests a particular syndrome.
  - Gene panels for isolated cardiac defects are available, but yield is low without a positive family history.
  - Consider exome sequencing when the pattern of anomalies is not diagnostic.
- Offer genetic counseling, and recommend starting daily 4 mg folic acid supplementation prior to next conception.

## Further Reading

Andersen TA, Troelsen Kde L, Larsen, LA. (2014) Of mice and men: Molecular genetics of congenital heart disease. Cell Mol Life Sci. 71:1327–52. PMID 23934094

Bahtiyar MO, Dulay AT, Weeks BP, et al. (2007) Prevalence of congenital heart defects in monochorionic/diamniotic twin gestations: A systematic literature review. J Ultrasound Med. 26:1491–8. PMID 17957043

Blue GM, Humphreys D, Szot J, et al. (2017) The promises and challenges of exome sequencing in familial, non-syndromic congenital heart disease. Int J Cardiol. 230:155–63. PMID 27989580

Chaix MA, Andelfinger G, Khairy P. (2016) Genetic testing in congenital heart disease: A clinical approach. World J Cardiol. 8:180–91. PMID 26981213

Dentici ML, Di Pede A, Lepri FR, et al. (2015) Kabuki syndrome: Clinical and molecular diagnosis in the first year of life. Arch Dis Child. 100:158–64. PMID 25281733

Egbe A, Uppu S, Stroustrup A, et al. (2014) Incidences and sociodemographics of specific congenital heart diseases in the United States of America: An evaluation of hospital discharge diagnoses. Pediatr Cardiol. 35:975–82. PMID 24563074

Matok I, Pupco A, Koren G. (2011) Drug exposure in pregnancy and heart defects. J Cardiovasc Pharmacol. 58:20–4. PMID 21499119

Morton S, Roberts AE. (2015) Genetic basis of congenital heart disease. Neoreviews. 16:c340–c350.

Roach ES. (2016) Applying the lessons of tuberous sclerosis: The 2015 Hower Award Lecture. Pediatr Neurol. 63:6–22. PMID 27543366

Zaidi S, Brueckner M. (2017) Genetics and genomics of congenital heart disease. Circ Res. 120:923–40. PMID 28302740

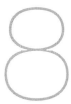

# Heterotaxy

## Clinical Consult

A 34-year-old pregnant woman with no known risk factors had a fetal ultrasound at 20 weeks' gestation that revealed an interrupted inferior vena cava and transposition of the great arteries. Family history was negative for consanguinity or similarly affected relatives. After delivery, asplenia and situs ambiguus were confirmed by abdominal ultrasound. An SNP chromosome microarray was normal. The baby girl initially did well, but on day 3, she had increasing requirements for supplemental oxygen with nasal discharge and radiographic findings of pneumonia. After her respiratory status failed to improve, she underwent a biopsy of the nasal epithelium that confirmed immotile cilia due to a **primary ciliary dyskinesia**. A multigene sequencing panel revealed a heterozygous de novo pathogenic variant in *DNAH6*. Immunology consultation provided guidance on a special plan for vaccination and prophylactic antibiotics. She was discharged home after a 6-week hospitalization, underwent cardiac repair at 9 months, and remains relatively well with normal development at age 18 months.

This vignette illustrates the contribution of genetic ciliary defects to the etiology of heterotaxy. Even sporadic cases can be caused by pathogenic variant, usually de novo.

## Definition

- Heterotaxy is synonymous with situs ambiguus for some, whereas others use the term for situs ambiguus with a cardiovascular defect, often a cardiac looping defect.
  - ○ Situs ambiguus (SA): intermediate body pattern that is neither the typical left–right body asymmetry pattern (situs solitus) nor the completely reversed (mirror image) body plan (situs inversus totalis).
- Incidence: 1/10,000 live births
  - ○ Heterotaxy is responsible for 3% of cardiac defects.
  - ○ Twice as common as situs inversus totalis
  - ○ 1.5 M:1 F
- Risk factors
  - ○ Assisted reproductive technology (ART)
  - ○ Hispanic, Black, Asian mothers
  - ○ Maternal cocaine use (OR 3.7)

- Maternal diabetes mellitus*, risk ≥3× for heterotaxy
- Maternal education <12 years
- Monozygotic twins* (OR 4.8)
- Inheritance
  - Most sporadic
    - Multifactorial inheritance
  - Familial 10%
    - Autosomal, X-linked, dominant and recessive inheritance
    - Incomplete penetrance in familial heterotaxy
      - Mild presentation may not be diagnosed: isolated dextrocardia.
- Etiology: Motile and nonmotile cilia at the embryonic node normally create leftward flow around the embryo. This initiates asymmetric gene expression and establishes the left–right body pattern (situs solitus). Heterotaxy is caused by disruption of normal embryonic nodal flow early in embryonic life.
  - The heart is the first organ to break symmetry in the developing embryo. By day 23, the symmetric cardiac tube forms a C-shaped or d (dextral) loop.

# Diagnosis

- Clinical features
  - Asplenia, "bilateral right sidedness," right-sided isomerism (**Ivemark syndrome**)
    - Cardiac defects 99%
  - Polysplenia, "bilateral left sidedness," left-sided isomerism
    - Cardiac defects 90%; many are rarely seen with asplenia.
      - Interrupted inferior vena cava (IVC)
      - Partial anomalous pulmonary venous return

*Pearl*: In heterotaxy with asplenia, cardiac defects are generally more severe and sepsis is more common. Prognosis for heterotaxy with polysplenia is better.

- Pulmonary isomerism
  - Trilobed (right-sided) or bilobed (left-sided) lungs
  - Useful sign, usually asymptomatic
- Intestinal malrotation ≥70%
  - Surgery may not benefit asymptomatic infants.

*Pearl*: A prophylactic Ladd procedure in heterotaxy patients can cause increased morbidity and mortality (Elder et al., 2014).

- Cardiac anomalies
  - DORV: most common
  - Tetralogy of Fallot, atrioventricular canal, transposition of the great arteries (TGA), aortic arch malposition, interrupted IVC

- Arrhythmias—onset ~4 years
- Reduced birth weight
  - Small for gestational age 16.95% versus 6.5% in controls
- Ciliary dysfunction 42%
  - Atelectasis, pneumonia increase perioperative and intraoperative morbidity and mortality
- Other anomalies >33%
  - Oral clefts, hydrocephalus, GI atresias, omphalocele, anomalies of the anus, gut, kidneys, spine, extrahepatic biliary atresia (with polysplenia)
  - Many are in **VATER/VACTERL association*** spectrum
- Genetic factors
  - CNV: abnormal chromosome microarray 20%
    - CNV positive group: 40% have additional sequence variants in heterotaxy genes.
  - Ciliary genes associated with laterality and cardiac looping defects (Deng et al., 2015)
    - Pathogenic variants in >15 genes cause <20% of heterotaxy.
      - *NODAL* (HTX5, MIM 270100) 5%
      - *ZIC3* (HTX1, MIM 306955) ~1% when sporadic; more when familial; both sexes affected
        - VATER-like anomalies are common.
      - *CFC1* (HTX2, MIM 605376) 2%
        - Laterality defects are not constant.

# Differential Diagnosis

- **Chromosome anomalies**
  - **Trisomy 13***
  - **2q21.1** deletions/duplications that involve *CFC1*
- **Maternal diabetes mellitus***
  - TGA (OR 61.87)
  - Situs ambiguus (OR 24.82)
- **Primary ciliary dyskinesias** (PCD)
  - Heterogeneous, usually autosomal recessive, disorders cause dysfunction or decreased numbers of motile cilia.
    - >30 known genes
    - **Kartagener syndrome** (MIM 244400): prototypic PCD
    - Heterozygotes (carrier parents) are usually unaffected, but heterozygous pathogenic variants in *DNAH6, DNAH5,* and *DNAI1* can cause PCD and heterotaxy.
  - Incidence 1/16,000
  - Clinical features: unexplained respiratory distress >75%, situs ambiguus/heterotaxy 6–12%
    - Among PCD with SA, 50% have cardiovascular defects

*Pearl*: Suspect a primary ciliary disorder in an infant with an unexplained oxygen requirement or lobar collapse, regardless of situs.

- ○ Syndromic Heterotaxy
    Nonmotile ciliary disorders can cause syndromic cardiac anomalies with situs inversus. Motile cilia functional normally.
- ○ **Agnathia-otocephaly complex** (MIM 202650)
    - ■ Usually de novo; occasionally recessive. One family with *PRRX1* pathogenic variant
    - ■ Clinical features: severe mandibular hypoplasia to absence, ears may meet in midline, microstomia, fused eyes or down-slanting fissures, hypoplasia of oropharynx, situs inversus, holoprosencephaly, absent corpus callosum
- ○ **Bardet–Biedl syndrome** (MIM 209900)
    - ■ Prototypic autosomal recessive ciliopathy, caused by pathogenic variants that affect intraflagellar transport
    - ■ Clinical features: polycystic kidneys, polydactyly, CNS anomalies, retinopathy, obesity
        - Neonatal respiratory distress 12%
- ○ **Total anomalous pulmonary venous return** (TAPVR1, scimitar syndrome, MIM 106700)
    - ■ Possible autosomal dominant trait, incomplete penetrance. No gene has been identified.
    - ■ Clinical features: respiratory distress, right lung hypoplasia, dextroposition of the heart, anomalous pulmonary venous drainage
        - Abnormal vessels resemble a scimitar radiographically.
        - Other syndromes with heterotaxy: **Ellis van Creveld syndrome** (MIM 225500), **renal-hepatic-pancreatic dysplasia** (MIM 208540, 615415), **short rib thoracic dysplasias** with or without polydactyly, **X-linked VACTERL-H** due to a pathogenic variant in *ZIC3* (MIM 314390)

## Evaluation and Management

- Seek a prenatal history of risk factors: ART, maternal diabetes mellitus, cocaine use
- Document family history: consanguinity, dextrocardia, cardiac defects, situs inversus, a/polysplenia
    - ○ Fetal loss, early childhood death, especially in males (X-linked inheritance)
- Evaluate for visceral and other anomalies: abdominal ultrasound, echocardiogram, skeletal survey, ECG; consider cardiac MRI.
    - ○ CBC: Howell–Jolly bodies, in asplenia
    - ○ Chest radiograph: pulmonary situs (best overpenetrated)
    - ○ Spine films: vertebral defects
- Watch for unexplained respiratory dysfunction.
    - ○ Consider primary ciliary dyskinesia.
        - ■ Diagnosis may require several testing modalities.
        - ■ Transmission electron microscopy of ciliary epithelium (nasal biopsy) 70% have an ultrastructural abnormality.
        - ■ Multigene panel detects 65–80%.
    - ○ May complicate surgery
        - ■ Avoid unnecessary surgery.
- Patients with asplenia: Anticipate infections, especially with encapsulated microorganisms; use long-term prophylactic antibiotics and a specific vaccine plan.
- Genetic testing
    - ○ Chromosome microarray
    - ○ *ZIC3* analysis, especially when VATER/VACTERL* spectrum anomalies are present
    - ○ Multigene panel, when family history is positive; lower yield in sporadic cases
    - ○ Consider research participation for genomic analysis, especially in familial cases: https://www.clinicaltrials.gov.

## Further Reading

Cowan JR, Tariq M, Shaw C, et al. (2016) Copy number variation as a genetic basis for heterotaxy and heterotaxy-spectrum congenital heart defects. Philos Trans R Soc B Biol Sci. 371(1710): pii 2015040. PMID 27821535

Deng H, Xia H, Deng S. (2015) Genetic basis of human left–right asymmetry disorders. Expert Rev Mol Med. 16:e19. PMID 26258520

Elder CT, Metzger R, Arrington C, et al. (2014) The role of screening and prophylactic surgery for malrotation in heterotaxy patients. J Pediatr Surg. 49:1746–8. PMID 25487475

Harrison MJ, Shapiro AJ, Kennedy MP. (2016) Congenital heart disease and primary ciliary dyskinesia. Paediatr Respir Rev. 18:25–32. PMID 26545972

Piano Mortari E, Baban A, Cantarutti N, et al. (2017) Heterotaxy syndrome with and without spleen: Different infection risk and management. J Allergy Clin Immunol. 139:1981–1984321. PMID 27864025

Versacci P, Pugnaloni F, Digilio MC, et al. (2018) Some isolated cardiac malformations can be related to laterality defects. J Cardiovasc Dev Dis. 5(2):E24. PMID 29724030

# Part III

## Craniofacial System

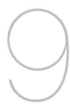

# Ear Anomalies

## Clinical Consult

A pregnant woman, who had a history of cardiac transplant, presented for a prenatal consultation in her second pregnancy because 8 years previously, her first child had been clinically diagnosed with Treacher–Collins syndrome with negative gene testing. The mother had taken CellCept (mycophenolate mofetil, MMF) as an immunosuppressant to prevent transplant rejection during her first pregnancy. Based on this exposure and the clinical features, the diagnosis in that child was revised to **mycophenylate mofetil (MMF) embryopathy**. The mother was not taking mycophenylate during the current pregnancy and later delivered a healthy baby.

Congenital anomalies have been reported in approximately 25% of live-born infants following in utero exposure to MMF. The features are variable, ranging from microtia to anotia, oral clefts, and cardiac, limb, and other anomalies. The diagnosis may be confused with other craniofacial syndromes. The developmental outcome is typically normal.

## Definition

- The external ear forms from the first branchial cleft during the 6th through 12th weeks of gestation.
- Malformed external ears with or without atresia of the external auditory canal or deafness occur in 1/8,000–1/10,000 births.
- Microtia is classified by severity, grade 1–4.
- Isolated microtia 70%
  - Unilateral ~80%; the right ear affected 60%
- 1.5 M:1 F
- Risk factors for isolated microtia
  - Advanced maternal age
  - Hispanic ethnicity
  - Low maternal education
  - Maternal obesity
  - Multiple gestation, fertility treatment
  - Pregestational diabetes: aOR 4.37

*Pearl*: Periconceptional folic acid supplementation reduces the risk for microtia, especially among offspring of non-obese women. The risk reduction for folic acid is greatest for isolated nonsyndromic microtia.

## Diagnosis

- Nonsyndromic microtia is usually sporadic.
  - Recurrence risk ~6% for isolated, nonsyndromic microtia
- Autosomal dominant families have markedly reduced penetrance and significant variability.
  - Autosomal dominant microtia and hearing loss can be due to heterozygous *HOXA2* pathogenic variant.
- Autosomal recessive inheritance is rare.
- Chromosome anomalies
  - Ear anomalies are common in **trisomies 13,\* 18,\* and 21\***
  - Microdeletions: **5p-, 18p-,** and **chromosome 22q11.2 deletion syndrome\***

*Pearl*: Isolated minor ear anomalies, such as preauricular pits or tags, are not associated with renal anomalies. A renal ultrasound is not necessary in the absence of a major ear or other anomaly.

## Differential Diagnosis

### Teratogens\*

- **Infant of a diabetic mother\***
  - Increased risk for ear anomalies: microtia, hearing loss, including hemifacial microsomia (mandibular hypoplasia) and oculoauricular vertebral syndrome (epibulbar dermoid, vertebral anomalies)
- **Isotretinoin (Accutane) embryopathy**
  - Accutane is a vitamin A derivative used to treat cystic acne.
  - In North America, ~2.5/1,000 women of childbearing age use isotretinoin.
    - Topical use of tretinoin (Retin-A) is not teratogenic.
    - Exposed pregnancies continue despite a pregnancy prevention program requiring negative pregnancy tests prior to starting the medication and two forms of birth control, direct-to-consumer education, and package insert warnings.
  - Embryopathy ~30% in exposures ≤28 days of gestation
  - Significantly increased risk for congenital anomalies, RR 25.6
  - Clinical features: characteristic microtia/anotia with a very small, slit-like ear (Figure 9.1), conotruncal and aortic arch anomalies
    - CNS anomalies, hydrocephalus, Dandy–Walker malformation

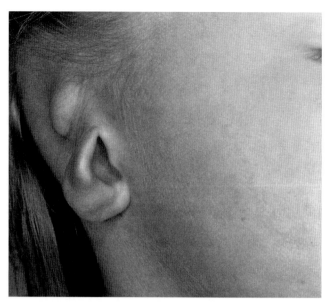

FIGURE 9.1  This child with Accutane embryopathy has characteristic microtia. She also has ipsilateral facial palsy and hypoplasia of the aortic arch.

- Retinal and optic nerve involvement, facial nerve palsy
- Cleft palate
- **Mycophenylate embryopathy** (mycophenolate mofetil, MMF, CellCept)
  - MMF is an immunosuppressive agent used after solid organ transplantation and for lupus nephritis, recurrent erythema multiforme, and bullous conditions.
  - Increased risk for microtia and other anomalies after first trimester MMF exposure
    - Spontaneous abortion ~40%
    - Among live-born exposed infants, ~25% have malformations.
  - Clinical features: bilateral moderate to severe microtia or anotia; 50%, external auditory canal atresia, micrognathia
    - Orofacial clefts (see Figure 6.4), hypertelorism
    - Eye anomalies: microphthalmia, colobomas, anophthalmia/microphthlamia
    - Cardiac 33%, commonly conotruncal defects
    - Less common anomalies: CNS, vertebral, distal limbs

### Syndromes

- **Auriculo-condular syndrome** (MIM 602483)
  - Autosomal dominant condition, due to heterozygous pathogenic variant in *GNAI3*, *PLCB4*, or *EDN1*.
  - Clinical features: cupped helix, "question mark" ear with a constriction between the upper two thirds and the lower third of the ear with an interruption in continuity between the base of the helix and the lobule, stenotic ear canals, microsomia, hypoplastic mandible with abnormal condyles, micrognathia, round face, prominent cheeks, hearing loss.
    - Question mark ears can also occur as an isolated finding

- **Branchio-oculo-facial syndrome** (BOFS, MIM 113620)
  - Autosomal dominant disorder, due to heterozygous pathogenic variant or deletion in *TFAP2A*
  - Clinical features: malformed auricles, cutis aplasia or hemangioma with or without a branchial sinus behind the ears
    - Eye anomalies: microphthalmia, anophthalmia, coloboma, cataract, lacrimal duct obstruction
    - Cleft or pseudo-cleft of the lip
    - Sebaceous cysts of the scalp and premature graying
- **Branchio-oto-renal syndrome** (MIM 113650)
  - Autosomal dominant syndrome, caused by heterozygous pathogenic variant in *EYA1* and, less often, *SIX1*, in ~40%
  - Incidence 1/40,000 deliveries
    - 2% of profoundly deaf children
  - The diagnosis is made clinically. Molecular testing is recommended when diagnostic criteria are met
  - Clinical features: variable unilateral or bilateral low-set, cup-shaped ears, preauricular pits, hearing loss
    - Branchial remnants, clefts and tags on anterior neck
    - Unilateral facial nerve palsy
    - Renal anomalies
- **CHARGE syndrome\*** (MIM 214800)
  - Autosomal dominant trait, due to a heterozygous *CHD7* pathogenic variant
  - Clinical features: characteristic microtia (Figure 9.2), primarily absence of the lower part of the external ear, absence of hypoplasia of the semicircular canals, deafness, colobomas, facial nerve paresis, choanal atresia

*Pearl*: The semicircular canals can be visualized on a lateral skull film in the newborn.

- **Hemifacial microsomia** (first and second branchial arch syndrome and **oculo-auriculo-vertebral syndrome**, OAVS, **Goldenhar syndrome**, MIM 164210)
  - Usually sporadic, typically multifactorial, disorder with a continuum of severity
    - Microarray abnormal ~10%, more in familial cases
    - Heterozygous pathogenic variants in *MYT1*, 1–2%
  - Clinical features: unilateral or bilateral asymmetric microtia (Figure 9.3) with middle and inner ear anomalies, 90%. Facial asymmetry and reduced buccal fat on the affected side. Asymmetric hypoplasia of the mandible causes a shift in the midline toward the more affected side.
    - Preauricular tags, facial tags, or dimples may occur in a line from the oral commissure to the ear.
    - Macrostomia, a lateral cleft through the oral commissure (usually unilateral, asymmetric), elongates the mouth on the affected side, 5%.

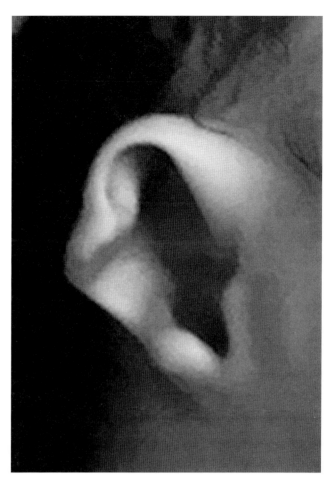

FIGURE 9.2 The external ear is simple and cupped in this child with CHARGE syndrome. There is a characteristic deficiency of the lobule and helix.
SOURCE: Courtesy of Antonio Perez-Aytes, MD, University and Polytechnic Institute La Fe, Valencia, Spain.

- Epibulbar dermoid, a fleshy nodule near the lateral canthus of the eye (see Figure 10.5); required for the diagnosis of OAVS/Goldenhar syndrome
- Other anomalies: cardiac, renal, vertebral (cervical), pulmonary agenesis
- **Hypertelorism microtia clefting syndrome** (HMC, MIM 239800)
  - Rare autosomal recessive disorder without a known genetic cause
  - Clinical features: microtia, oral clefting, hypertelorism, micrognathia, microcephaly, congenital heart and renal malformations
- **Mandibulofacial dysostosis syndromes**
  - **Diamond–Blackfan anemia 15 with mandibulofacial dysostosis** (MIM 606164)
    - Autosomal dominant due to pathogenic variants in *RPS28* involved in ribosomal biogenesis
    - Clinical features: micrognathia, down-slanting palpebral fissures, submucosal cleft palate or bifid uvula, malar hypoplasia, microtia

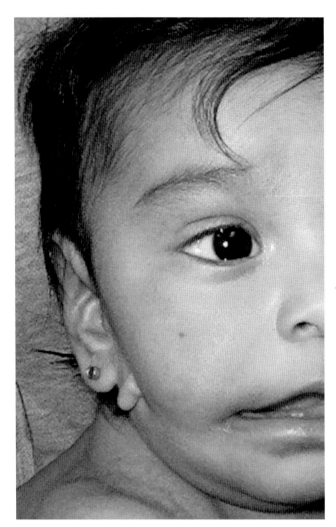

FIGURE 9.3 This baby with oculo-auriculo-vertebral syndrome has macrostomia with a cleft in the lateral commissure. Note the epibulbar dermoid and cheek tag.

- Mixed hearing loss, developmental delay, short stature
- Steroid responsive macrocytic anemia in infancy
- **Mandibulofacial dysostosis with microcephaly** (MFD Guion–Ameida type, MIM 610536)
  - Autosomal dominant disorder, caused by heterozygous pathogenic variants in *EFTUD2*
  - Clinical features: facial features of mandibulofacial dysostosis, similar to both Treacher–Collins syndrome and hemifacial microsomia
    - Microtia (Figure 12.4), sensorineural hearing loss, micrognathia, cleft palate, choanal atresia
    - Cardiac defects, esophageal atresia
    - Microcephaly and developmental delay distinguish this type.
- **Miller syndrome** (MIM 263750)
  - Autosomal recessive, caused by biallelic pathogenic variants in *DHODH*
  - Clinical features: facial features of mandibulofacial dysostosis, postaxial defects of the fourth or fifth rays of the hands and feet

- **Nager acrofacial dysostosis syndrome** (MIM 154400)
  - Autosomal dominant disorder, due to heterozygous pathogenic variant in *SF3B4* in half of the patients
  - Clinical features: facial features of mandibulofacial dysostosis
    - Hypoplasia or aplasia of the radius and/or thumb
    - Gastrointestinal, renal, and genital anomalies
- **Treacher-Collins syndrome** (MIM 248390)
  - Most autosomal dominant
    - Caused by pathogenic variants in three genes: *TCOF1* 80–90%; *POLR1C, POLR1D* 8%.
  - Family history
    - 40% have an affected parent.
    - The presentation can range from severe to mild even within the same family.
      - Subtle manifestations in undiagnosed carrier parents
  - Clinical features
    - Hypoplasia of the zygomatic arches, mandible, and external ears; conductive hearing loss
    - Less commonly, cleft palate and choanal stenosis
  - Airway management and intubation can be challenging and ultimately life-threatening.
    - Laryngeal mask airway should be available at delivery. Tracheostomy or mandibular distraction is sometimes needed (Figure 9.4).
- **Townes–Brocks syndrome** (MIM 107480)
  - Autosomal dominant disorder, caused by a heterozygous pathogenic variant in *SALL1*
  - Clinical features: anal atresia, ear anomalies (see Figure 24.2), various thumb anomalies (Figure 24.2)
    - Consider in the differential diagnosis of VATER/VACTERL association*.

# Evaluation and Management

- Review pregnancy history: request results of first trimester HbA$_{1c}$ when there is a history of maternal diabetes, medication use.
- Take family history: consanguinity, hearing loss, ear, other congenital anomalies.
- Examine the parents: ear anomalies, mandibular hypoplasia, facial asymmetry, down-slanting palpebral fissures, zygomatic notches, irregular eyelashes on lower lids, preauricular pits, tags, hearing loss, branchial remnants, hand anomalies.
- Stabilize the airway
  - Micrognathia can compromise the airway, and intubation can be difficult.
    - Keep laryngeal mask airways at the ready.
    - An ex utero intrapartum treatment (EXIT) procedure at delivery may be necessary in the most severe cases.
- Evaluate for anomalies in other organ systems: cardiac, renal.

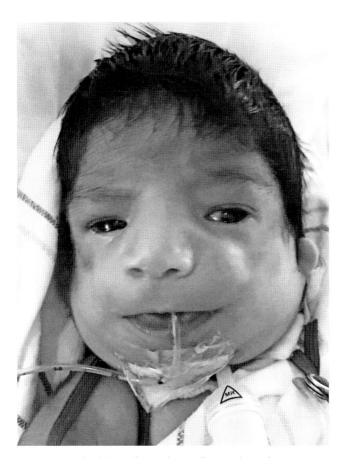

FIGURE 9.4 This baby with Treacher–Collins syndrome has a tracheostomy due to severe mandibular hypoplasia and airway inadequacy. He has the classic features of lower lid colobomas, zygomatic hypoplasia, and ear dysplasia. Note the patch of hair extending onto the face below the right eye.

- Order a formal audiology evaluation for infants with microtia.
  - Passing the newborn hearing screen is not sufficient.
- Genetic studies
  - Chromosome microarray studies are indicated when there are multiple congenital anomalies without a clear etiology.

- Choose chromosome analysis when a trisomy is suspected.
- When a syndrome is suspected, perform appropriate genetic testing single gene, gene panel or exome.
- Recommend genetic counseling.
- Refer to a multidisciplinary craniofacial team where available.
- Recommend daily supplemental folic acid (4–5 mg/day) prior to and throughout first trimester of subsequent pregnancies.

## Further Reading

Alasti F, Van Camp G. (2009) Genetics of microtia and associated syndromes. J Med Genet. 46:361–9. PMID 19293168

Beleza-Meireles A, Clayton-Smith J, Saraiva JM, Tassabehji M. (2014) Oculo-auriculo-vertebral spectrum: A review of the literature and genetic update. J Med Genet. 51:635–45. PMID 25118188

Chang EU, Menezes M, Meyer NC, et al. (2004) Branchio-oto-renal syndrome: The mutation spectrum in EYA1 and its phenotypic consequences. Hum Mutat. 23:582–589. PMID 15146463

Deshpande SA, Watson H. (2006) Renal ultrasonography not required in babies with isolated minor ear anomalies. Arch Dis Child Fetal Neonatal Ed. 91:F29–F30. PMID 16223753

Gripp KW, Curry C, Olney AH (2014) Diamond–Blackfan anemia with mandibulofacial dystostosis is heterogeneous, including the novel DBA genes *TSR2* and *RPS28*. Am J Med Genet A. 164A(9):2240–9. PMID 24942156

Huang L, Vanstone MR, Hartley T, et al. (2016) Mandibulofacial dysostosis with microcephaly: Mutation and database update. Hum Mutat. 37:148–54. PMID 26507355

Lehalle D, Wieczorek D, Zechi-Ceide RM, et al. (2015) A review of craniofacial disorders caused by spliceosomal defects. Clin Genet. 88:405–15. PMID 25865758

Ma C, Carmichael SL, Scheuerle AE, et al.; National Birth Defects Prevention Study. (2010) Association of microtia with maternal obesity and periconceptional folic acid use. Am J Med Genet A. 152A:2756–61. PMID 20949601

Perez-Aytes A, Marin-Reina P, Boso V, et al. (2017) Mycophenolate mofetil embryopathy: A newly recognized teratogenic syndrome. Eur J Med Genet. 60:16–21. PMID 27639443

# 10

## Eye Anomalies

### Clinical Consult

A 9-day-old male, one of unlike-sex 33-week gestation twins conceived by in vitro fertilization, had prenatally diagnosed IUGR and hydronephrosis. The genetics consultant noted bilateral microphthalmia, opaque corneas, and mildly unusual ears and toes. The patient's mother and the maternal grandmother were asymptomatic, but the family history suggested X-linked inheritance. The maternal grandmother's sister had a retinal coloboma with normal vision; her 33-year-old legally blind son was "slow" with bilateral retinal and iris colobomas, cataracts, severe hearing loss, and a hydronephrotic kidney. The maternal grandmother's brother died of renal failure at age 13 years.

The diagnosis of **Lenz microphthalmia syndrome** (MIM 309800) was made clinically, but no pathogenic variants were detected in a gene panel for eye disease that included *BCOR* and *NAA10*. He had postnatal growth failure and severely delayed development (Figure 10.1). He could not sit at 18 months. He was fed entirely by gastrostomy tube. His hearing was normal. Later, he developed large retro-orbital cysts. He required renal dialysis at 1 year of age. Genome sequencing is in process on a research basis.

### Definition

- Prevalence of all types of congenital ophthalmic anomalies is 7.5/10,000: 1.8/10,000 for microphthalmia, 0.3/10,000 for anophthalmia, 2.3/10,000 for cataract, 0.7/10,000 for coloboma, 0.3/10,000 for congenital corneal opacities, 0.2/10,000 for aniridia.
- Consanguinity is more frequent than in controls.
- Non-ocular malformations are present in ~50%: clubfeet, microcephaly, hydrocephaly, dysmorphic features.
- At birth, infants with eye anomalies have lower average birth weights and smaller head circumferences.
- Five eye anomalies that are commonly encountered in the newborn period are reviewed in this chapter: anterior chamber disorders, microphthalmia/anophthalmia/coloboma (MAC), cataract, ptosis, and miscellaneous syndromes with ocular manifestations.
  - Cranial dysinnervation disorders (e.g., Moebius syndrome) are discussed in Chapter 6 (Gutowski and Chilton, 2015).

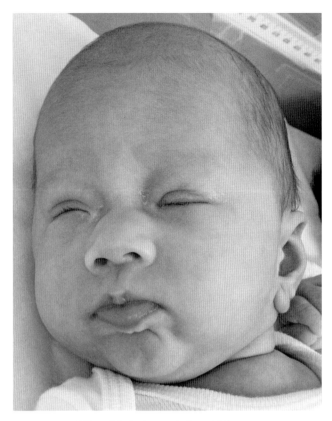

FIGURE 10.1 Microphthalmia in an infant with Lenz microphthalmia. Note micrognathia, prominent antihelix, and minor ear anomalies.

○ For a full discussion of retinoblastoma, see Lohmann and Gallie (2015).

# Anterior Chamber Anomalies

- Anterior chamber defects, which affect the lens, iris, ciliary body, and pupil, range from mild iris hypoplasia, presenting with a displaced pupil, to significant disorders limiting vision and associated with glaucoma.
- These disorders represent a spectrum of related phenotypes with overlapping findings among affected family members.
- Most are autosomal dominant traits with variable expression and incomplete penetrance.

## Isolated Anterior Chamber Anomalies

- **Aniridia** (MIM 106210)
  ○ Autosomal dominant, heterozygous pathogenic variants in *PAX6* account for two-thirds of isolated bilateral iris hypoplasia or aplasia.
  ○ Clinical features: diminished visual acuity due to foveal dysplasia and early onset nystagmus (usually by 6 weeks). Early onset glaucoma is common.
    ■ Photophobia and cataract occur occasionally.

*Pearl*: In sporadic aniridia, 25–30% develop Wilms' tumor. Consider tumor surveillance with renal ultrasound every 6 mos.

## Syndromic Anterior Chamber Anomalies

- **Axenfeld–Rieger syndrome** (MIM 602482, 180500)
  ○ Autosomal dominant disorder, caused by a heterozygous pathogenic variant in *FOXC1* or *PITX2* and, less commonly, *PAX6* and *FOXO1A*
  ○ Prevalence 1 in 200,000 live births
  ○ Clinical features: variable anterior chamber dysgenesis (iris hypoplasia, iridocorneal adhesions, posterior embryotoxon, Peters anomaly)
    ■ Non-ocular anomalies: characteristic umbilicus with excess periumbilical skin, hypertelorism, hypodontia, microdontia, hearing loss, cardiac anomalies
- **Peters plus syndrome** (MIM 261540)
  ○ Autosomal recessive disorder of protein O-glycosylation, caused by biallelic pathogenic variants in *B3GALTL*
  ○ Clinical features: central corneal opacity, adhesion of the iris to the cornea and variable other anterior chamber anomalies, usually bilateral, congenital glaucoma
    ■ Non-ocular anomalies include prenatal-onset disproportionate short stature, abnormal ears, cleft lip and palate, hydrocephalus, and genitourinary and cardiac anomalies.
      • Intellectual disability in some
- **WAGR syndrome** (*W*ilms tumor, *a*niridia, *g*enitourinary anomalies, and mental *r*etardation syndrome, MIM 194072)
  ○ Usually a sporadic interstitial contiguous gene syndrome, due to deletion of varying length, at chromosome 11p13, including both *PAX6* and *WT1*
    ■ Deletions in 50% of patients
    ■ Somatic mosaicism explains some without a pathogenic variant
  ○ Clinical features: aniridia, bilateral ptosis ≤10%; genitourinary abnormalities: cryptorchidism, streak ovaries, bicornuate uterus
    ■ Later findings: Wilms tumor ages 1–8 years; learning, behavioral, and psychiatric symptoms such as anxiety, obsessive–compulsive disorder, depression
      • Abdominal US every 3m until age 8 years for tumor risk

# Microphthalmia/ Anophthalmia/Coloboma

- Microphthalmia (a small eye), anophthalmia, and coloboma (MAC) occur singly or in combination in isolated and syndromic disorders that are largely genetic.

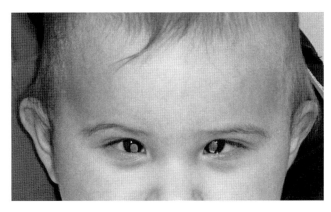

FIGURE 10.2 Typical inferionasal iris colobomas cause an oval or keyhole-shaped pupil.

- Incidence 1/7,000 live births
- Coloboma, caused by failure of closure of the optic fissure, occurs in 1/5,000 live births (Figure 10.2).
- Clinical anophthalmia, the apparent complete absence of a globe, occurs in 1/30,000 live births.

*Pearl*: True or primary anophthalmia is a histologic diagnosis that is incompatible with life because of severe CNS anomalies. The term anophthalmia is used here to mean clinical anophthalmia, where there is no apparent globe.

## Nonsyndromic MAC

- Teratogens*
  - **Vitamin A deficiency** due to malnutrition or in the context of gastric bypass surgery
  - Intrauterine exposure to **alcohol,** * **retinoic acid, thalidomide**, or **rubella**.
- Chromosome anomalies*
  - **Trisomy 13** * and **mosaic trisomy 9**
  - Copy number variants 17%
  - Balanced chromosome rearrangements
- Pathogenic variants in known genes explain only ~40% of cases of microphthalmia or anophthalmia.
  - Variants in ≥20 genes have been identified; most commonly *SOX2* and *OTX2*.
  - Some cause both nonsyndromic and syndromic MAC.

## Syndromic MAC

- *Anophthalmia–esophageal atresia–genital syndrome* (AEG, MIM 206900)
  - Usually a sporadic disorder, caused by heterozygous loss-of-function pathogenic variant in *SOX2*, or *de novo* chromosome 3q27 alterations
  - Clinical features: anophthalmia, microphthalmia
    - Non-ocular findings: esophageal atresia with or without tracheoesophageal fistula, genital anomalies,

hypogonadotropic hypogonadism, cryptorchidism, micropenis, sensorineural deafness, renal and cardiac anomalies
    - Growth failure, learning disabilities
- **Bosma arhinia microphthalmia syndrome** (MIM 603457)
  - Autosomal dominant disorder, caused by a heterozygous pathogenic variant in *SMCHD1*
  - Clinical features: microphthalmia, coloboma, absent nose (arhinia), choanal atresia, cleft palate, normal CNS and intelligence. Hypogonadotrophic hypogonadism in males
- **CHARGE syndrome** * (MIM 214800)
  - Autosomal dominant disorder caused by a pathogenic variant or deletion of *CHD7*
  - Clinical features: retinal coloboma, choanal atresia, facial nerve palsy and ear and heart defects, renal and genital anomalies
- **COMMAD syndrome** (*c*oloboma, *o*steopetrosis, *m*icrophthalmia, *m*acrocephaly, *a*lbinism, and *d*eafness, MIM 617306)
  - Rare autosomal recessive syndrome, due to compound heterozygous pathogenic variants in *MITF*, the gene responsible for Waardenberg syndrome type 2
    - Parents have Waardenberg syndrome type 2A: congenital sensorineural hearing loss, blue irides, fair skin, premature graying of the hair, but no dystopia canthorum
  - Clinical features: macrocephaly, coloboma, microphthalmia, deafness, albinism, osteopetrosis
- **Goltz syndrome** (focal dermal hypoplasia syndrome, MIM 305600)
  - X-linked dominant disorder seen predominantly in females (1 M:9 F)
    - Presumed lethal *in utero* in males, unless they are mosaic
    - Rare affected males who survive are generally less severely affected than females.
  - Caused by a pathogenic variant or a large deletion of *PORCN* on Xp11.23
    - Most are *de novo*, but 5% are inherited from a mother, who may have linear or reticular skin defects.
    - Somatic mosaicism for a pathogenic variant can be detected only in affected tissues, not in lymphocytes.
  - Clinical features: ocular anomalies often asymmetric: strabismus, coloboma, microphthalmia, anophthalmia
    - Non-ocular findings: dermatologic features— streaks of atrophic or hyperpigmented skin follow Blaschko's lines, cutis aplasia, patchy punched-out defects of the dermis that allow fatty herniation; digital anomalies—syndactyly, oligodacty; microcephaly, developmental disability
      - Abdominal wall defects, cleft lip and palate, diaphragmatic hernia, renal anomalies
      - Osteopathica striata on plain radiographs is a diagnostic sign.

- **Lenz microphthalmia** (syndromic microphthalmia type 1, MCOP1, MIM 309800; see Clinical Consult)
  - X-linked disorder caused, in some, by hemizygous pathogenic variant in *NAA10* (MCOPS1) or *BCOR* (MCOPS2)
  - Clinical features: bilateral microphthalmia, coloboma, anophthalmia
    - Non-ocular anomalies: ear 63%—simple or cupped ears, hearing loss; genitourinary 77%—renal aplasia, hydronephrosis, hydroureter, cryptorchidism, hypospadias; skeletal and limb 44%—sloping shoulders, oligodactyly, syndactyly, clinodactyly, polydactyly (duplicated thumbs), brachydactyly
  - Intellectual disability, seizures and self-mutilating behavior (eye poking) 60%
- **Matthew–Wood syndrome** (MIM 601186)
  - Rare, autosomal recessive disorder; usually lethal, caused by biallelic pathogenic variants in *STRA6*
  - Clinical features: microphthalmia or anophthalmia a constant finding
    - Non-ocular findings: pulmonary agenesis or hypoplasia 44%, cardiac defects 53%, diaphragmatic hernia 25%, renal anomalies 20%
- *Microphthalmia with linear skin defects* (*m*icrophthalmia–*d*ermal *a*plasia–*s*clerocornea syndrome, MIDAS/MLS, MIM 309801)
  - X-linked disorder with a variable phenotype, primarily affects females; presumed lethal in males
  - Affected females have an Xp22.3 deletion, the locus for *HCCS*.
    - Almost all affected females have skewed X-inactivation with preferential activation of the abnormal chromosome.
  - Clinical features: microphthalmia, anophthalmia, sclerocornea, orbital cysts, glaucoma, cataracts, aniridia, coloboma
    - Non-ocular findings: linear skin defects of face and neck, microcephaly, CNS anomalies, infantile seizures
- **Renal–coloboma syndrome** (papillorenal syndrome, MIM 167409, 120330)
  - Autosomal dominant disorder, caused by a heterozygous pathogenic variant in *PAX2* in 50%
  - Clinical features: optic nerve dysplasia, retinal coloboma, small cornea
    - Non-ocular findings: small malformed kidneys, renal anomalies often identified before eye anomalies; can progress to renal failure
- **Waardenburg anophthalmia** (ophthalmoacromelic syndrome, MIM 206920)
  - Autosomal recessive disorder, caused by biallelic pathogenic variants in *SMOC1* or *FNBP4*
  - Clinical features: bilateral anophthalmia, syndactyly
  - Non-ocular findings: limb anomalies, oligodactyly, split hand, polydactyly.

# Congenital Cataracts

- Congenital cataract is a lens opacity that presents in the first year of life.
- Incidence is ~3/10,000 live births in industrialized nations.
  - Incidence is higher, 5–15/10,000 live births, in developing countries due to infectious diseases during pregnancy, especially rubella.
- Male > female
- Etiology is heterogeneous: inherited, sporadic, environmental.
  - Morphologic types are defined by anatomic location and appearance.
  - Can be unilateral, bilateral, isolated, associated with other ophthalmic disorders, or part of multisystem syndromes.
    - Bilateral cataracts are more likely to have associated birth defects, low birth weight, and a positive family history. Inherited cataracts are almost always bilateral.
- Intrauterine infections with **toxoplasmosis, rubella, cytomegalovirus, syphilis, Herpes simplex, HIV, Coxsackie virus**, and **Zika virus** are known causes.

*Pearl*: Heterozygous pathogenic variants of *COL4A1* or *COL4A2* can cause congenital cataracts and a clinical picture similar to congenital TORCH infection: variable growth retardation, microcephaly, epilepsy, periventricular calcifications, schizencephaly, porencephaly, fetal intracranial hemorrhage, or perinatal stroke.

- Chromosome disorders include **Down syndrome**\* and **trisomies 13**\* **and 18.**\*
  - Among children with Down syndrome, <1% have a dense cataract.
  - Among children undergoing surgery for cataract, 7% have Down syndrome.

## Single Gene Disorders Associated with Cataract

- More than 100 genes are associated with cataracts. Large gene panels identify gene pathogenic variants in 75% of patients with congenital cataract. Some disorders require exome sequencing.

## Isolated Cataracts

- Single gene disorders: Approximately one-third of isolated bilateral congenital cataracts are encoded by ~25 genes.
  - Most isolated cataracts are caused by autosomal dominant traits, but X-linked and recessive forms exist.

○ Genes responsible for isolated cataract encode the major proteins of the lens, in three main groups: crystallins (alpha, beta, gamma), lens-specific connexin gap junction proteins, and cytoskeletal proteins.

○ Genotype–phenotype correlation: Pathogenic variants in the same gene may lead to different cataract phenotypes, but some cataract types predict a specific genotype.

- **Hyperferritinemia cataract syndrome** (MIM 600886)
  ○ Autosomal dominant congenital nuclear "bread crumb-like" cataracts are caused by a heterozygous pathogenic variant in *FTL*.
    ▪ The cataract is not necessarily congenital in all affected family members.
  ○ Defective iron-responsive element of the ferritin light chain interferes with binding of the iron regulatory protein causing overproduction of ferritin unrelated to iron overload.
    ▪ Normal serum iron and iron saturation
    ▪ High levels of ferritin crystallize in the lens

## Syndromic Cataracts

- Syndromic and metabolic disorders account for ~15% of congenital cataracts.
  ○ The genetic cause of syndromic congenital cataract can be detected in 63%.

*Pearl*: Patients with presumed syndromic forms of cataract have had pathogenic variants in genes that cause nonsyndromic congenital cataract. In these patients, consider the possibility of two separate and distinct genetic disorders—one responsible for the cataracts and the other for the non-ocular phenotype.

- A few syndromes associated with cataract are discussed here.
- **Cockayne syndrome** (MIM 216400)
  ○ Rare, progressive multisystem autosomal recessive disorder of defective DNA repair, caused by biallelic pathogenic variants in *ERCC6*, in two-thirds of patients, and *ERCC8*, in one-third
  ○ Clinical features: cataracts, seen in half of the patients, may be only feature in the newborn period; sunken eyes, "salt-and-pepper" retinopathy
    ▪ Non-ocular findings: progressive microcephaly, neurological problems, and failure to thrive usually evident after a period of normal growth and development
  ○ Prenatal growth deficiency, congenital microcephaly, cataracts, joint contractures occur in the severe form: **cerebro-*oculo*-*facio*-*skeletal* syndrome** (COFS, MIM 214150)
- **Galactosemia** (MIM 230400)
  ○ Autosomal recessive disorder, due to biallelic pathogenic variants in *GALT* (galactose-1-phosphate uridyltransferase); usually diagnosed with newborn screening test

○ Clinical features: cataracts may be visible only with a slit lamp, not an ophthalmoscope
    ▪ Non-ocular findings: jaundice, hepatosplenomegaly, hypotonia, hypoglycemia and fulminant *Escherichia coli* sepsis, failure to thrive, vomiting and diarrhea after ingestion of lactose

*Pearl*: Lactating heterozygote mothers of babies with galactosemia can develop rapidly progressive cataracts, presumably through self-intoxication from their own lactose.

- **Galactokinase deficiency** (MIM 230200)
  ○ Autosomal recessive disorder, due to biallelic pathogenic variants in *GALK1*
  ○ Clinical features: cataracts 75%
- **Knobloch syndrome** (MIM 267750)
  ○ Autosomal recessive trait, caused by biallelic pathogenic variants in *COL18A1*
  ○ Clinical features: cataract, high myopia, glaucoma, dislocated lenses, vitreoretinal degeneration, retinal detachment
    ▪ Non-ocular findings: polymicrogyria, cerebral and cerebellar atrophy
    ▪ Variable occipital defects—encephalocele, dermal sinus, skull defects, alopecia, cutis aplasia of the scalp
- **Lowe syndrome** (oculocerebrorenal syndrome, MIM 309000)
  ○ Rare X-linked disorder, caused by a pathogenic variant in *OCRL*
    ▪ Carrier females usually have cataracts; some are asymptomatic.
  ○ Incidence is 1/500,000
  ○ Clinical features: bilateral congenital cataract, neonatal glaucoma
    ▪ Non-ocular findings: hypotonia, areflexia, renal tubular acidosis, may be asymptomatic at birth
- **Muscular dystrophy–dystroglycanopathy type A1** (MDDGA1, Walker–Warburg syndrome, HARD+/E, MIM 236670)
  ○ Rare autosomal recessive congenital muscular dystrophy with early lethality
    ▪ Severe autosomal recessive disorder of glycosylation of α-dystroglycan, caused by biallelic pathogenic variant in *POMT1, POMT2, POMGNT1, FKTN*, and others
    ▪ Less severe dystroglycanopathy phenotypes are described in Chapter 1.
  ○ Incidence 1.2/100,000
  ○ Clinical features: microcornea, microphthalmia, cataract, and retinal dysplasia with or without detachment, optic nerve hypoplasia, coloboma
    ▪ Non-ocular features: severe hypotonia, hydrocephalus, encephalocele, hypoplasia or absence of the corpus callosum, complete agyria to severe lissencephaly (type II), severe cerebellar anomalies, occipital encephalocele
    ▪ Elevated creatine kinase level is a helpful finding.

- **Nance–Horan syndrome** (MIM 302350)
  - X-linked recessive disorder, caused by hemizygous pathogenic variant in *NHS* or deletion of its locus on Xp22.13
  - Clinical features: central cataracts, microcornea
    - Non-ocular findings: simple anteverted ears, short metacarpals
    - Later: intellectual disability, dental anomalies (Hutchinsonian incisors)
  - Consider other X-linked disorders that cause congenital cataract: **Alport syndrome** (MIM 301050), **Conradi–Hünermann–Happle syndrome** (MIM 302960), **oculo-facial-cardio-dental syndrome** (MIM 300166).
- **Sengers syndrome** (MIM 212350)
  - Autosomal recessive trait, caused by pathogenic variants in the *AGK* gene
  - Clinical features: cataract and hypotonia
    - Non-ocular features: hypertrophic cardiomyopathy can cause early death; lactic acidosis with exercise or stress, mitochondrial depletion on muscle biopsy

*Pearl*: Order an echocardiogram prior to surgery for congenital cataracts. Undiagnosed cardiomyopathy has led to postoperative death after elective cataract surgery.

- **Warburg micro syndrome** (MIM 600118)
  - Autosomal recessive trait, caused by biallelic pathogenic variants in *RAB3GAP1, PAB3GAP2,* or *RAB18*
  - Clinical features: microphthalmia, microcornea, congenital cataract, corneal opacity, optic atrophy
    - Non-ocular features: dysmorphic features, postnatal microcephaly, spasticity, agenesis of the corpus callosum, seizures, hypogenitalism
    - Later onset: intellectual disability, hormonal dysfunction

- Non-ocular findings: microcephaly, anterior predominant lissencephaly, seizures, hearing loss
- ***Blepharophimosis ptosis epicanthus inversus syndrome*** (BPES, MIM 110100)
  - Autosomal dominant disorder of the eyelids, caused by heterozygous pathogenic variant in *FOXL2*
    - Syndromic blepharophimosis is also caused by pathogenic variants in *UBE3B, MED12,* and *KAT6B.*
  - Clinical features: short palpebral fissures, ptosis, inverse epicanthal folds, telecanthus (lateral deviation of the median canthus, covering the caruncula) (Figure 10.3)
    - Non-ocular features: renal anomalies, hypotonia
    - In BPES type I, females have premature ovarian failure and infertility; in BPES type II, they do not.

- **Noonan syndrome and other RASopathies*** (MIM 163950)
  - Relatively common autosomal dominant disorder, caused by heterozygous pathogenic variant in *PTPN11* and other genes in the MAPK pathway
- **Saethre–Chotzen syndrome** (MIM 101400)
  - Autosomal dominant syndrome, caused by a heterozygous pathogenic variant in *TWIST1* or *FGFR2*
  - Clinical features: ptosis, low frontal hairline, prominent ear crus, coronal craniosynostosis
- **Smith–Lemli–Opitz syndrome*** (MIM 270400)
  - Autosomal recessive disorder of cholesterol biosynthesis with variable phenotype, caused by biallelic pathogenic variants in *DHCR7*
  - Clinical features: cataract, microphthalmia, coloboma

# Ptosis

- Ptosis in the newborn is usually unilateral, due to congenital fibrosis or dysfunction of the levator palpebrae superioris muscle.
- Other causes: neurogenic (including defects of axon guidance), aponeurotic, autoimmune (congenital myasthenia gravis), myopathic, mechanical, traumatic, chromosomal
- Some syndromes are described next.

## Syndromic Ptosis

- **Baraitser–Winter syndrome** (MIM 243310, 614583)
  - Autosomal dominant disorder, caused by heterozygous pathogenic variant in actin genes: *ACTB* or *ACTG1*
  - Clinical features: ptosis (most consistent ocular finding), high arched eyebrows, epicanthal folds, hypertelorism, iris colobomata

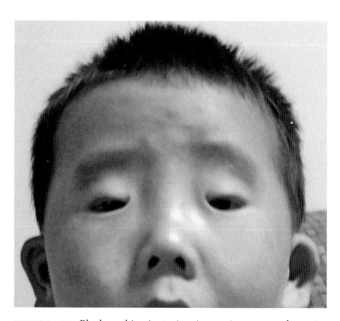

FIGURE 10.3 Blepharophimois ptosis epicantus inversus syndrome in a boy with short palpebral fissures, ptosis, and inverse epicanthal folds that arise from the lower lid.

# Other Syndromes with Major Ocular Involvement

- **De Barsy syndrome** (MIM 219150)
  - Autosomal recessive syndrome caused by biallelic pathogenic variants in *ALDH18A1*
  - Clinical features: cloudy corneas, cataracts, cutis laxa, progeriod features
- **Fraser syndrome** (cryptophthalmos–syndactyly syndrome, MIM 219000)
  - Autosomal recessive disorder caused by truncating pathogenic variants in *FRAS1, GRIP1,* and *FREM2*
    - Missense pathogenic variants in the same genes cause congenital anomalies of the kidney and renal tract.
  - Consanguinity and/or a positive family history are common.
  - Clinical features: classically presents with fusion of the eyelids without eyelashes, but cryptophthalmos is not obligatory—it can be unilateral, incomplete with an area of scalp hair extending from the lateral forehead onto the upper lateral eye area, or absent altogether; microphthalmia (Figure 10.4)
    - Non-ocular findings: cutaneous syndactyly, genitourinary malformations ranging from bilateral renal agenesis to ambiguous genitalia, ear anomalies, laryngeal and tracheal stenosis, imperforate anus, cleft lip and palate

- **Fryns syndrome** (MIM 229850)
  - Autosomal recessive disorder, caused by biallelic pathogenic variants in *PIGN* in some patients
  - Clinical features: cloudy corneas, congenital diaphragmatic hernia, coarse facial features, broad nasal bridge, cleft palate, absent lung lobation, nail hypoplasia, hypoplasia of fingertips, duodenal atresia; other GI, CNS, renal, and genital anomalies
- **Norrie syndrome** (MIM 310600)
  - X-linked disorder, caused by a pathogenic variant in *NPD* in 95% of affected males
  - Clinical features: retinal degeneration, retrolental masses (retrolental fibroplasia, pseudoglioma) cause congenital blindness, microphthalmia, vitreoretinal hemorrhages, cataracts, leukocoria, phthisis bulbi
    - Non-ocular findings: sensorineural hearing loss, progressive intellectual disability 50%
- ***Oculo-auricular-vertebral spectrum*** (OAVS, Goldenhar syndrome, hemifacial macrosomia, MIM 164210)
  - Relatively common, usually sporadic, disorder that represents a phenotypic spectrum
  - Incidence 1/3,500 newborns
  - Recurrence risk 2–3% without a chromosome anomaly or positive family history
  - Common in infants of diabetic mothers
  - Clinical features: notching of the upper eyelid, microphthalmia (rare), asymmetric palpebral fissures. When an epibulbar dermoid is present (Figure 10.5), the diagnosis is Goldenhar syndrome.
    - Non-ocular findings: preauricular pits and tags, ear malformations including microtia, facial asymmetry, macrostomia, hearing loss, torticollis, vertebral anomalies, especially cervical spine fusions, cardiac defects

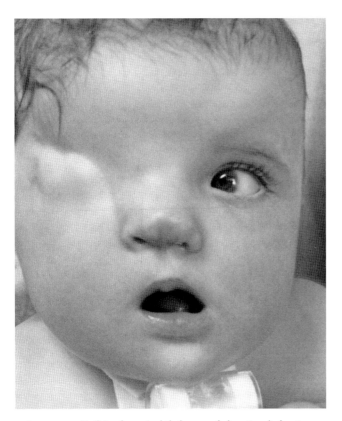

FIGURE 10.4 Unilateral cryptophthalmos and absent eyelashes in a child with Fraser syndrome. Note the broad nasal tip.

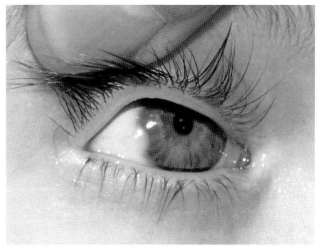

FIGURE 10.5 An epibulbar dermoid in a child with Goldenhar syndrome or OAVS.

- **Oculo-dento-digital dysplasia** (MIM 164200)
  - Autosomal dominant disorder caused by a heterozygous pathogenic variant in *GJA1*, which encodes connexin-43, a gap junction protein
  - Clinical features: microphthalmia, microcornea, iris coloboma, congenital cataract, glaucoma, epicanthal folds, short palpebral fissures
    - Non-ocular findings: pinched nose, small thin hypoplastic alae nasi (Figure 33.1), prominent columella, syndactyly of ring and little fingers, camptodactyly of little fingers, missing middle phalanges of toes 2–5
    - Cardiac arrhythmias
      - Connexin-43 is an integral component of the cardiac conduction system.
      - *GJA1* pathogenic variants were identified in 2/292 infants with SIDS.
    - Hearing loss, variable neurological sequelae (spasticity, ataxia, nystagmus, gaze palsy), slow hair growth
    - Later: dental anomalies
- **Stickler syndrome** (MIM 108300)
  - Autosomal dominant disorder, caused by heterozygous pathogenic variant in *COL2A1* or other collagen genes, affecting primarily the vitreous jelly
  - Clinical features: vitreous anomaly, high myopia, cataracts
    - Non-ocular findings: cleft palate 25%. Pierre–Robin sequence (micrognathia and retroposition of the tongue) can cause respiratory distress, poor saturation, and increased work of breathing when supine. The face can have a flat profile, prominent eyes, and depressed nasal bridge.

*Pearl*: Although an ophthalmologist may not be able to diagnose high myopia at a bedside exam in the nursery, any degree of myopia in a newborn is abnormal and deserves further investigation.

## Evaluation and Management

- Take a detailed family history: for relatives with ocular and other anomalies, consanguinity, infertility, premature ovarian failure, miscarriages.
- Inquire about pregnancy history: teratogen exposure, diabetes mellitus, TORCH infections, especially when there are cataracts.
- Examine the parents: ocular anomalies, poor visual acuity, thick eyeglasses, other congenital anomalies.
- Carefully delineate the ocular defect with a detailed ophthalmologic assessment by a pediatric ophthalmologist. It is best to do this early in the clinical course because some signs that are not clinically apparent are treatable (e.g., glaucoma).

- Determine if ocular defect is isolated or syndromic by searching for anomalies in other organ systems.
  - Undress the baby completely and examine the infant carefully for ocular and non-ocular anomalies. Assess the neurologic status.
  - Further investigations depend on clinical findings and may include brain imaging, hearing screening, abdominal ultrasound, skeletal radiographic survey, and echocardiogram.
  - Construct a differential diagnosis based on the rarest feature present in the patient or on a distinctive pattern of anomalies.
- Laboratory studies will be determined by the differential diagnosis.
  - Cataracts: Check ferritin, urine for reducing substance, newborn screening tests, urine quantitative amino acids, and creatine phosphokinase (CPK).
    - Consider TORCH titers/PCR, VDRL, and Coxsackie and Zika titers in the mother and infant.
  - Check for elevated 7-dehydrocholesterol to diagnose **Smith–Lemli–Opitz syndrome** when ptosis and/or cataracts occur in association with ambiguous genitalia, syndactyly of the toes, or polydactyly.
  - A chromosome microarray is the preferred first test when ocular signs present with other dysmorphic features and/or congenital anomalies.
  - When aneuploidy is suspected (e.g., **trisomy 18**), chromosome analysis is the preferred first test.
  - Molecular testing: Test for a single gene when there is a high degree of clinical suspicion for a specific syndrome. Otherwise, choose a gene panel designed for the ocular anomaly, or exome sequencing.
- Refer for genetic counseling.

## Further Reading

Beleza-Meireles A, Clayton-Smith J, Saraiva JM, Tassabehji M. (2014) Oculo-auriculo-vertebral spectrum: A review of the literature and genetic update. J Med Genet. 51:635–45. PMID 25118188

George, A, Zand, DJ, Hufnagel, RB, et al. (2016) Biallelic mutations in MITF cause coloboma, osteopetrosis, microphthalmia, macrocephaly, albinism, and deafness. Am J Hum Genet. 99:1388–94. PMID 27889061

Gutowski NJ, Chilton JK. (2015) The congenital cranial dysinnervation disorders. Arch Dis Child. 100:678–81. PMID 25633065

Haghighi A, Haack TB, Atiq M, et al. (2014) Sengers syndrome: Six novel AGK mutations in seven new families and review of the phenotypic and mutational spectrum of 29 patients. Orphanet J Rare Dis. 9:119. PMID 25208612

Hull S, Arno G, Ku CA, et al. (2016) Molecular and clinical findings in patients with Knobloch syndrome. JAMA Ophthalmol. 134:753–62. PMID 27259167

Lee HJ, Colby KA. (2013) A review of the clinical and genetic aspects of aniridia. Semin Ophthalmol. 28:306–12. PMID 24138039

Lohmann DR, Gallie BL. Retinoblastoma. In: Pagon RA, Adam MP, Ardinger HH, et al., editors. GeneReviews [Internet]. Seattle, WA: University of Washington, Seattle; 1993–2016. PMID 20301625

Pichi F, Lembo A, Serafino M, Nucci P. (2016) Genetics of congenital cataract. Dev Ophthalmol. 57:1–14. PMID 27043388

Schanilec P, Biernacki R. (2014) Aniridia: A comparative overview. Am Orthopt J. 64:98–104. PMID 25313118

Slavotinek AM, Garcia ST, Chandratillake G, et al. (2015) Exome sequencing in 32 patients with anophthalmia/microphthalmia and developmental eye defects. Clin Genet. 88:468–73. PMID 25457163

# 11

## Cleft Lip

## Clinical Consult

A genetics consultation was requested for a 2-day-old AGA female infant for significant nasopharyngeal regurgitation. An oral examination revealed a cleft palate. No other abnormalities were noted. The maternal family history was positive for both cleft lip and cleft palate in different relatives. The mother had a cleft lip repaired in infancy, and her father had a cleft palate. The geneticist noted bilateral paramedian pits on the buccal surface of the mother's lower lip. Careful re-examination of the infant revealed bilateral subtle lip mounds on the lower lip, establishing the clinical diagnosis of autosomal dominant **Van der Woude syndrome** (Figure 11.1). This variable autosomal dominant condition is responsible for approximately 2% of oral clefts.

*Pearl*: Van der Woude syndrome is one of the few disorders in which cleft lip with or without cleft palate occurs in the same family as cleft palate alone.

## Definition

- Cleft lip (CL) occurs when the lateral maxillary processes fail to fuse with the midline frontonasal process at 7–12 weeks' gestation. CL occurs with or without cleft palate (CL/P). Cleft palate only without cleft lip (CP) is reviewed in Chapter 12.
- Prevalence 1/700; varies with racial group: Asian and Native American 1/500, Caucasian 1/1,000, African American 1/2,500
  - Prevalence is not increased in twins.
  - Monozygotic twins can have mirror image defects.
- CL can be variable and subtle. Classic unilateral or bilateral forms are easily recognized, but milder defects can be missed.
  - In a *complete* CL, a defect in the upper lip and philtrum extends into the nostril with or without an ipsilateral cleft in the alveolar ridge. The premaxilla is attached to the columella (Figure 11.2).
  - An *incomplete* CL does not extend completely into the nostril and the defect may be bridged by a band of tissue (Figure 11.3).

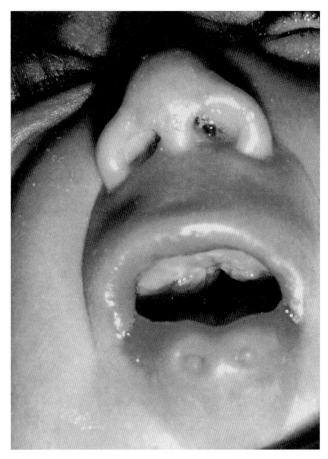

FIGURE 11.1 This infant with Van der Woude syndrome has a cleft palate and bilateral paramedian lower lip pits. Lip pits are accessory salivary glands.

o In the mildest *microform*, a prominent unilateral or bilateral philtral ridge resembles a scar; a notch in the vermillion border or a small "whistle" gap occurs in the midline where the lips should meet.

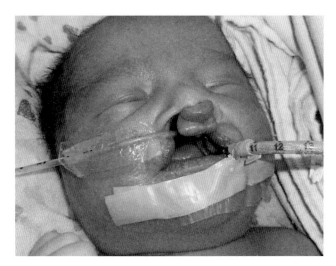

FIGURE 11.2 Bilateral cleft lip in a child. Note the short columella and prominent premaxilla. The premaxilla is always present in a bilateral cleft lip.

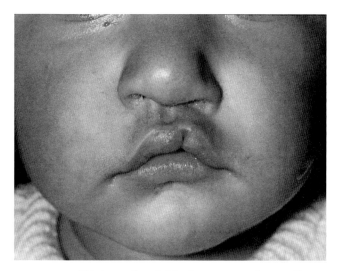

FIGURE 11.3 This incomplete cleft lip does not cross the vermillion border.

o In *subclinical* forms, small, fused, or missing upper lateral incisors or defects in the orbicularis oris muscle may be present in family members.

• Premaxillary agenesis is a wide defect in the upper lip with absence of the premaxilla, columella, and central portion of the maxillary alveolar ridge. It is distinct from bilateral cleft lip and has a different etiology.

o The premaxilla develops from the frontonasal process, which is induced by midline brain structures.

o Premaxillary agenesis implies a midline brain anomaly.

■ It should prompt imaging studies of the brain.

o Common in **trisomy 13**\* syndrome and **holoprosencephaly**\*

• Isolated nonsyndromic CL/P

o Most common type, occurs in ~70%

o 2 M:1 F; males predominate

o CL with cleft palate is twice as common as CL without cleft palate.

o Unilateral 75%; left-sided 2 L:1 R

o Mild hypertelorism (increased intercanthal distance) 7%

o Inheritance pattern is typically multifactorial and non-Mendelian.

■ Genetic contribution

• Familial clustering

• Higher concordance rate in monozygotic twins (40–60%) than dizygotic twins (3–5%)

■ Uncommonly, familial nonsyndromic CL/P occurs as an autosomal dominant trait with incomplete penetrance, caused by heterozygous pathogenic variant in *IRF6*.

■ CL/P and CP typically do not segregate in the same families.

• When they do occur in the same family, consider **Van der Woude syndrome** (MIM 119300; see Clinical Consult).

- o Recurrence risk 3–5%
  - ■ Higher when the proband has bilateral cleft lip, is female, or when unaffected parents are consanguineous
  - ■ When another first-degree relative (parent or sibling) is affected, the risk increases to 5–9%
- • Risk factors
  - o Assisted reproductive technology
  - o Maternal smoking, including passive smoking (aOR 1.24–1.8)
    - ■ A positive dose–response effect has been observed.
  - o Folic acid supplementation reduces the incidence of CL/P.
    - ■ This was noted following folic acid fortification of grain in the United States.
    - ■ Preconceptional supplementation with high-dose folic acid (2–5 mg/day) may decrease risk by 25%.

## Differential Diagnosis

- • Teratogens*
  - o Anti-epileptic medication, especially phenytoin, use during pregnancy increases the incidence of CL/P in exposed infants.
    - ■ Approximately 4–5% of babies exposed to phenytoin have congenital anomalies, approximately double the rate in the general population.
  - o **Fetal alcohol spectrum disorder***
  - o **Diabetic embryopathy***
- • Chromosomal anomalies
  - o Rare in isolated CL/P with no associated anomalies
    - ■ Almost all CL/P patients with chromosome abnormalities also have associated abnormalities.

*Pearl*: Chromosome anomalies, including microdeletions, occur more often Rare in isolated CL/P with no associated anomalies in patients with cleft lip *with* palate (CLP) than in patients with cleft lip *without* cleft palate (CL).

- o Common chromosome anomalies with CL/P
  - ■ **Deletion 1p36 syndrome** (MIM 607872)
    - • Clinical features: microcephaly, late closing fontanelles, straight eyebrows, deep-set eyes, noncompaction cardiomyopathy and other heart defects, eye, skeletal, genitourinary, and CNS anomalies, seizures. CL/P 5%
  - ■ **Wolf–Hirschhorn syndrome*** (4p minus, MIM 194190)
  - ■ **Trisomy 13*** and **trisomy 18***
- • Syndromic CL/P
  - o Accounts for 20% of patients with CL/P
  - o Associated anomalies occur more often with CLP (25%) than with CL- (10%).
    - ■ Cardiac anomalies are the most common associated malformation. Also, limb deficiencies, anal atresia, hydronephrosis

- o Females with CL/P are more likely to have a syndrome.
- o CL/P is a feature of hundreds of genetic syndromes, but only a few are discussed here. See Setó-Salvia and Stanier (2014) and Leslie and Marazita (2013).
- • **Bohring–Opitz syndrome** (Opitz C syndrome, MIM 605039)
  - o Autosomal dominant disorder, caused by heterozygous pathogenic variant in *ASXL1*
  - o Clinical features: IUGR, failure to thrive, poor feeding, trigonocephaly, microcephaly, hypertelorism, shallow orbits, prominent eyes, up-slanting palpebral fissures, nevus flammeus on forehead, CL/P, hypertrichosis, flexed elbows and wrists (Figure 11.4)
- • **Branchio-oculo-facial syndrome** (MIM 113620)
  - o Autosomal dominant disorder, caused by heterozygous pathogenic variant in *TFAP2A*
  - o Clinical features: CL/P, microform cleft lip, external and middle ear anomalies, branchial cleft sinus with hemangiomatous component, characteristic nose, microphthalmia, cataract, iris coloboma, lacrimal duct obstruction
- • **Craniofrontonasal syndrome** (MIM 304110)
  - o X-linked dominant disorder, caused by pathogenic variant in *EFNB1*
  - o Clinical features: females more severely affected; coronal craniosynostis, hypertelorism, broad bifid nasal tip, CL/P, microform of cleft lip, wiry hair, corpus callosum

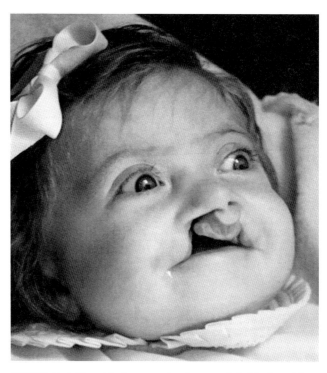

FIGURE 11.4 Hypertelorism, prominent eyes, and cleft lip in a girl with Bohring–Opitz syndrome.

agenesis, syndactyly, axillary pterygia, pectus excavatum, diaphragmatic hernia

- **Ectrodactyly–ectodermal dysplasia–clefting syndrome** (EEC3, MIM 603273)
  - ○ Autosomal dominant disorder, caused by heterozygous pathogenic variant in *TP63*
  - ○ Clinical features: variable limb anomalies, cleft hands and/or feet, ectodermal dysplasia affecting hair, sweat glands, teeth, CL/P (Figure 11.5)
    - ■ The following primarily dermatologic syndromes are also caused by heterozygous pathogenic variants in *TP63* and feature CL/P:
      - **Rapp–Hodgkin syndrome** (MIM 129400)
      - **Hay–Wells syndrome** (MIM 106260).
- **Hypertelorism, microtia, clefting syndrome** (HMC, MIM 239800)
  - ○ An apparently autosomal recessive disorder. A causative gene has not been identified.

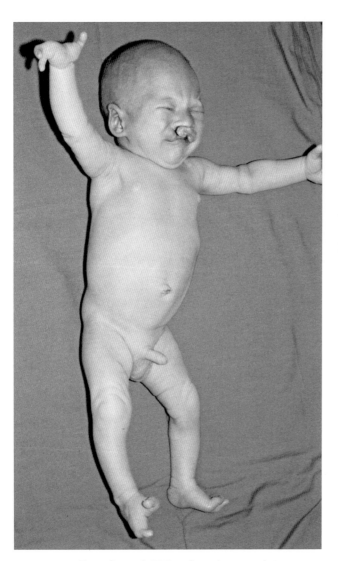

FIGURE 11.5  This infant with EEC syndrome has sparse hair, a bilateral cleft lip, and cleft hands and feet.

- ○ Clinical features: hypertelorism, microtia, CL/P, broad bifid nose, psychomotor retardation, conductive hearing loss, microcephaly, atretic auditory canals, cardiac malformation
- **Kallmann syndrome 1** (MIM 308700)
  - ○ X-linked recessive disorder, caused by pathogenic variant in *KAL1*
    - ■ Many autosomal dominant forms also exist (MIM 147950).
  - ○ Clinical features: CL/P, cleft palate only is uncommon), renal agenesis. Affected males can have small phallus and cryptorchidism.
    - ■ Hypogonadotropic hypogonadism with or without anosmia is usually recognized at puberty.
- **Roberts syndrome** (SC phocomelia syndrome, MIM 268300)
  - ○ Autosomal recessive disorder, caused by biallelic pathogenic variants in *ESCO2*
  - ○ Clinical features: CL/P, tetraphocomelia, absent long bones, corneal opacities
    - ■ Puffing and premature separation of centromeres on chromosome analysis
- **Van der Woude syndrome** (OMIM 119300)
  - ○ Autosomal dominant disorder, caused by heterozygous pathogenic variant in *IRF6*
  - ○ Most common syndrome associated with cleft lip or palate
    - ■ Accounts for 2% of all oral clefts
  - ○ Clinical features: variable combinations of oral clefts (CL/P, CP) and lower lip pits
    - ■ Paramedian fistulae, lip mounds, or lip pits are paired accessory salivary glands in the mucosal surface or on the lower lip. (Figure 11.1)

*Pearl*: To examine for lip pits or mounds, dry the lower lip and adjacent buccal surface with a paper towel and watch for the appearance of two tiny paramedian dots of saliva.

- - ■ Lip pits may be the only expression of the syndrome. Penetrance for lip pits is 86%.
  - ○ Lip pits also occur with oral clefts in other syndromes.
    - ■ **Popliteal pterygia syndrome** (MIM 119500), also caused by a pathogenic variant in *IRF6*
    - ■ **Kabuki syndrome** (MIM 147920. 300867), a dysmorphic multiple congenital anomaly syndrome, due to a pathogenic variant in *KMT2D* or *KDM6A*
      - Clinical features: long, everted palpebral fissures, large prominent ears, hypoplastic lateral eyebrows; cleft palate; prominent fetal pads on the fingertips and cardiac, vertebral, and limb anomalies. (Figures 7.4, 12.3)
- Midline cleft lip, almost always syndromic
  - ○ **Oral–facial–digital syndrome type 1** (OFD1; MIM 311200)
    - ■ X-linked dominant ciliopathy; lethal in males
    - ■ The responsible gene, *OFD1*, codes for a component of the basal body of the primary cilia.

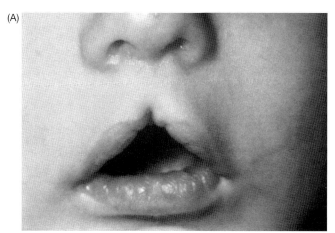

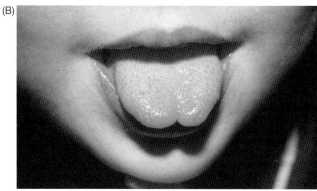

FIGURE 11.6 (A) A midline cleft lip is characteristic of oral–facial–digital syndrome (OFD). Note the presence of milia on the nose. (B) This child with a bifid tongue has OFD.

- Clinical features: median cleft lip (Figure 11.6A), anomalous oral frenulae, lobulated or cleft tongue (Figure 11.6B), facial milia, broad thumbs and great toes, finger syndactyly, postaxial polydactyly, renal cysts
  - **Pai syndrome** (MIM 155145)
    - Autosomal dominant trait with incomplete penetrance. The genetic cause has not been identified.
    - Clinical features: mild hypertelorism, mildline cleft lip, facial and nasal septum polyps, ocular anomalies, lipoma of corpus callosum, normal intellectual development
- Atypical oral clefts
  - **Amniotic band disruption sequence** (MIM 217100)
    - Usually sporadic and not hereditary. No responsible gene has been identified.
    - Clinical features: asymmetric distal constriction rings with distal swelling and amputations, amniotic bands attached to limbs and cranium. Oblique facial clefts, usually of the nasoocular type, can extend from around the ala nasi into the orbit(s). May have typical oral clefting.
  - **Oblique facial clefts** (MIM 600251)
    - Nasoocular or oroocular oblique facial clefts are very rare: 0.25% of all oral clefts.
    - Heterozygous pathogenic variant in the *SPECC1L* gene

- Consider this condition when oblique facial clefts are bilateral.
  - **Oculo-auriculo-vertebral syndrome** (OAVS, hemifacial microsomia, Goldenhar syndrome, MIM 164210)
    - Sporadic, multifactorial disorder
      - Uncommonly, occurs as an autosomal dominant trait.
      - Heterozygous pathogenic variant in *MYT1* is rare.
    - More common in the offspring of diabetic mothers* (OR 2.28)
    - Clinical features: asymmetric dysplasia of the ear(s), preauricular tags, hemifacial microsomia, epibulbar dermoids, micrognathia, cervical vertebral anomalies, cardiac defects
      - A lateral (horizontal) cleft through the oral commissure can cause macrostomia, usually on the more severely affected side. (Figure 9.3)
      - Intrauterine constraint can restrict mandibular growth on one side, creating a phenocopy of hemifacial microsomia (Figure 11.7).

## Evaluation and Management

- Take a pregnancy history: anti-epileptic medications, smoking, other teratogenic or environmental exposures, maternal diabetes mellitus.
- Document family history: consanguinity, other relatives with oral clefts, lip pits.
- Examine the parents for microforms of cleft lip, missing teeth, bifid, wide or deviated uvula, and lip pits or mounds.
- Prenatal management
  - Consider fetal echocardiogram.
  - When other anomalies are present, offer cfDNA or amniocentesis for chromosomal microarray.
  - Refer to craniofacial team for prenatal consult and parental support if available.
- Evaluate the extent of clefting, lip pits, dysmorphic features, and associated malformations in other organs.
  - Echocardiogram, abdominal ultrasound, head imaging
  - Hygoglycemia and other endocrine abnormalities. Various hormone deficiencies (growth hormone, thyroid, ACTH) are more common in infants with oral clefts.
- Genetic testing
  - Chromosome microarray is indicated in CL/P patients who have other malformations, IUGR, dysmorphic features, hypotonia, or severe feeding difficulties.
  - Consider gene panel or genomic testing if a nonchromosomal syndrome is suspected.
- Ensure adequate oral intake before discharge.
  - Offer occupational therapy consult for issues with oral feeding.
    - Utilize special nipples (pigeon nipple, Haberman).

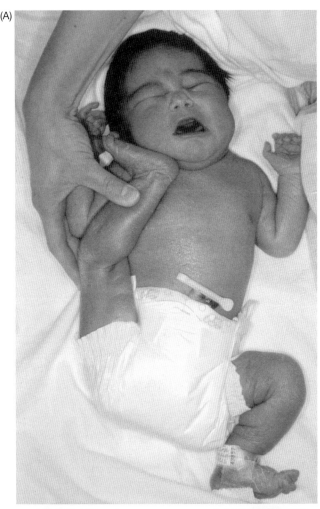

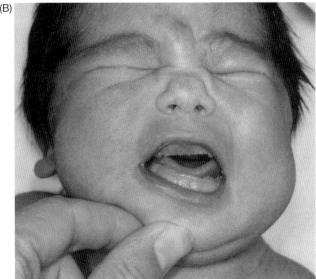

o Poor oral feeding can indicate an underlying syndrome or CNS anomaly.
• Refer to a multidisciplinary craniofacial team for coordinated outpatient management and therapy to include plastic surgery, genetics, ENT, audiology, developmental and speech therapy, and dental and orthodontic specialists.
• Schedule early and frequent pediatric visits post discharge.
• Refer for genetic counseling.

## Further Reading

Leslie EJ, Koboldt DC, Kang CJ, et al. (2016). IRF6 mutation screening in non-syndromic orofacial clefting: Analysis of 1521 families. Clin Genet. 90:28–34. PMID 26346622

Leslie EJ, Marazita ML. (2013) Genetics of cleft lip and cleft palate. Am J Med Genet C Semin Med Genet. 163C:246–58. PMID 24124047

Milunsky JM, Maher TM, Zhao G, et al. (2011) Genotype–phenotype analysis of the branchio-oculo-facial syndrome. Am J Med Genet A. 155A:22–32. PMID 21204207

Pengelly RJ, Upstill-Goddard R, Arias L, et al. (2015) Resolving clinical diagnoses for syndromic cleft lip and/or palate phenotypes using whole-exome sequencing. Clin Genet. 88:441–9. PMID 25441681

Rojnueangnit K, Mikhail FM, Cui X, et al. (2015) Predictor(s) of abnormal array comparative genomic hybridization results in patients with cleft lip and/or palate. Cleft Palate Craniofac J. 52:724–31. PMID 25489768

Setó-Salvia N, Stanier P. (2014) Genetics of cleft lip and/or cleft palate: Association with other common anomalies. Eur J Med Genet. 57:381–93. PMID 24768816

Rittler M, Cosentino V, López-Camelo JS, et al. (2011) Associated anomalies among infants with oral clefts at birth and during a 1-year follow up. An J Med Genet. 155A:1588–96. PMID 21671378

FIGURE 11.7 (A) This infant's breech position *in utero* deformed his right mandible, creating the appearance of hemifacial microsomia. (B) Pressure from his foot restricted the growth of his right mandibular ramus, causing an occlusal cant. Within a few months, the mandible had grown and the asymmetry resolved without other treatment.

# 12

# Cleft Palate

## Clinical Consult

A 4-day-old term male infant had micrognathia, feeding difficulties, respiratory distress, and desaturations that were worse when he was supine. Pregnancy and family histories were noncontributory. With a tongue blade and penlight, a cleft of the soft palate was visible. The retropositioned tongue obstructed the posterior pharynx, confirming the diagnosis of Pierre–Robin sequence (Figure 12.1). Feeding improved with occupational therapy, a suitable nipple, and upright positioning. Desaturations resolved when he was prone or on his side. At 2 weeks, he went home with an apnea monitor to be followed in the craniofacial specialty clinic. An ophthalmology examination was scheduled to rule out myopia.

Approximately half of infants with Pierre–Robin sequence have a syndrome, of which **Stickler syndrome** is the most common. In Stickler syndrome, abnormal vitreous gel and high myopia predispose patients to retinal detachment.

*Pearl:* Any degree of myopia is abnormal in the newborn.

## Definition

- Cleft palate alone (CP) is genetically separate from cleft lip with or without cleft palate (CL/P). This chapter focuses on CP without cleft lip. See Chapter 11 for a review of cleft lip with cleft palate.
- CP can be complete, extending from the primary or hard palate through the secondary or soft palate, or it can cause a V- or U-shaped posterior defect in the secondary, soft palate.
  - A bifid uvula is the mildest expression of cleft palate, and it is often undiagnosed in the newborn period (possibly due to a pervasive lack of tongue blades at the bedside).
- Milder forms of CP can be difficult to diagnose: Submucous CP may present with nasal regurgitation during feeding or later with frequent otitis media and speech problems.
- CP can be missed in the NICU when secretions limit the exam, when an oral tracheal tube obscures the palate or a tongue blade is not used because the baby's mouth is small or the baby is too unstable.

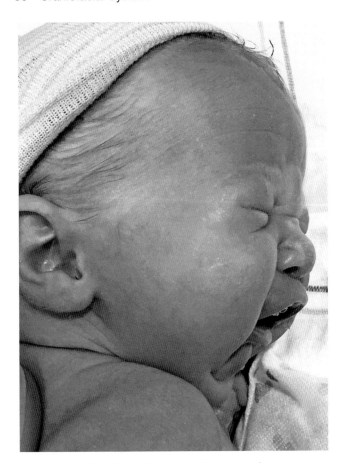

FIGURE 12.1 This infant with Pierre–Robin sequence has micrognathia, cleft palate, and glossoptosis that causes upper airway obstruction when he is supine.

*Pearl*: Visualize the palate and uvula directly with a small tongue blade and penlight. Digital palpation may not detect a cleft of the soft palate. CP can be missed in the NICU when secretions limit the exam, when an oral tracheal tube obscures the palate or a tongue blade is not used because the baby's mouth is small or the baby is too unstable.

- Incidence 1:2,500 births
  - CP is less common than CL/P.
  - Incidence varies with racial and ethnic background; it is more frequent among non-Hispanic Caucasians, some Filipino groups, Hmong, and Native American populations.
- 1 M:2 F; females with isolated CP predominate
- Etiology
  - The palatal shelves fail to fuse in the first trimester
- Multifactorial inheritance; both genetic and environmental factors contribute to isolated CP
- Recurrence risk 2–3%
  - Higher for male probands, or positive family history
- Risk factors
  - Maternal smoking in first trimester
  - Heavy maternal alcohol use (five or more drinks at one time) in the first trimester

## Differential Diagnosis

- Associated malformation or syndrome ~50%
  - Cardiac defects: the most common second malformation in patients with CP
  - Choanal atresia: a common second malformation in Pierre–Robin sequence
  - Hundreds of single gene disorders include CP. Some common causes of syndromic CP are summarized later.
- Teratogens*
  - **Diabetic embryopathy***
  - **Fetal alcohol spectrum disorder***
  - **Valproic acid embryopathy**
    - Isolated CP is increased 11.3-fold compared to the general population.
- Chromosome disorders: CP occurs in autosomal aneuploidies and many microdeletions and microduplications.
  - **Deletion 1q41–42** (MIM 612530)
    - Clinical features: short stature, frontal bossing, deep-set eyes, cleft palate, diaphragmatic hernia, clubfeet, developmental delay, seizures
  - **Tetrasomy 12p mosaicism** (Pallister–Killian syndrome, MIM 601803)
    - Rare, tissue-specific mosaicism for an additional isochromosome containing two copies of chromosome 12p
      - Clinical severity does not correlate with the percentage of mosaicism.
      - The extra chromosome is found in amniotic fluid cells and skin fibroblasts but less often in blood.
    - Clinical features: CP ~20%. LGA, frontal balding, sparse eyebrows, hypertelorism, short upturned nose, long philtrum, coarse facies, cardiac defects, diaphragmatic hernia, imperforate anus, streaky pigmentation, feeding problems. (Figure 3.2)
  - **Chromosome 22q11.2 deletion syndrome*** (MIM 188400)
    - Palatal defects >70%, velopharyngeal incompetence 90% (Figure 12.2)
  - **Chromosome 22q11.2 duplication syndrome** (MIM 608363)
    - Clinical features: similar to the more common deletion; palatal anomalies 69%: bifid uvula, submucous CP, velopharyngeal incompetence, cardiac anomalies
- Syndromes
  - **Cornelia de Lange syndrome*** (MIM 122470)
    - A spectrum of disorders caused by pathogenic variants in genes associated with sister chromatin cohesion: *NIPBL, SMC1A, SMC3, HDAC8, RAD21.*

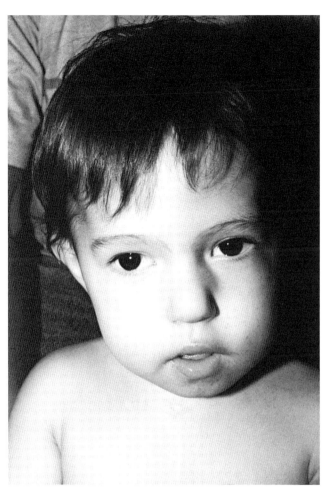

FIGURE 12.2 Child with chromosome 22q deletion who has the characteristic broad nose with unmodeled lateral margins, long face, and cardiac anomalies of this disorder.

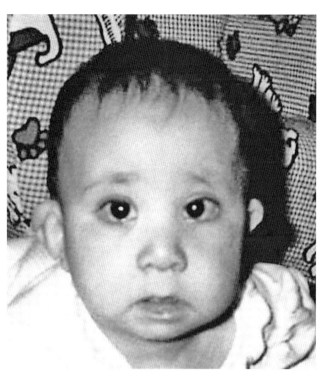

FIGURE 12.3 This child with Kabuki syndrome has long palpebral fissures with eversion of the lower lids, hypoplastic "interrupted" eyebrows, and large prominent ears. The sclerae are blue.

- ■ Clinical features: CP, or submucous CP, 20%. Distinctive facial features with arched eyebrows, synophrys, prominent and thin upper lip, and microcephaly, poor growth, hypertrichosis, upper limb defects. (Figure 21.2)
- o **Femoral facial syndrome** (femoral hypoplasia unusual facies syndrome, MIM 134780)
  - ■ Sporadic, associated with maternal diabetes* in ≤50%
  - ■ Clinical features: long philtrum, micrognathia, small mouth, femoral hypoplasia, radiohumeral synostosis, sacral dysgenesis, renal dysplasia. CP ~20% (Figure 12S.1)
- o **Gordon syndrome** (distal arthrogryposis type IIIA, MIM 114300)
  - ■ Autosomal dominant disorder, caused by heterozygous pathogenic variant in *PIEZO2*
  - ■ Clinical features: short stature, CP, distal limb contractures distal limbs, clubfoot, camptodactyly of fingers
- o **Kabuki syndrome** (MIM 147920)
  - ■ Autosomal dominant disorder, caused by a pathogenic variant in *KMT2D*, usually de novo

- • X-linked form, due to pathogenic variant in *KDM6A* (MIM 300867)
  - ■ Clinical features: poor growth, long palpebral fissures, interrupted eyebrows, everted lower lids (Figure 12.3), CP, prominent ears, persistent prominent fingerpads, brachydactyly of the little finger; vertebral, skeletal, and cardiac defects
- o **Loeys–Dietz syndrome** (MIM 609192)
  - ■ Autosomal dominant connective tissue disorder, caused by heterozygous pathogenic variant in *TGFBR1, TGFBR2, SMAD3, TGFB2, TGFB3*
    - • Germ line mosaicism has been reported in clinically unaffected parents.
  - ■ Clinical features: Marfan-like phenotype, bifid uvula, CP, hypertelorism, sagittal craniosynostosis, camptodactyly, arachnodactyly, pectus deformities, clubfeet, hip dislocation
    - • Aortic dilatation, severe arterial tortuosity, and aneurysms warrant aggressive therapy.
- o **Lymphedema distichiasis syndrome** (MIM 153400)
  - ■ Autosomal dominant trait, caused by a heterozygous pathogenic variant in *FOXC2*
  - ■ Clinical features: CP, distichiasis (double row of eyelashes), increased tearing, webbed neck, lymphedema of the legs
    - • Variable phenotype, decreased penetrance
- o Mandibulofacial dysostosis syndromes

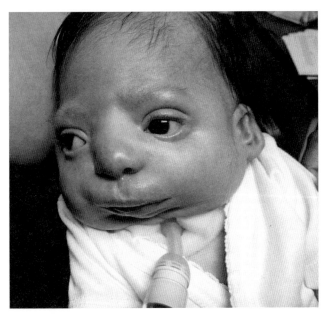

FIGURE 12.4 This child has cleft palate and severe mandibular hypoplasia due to mandibulofacial dysostosis with microcephaly, Guion–Ameida type. Note the small dysplastic ear and the coloboma in the upper eyelid.

- **Mandibulofacial dysostosis with microcephaly, Guion–Ameida type** (MIM 610536)
  - Autosomal dominant trait, due to heterozygous pathogenic variant in *EFTUD2*
  - Clinical features: microcephaly, CP, dysplastic ears, zygomatic arch hypoplasia, micrognathia, choanal atresia, esophageal and other GI atresias, cardiac defects, thumb and digital anomalies (Figure 12.4)
- **Nager syndrome** (acrofacial dysostosis, MIM 154400)
  - Autosomal dominant disorder, caused by heterozygous pathogenic variant in *SF3B4*
  - Clinical features: similar to Treacher–Collins syndrome; radial ray anomalies: small or absent thumbs, radial hypoplasia or aplasia, upper limb phocomelia
- **Treacher–Collins syndrome** (MIM 154500)
  - Autosomal dominant disorder, caused by a heterozygous pathogenic variant in *TCOF1, POLR1D*
    - An autosomal recessive form is caused by biallelic pathogenic variants in *POLR1C*.
  - Clinical features: palpebral fissures slant downward, lower lid coloboma, missing lateral eyelashes, depression or notch in the zygomatic arch, microtia, hearing loss, micrognathia. CP 20% (Figure 9.4)
  - Variable severity, incomplete penetrance
    - Carrier parents may appear unaffected.
- **Oculo-auriculo-vertebral syndrome** (OAVS, hemifacial microsomia, MIM 164210)
  - Multifactorial disorder, usually sporadic, more common in **infants of diabetic mothers**\* (Figures 9.3, 10.5)

- Clinical features: unilateral or bilateral asymmetric ear dysplasia, mandibular midline shift to one side, epibulbar dermoid in the lateral canthus of the eye, facial pits or tags from the ear to the corner of the mouth, macrostomia. Cervical vertebral defects and cardiac anomalies are common. CP is occasional.
- **Otopalatodigital syndrome** (OPD1, MIM 311300)
  - X-linked disorder, caused by hemizygous gain-of-function pathogenic variant in *FLNA*
    - Variable expression in carrier females
    - OPD2 more severe, sometimes lethal; also caused by *FLNA* pathogenic variant
  - Clinical features: short stature, hypertelorism, broad nasal root, coarse "pugilistic" face, CP, broad thumbs and great toes, widely spaced and bulbous ("tree frog") toes, short fingernails, conductive deafness, mild skeletal dysplasia: scoliosis, pectus deformities

*Pearl*: Pierre–Robin sequence is a "sequence," not a "syndrome," because CP is hypothesized to be secondary to a small mandible and a posteriorly placed tongue that obstructs closure of the palatal shelves.

- **Pierre–Robin sequence** (MIM 261800; see Clinical Consult)
  - Incidence 1/8,500 to 1/14,000
  - Heterogeneous disorder: Affected siblings and parents been reported.
    - Approximately half are syndromic. Some syndromes are summarized next.
  - Clinical features: classic triad of micrognathia (Figure 12.1), glossoptosis, and upper airway obstruction. CP is not a constant feature.
    - The original case description did not include CP.
- **Catel–Manzke syndrome** (MIM 616145)
  - Autosomal recessive disorder, caused by biallelic pathogenic variants in *TGDS*
  - Clinical features: Pierre–Robin sequence, hyperphalangy (additional phalanx between the proximal phalanx and the metacarpal), radial deviation of the index finger
- **Stickler syndrome** (MIM 108300)—most common syndrome associated with Pierre–Robin sequence
  - Autosomal dominant disorder, due to heterozygous pathogenic variant in *COL2A1, COL11A1, COL11A2*
    - Rare autosomal recessive forms are caused by biallelic pathogenic variants in *COL9A1, COL9A2*.
    - Affected parents with high myopia are often undiagnosed.
  - Clinical features: Pierre–Robin sequence, CP 25%, congenital myopia, flat midface (Figure 12.5), hearing loss, mitral valve prolapse 50%, mild spondyloepiphyseal dysplasia, early degenerative joint changes

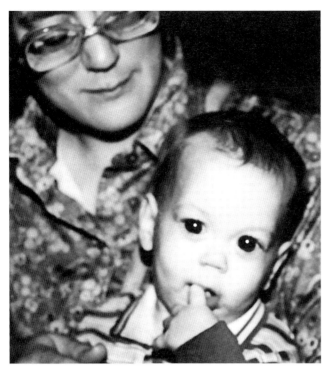

FIGURE 12.5 This mother and child are both affected with Stickler syndrome. The baby has prominent eyes, a short nose, and a long philtrum. Note the mother's thick glasses.

- Increased risk of retinal detachment, glaucoma
- **Talipes equinovarous–atrial septal defect–Robin sequence–persistence of left superior vena cava syndrome** (TARP syndrome, MIM 311900)
  - X-linked disorder, caused by hemizygous pathogenic variant in *RBM10,* often de novo
    - Mosaicism reported in unaffected mothers of affected siblings
    - Early lethality in affected males
  - Clinical features: short palpebral fissures, small ears, wide mouth, cleft palate, micrognathia, cardiac anomalies, left superior vena cava, ASD, cutaneous syndactyly of fingers or toes (including Y-shaped 2–3 toe syndactyly), postaxial toe polydactyly, clubfeet, partial agenesis of corpus callosum, hypoplastic cerebellum, hypotonia. No feature is obligatory.
- **Toriello–Carey syndrome** (MIM 217980)
  - Heterogeneous: 20% have a chromosome anomaly.
  - No causative gene has been identified. Autosomal recessive inheritance is suggested by reports in consanguineous families, affected siblings and concordant MZ twins.
  - Clinical features: IUGR, poor postnatal growth, hypertelorism, telecanthus, short palpebral fissures, flat nasal bridge, agenesis of corpus callosum, cardiac (usually septal) defects, congenital tracheal stenosis, hypotonia, developmental delay. Pierre–Robin sequence is common.

- ○ Skeletal dysplasias*: Many skeletal dysplasias have CP, especially type II collagenopathies.
  - **Campomelic dysplasia** (MIM 114290)
    - Autosomal dominant trait, caused by heterozygous pathogenic variant in *SOX9*
    - Clinical features: CP, bowing of the long bones (especially lower extremity), sex reversal among cytogenetic males, 46,XY
      - Tracheobronchial hypoplasia and small chest size contribute to respiratory compromise.
  - **Diastrophic dysplasia** (MIM 222600)
    - Autosomal recessive disorder, caused by biallelic pathogenic variants in *SLC26A2* (Figure 29.4)
    - Clinical features: CP >40%; submucous CP or microform in an additional 30% short stature, cystic ear swelling, "hitchhiker" thumbs, clubfeet.
  - **Kniest syndrome** (MIM 156550)
    - Autosomal dominant disorder, due to a heterozygous pathogenic variant in *COL2A1,* usually sporadic
    - Clinical features: CP, depressed midface, prominent eyes, congenital severe myopia, joint contractures, deafness, short stature.
  - **Spondyloepiphyseal dysplasia congenita** (MIM 183900)
    - Autosomal dominant disorder, due to a heterozygous pathogenic variant in *COL2A1*
    - Clinical features: CP, severe myopia, hearing loss, disproportionate short stature, short trunk, delayed ossification, platyspondyly.
- ○ **Smith–Lemli–Opitz syndrome*** (MIM 270400)
  - Autosomal recessive disorder, caused by biallelic pathogenic variants in *DHCR7*. Elevated 7-dehydrocholesterol is a reliable sign.
  - Clinical features: microcephaly, ptosis, anteverted nares, CP, polydactyly, thumb anomalies, Y-shaped syndactyly of toes 2–3, cardiac defects, undervirilized male genitalia, hypotonia, developmental delay (Figure 17S.1)
- ○ **Van der Woude syndrome** (MIM 119300)
  - Autosomal dominant disorder, caused by heterozygous pathogenic variant in *IRF6* (Figure 11.1)
    - Often familial, and unrecognized, with paramedian lip pits in the lower lip of undiagnosed parents
  - Clinical features: variable combinations of cleft lip, CP, and paramedian lower lip pits (accessory salivary glands)
- ○ **X-linked cleft palate with or without ankyloglossia** (MIM 303400)
  - X-linked disorder, caused by a hemizygous pathogenic variant in *TBX22*
    - More common in Iceland and in native people of North America, including Hispanic Americans
  - Clinical features: CP or submucous CP, ankyloglossia; milder phenotype in carrier females: bifid uvula or CP
    - Ankyloglossia can be the sole feature: males 4%, females 45%.

# Evaluation and Management

- Take a pregnancy history: anti-epileptic drugs or other teratogen exposures, maternal diabetes.
- Document family history: ethnicity, consanguinity, oral clefts, lip pits, ankyloglossia, myopia, retinal detachment, distichiasis, lymphedema, cardiac and vascular anomalies.
- Examine parents for microforms and associated malformations: bifid uvula, submucous CP, lower lip pits, ankyloglossia, high myopia.
- Evaluate infant carefully for other malformations.
  - Use a tongue blade and a flashlight to visualize the infant's palate directly.
  - Consult ophthalmology to identify myopia early.
    - *Any* degree of myopia is abnormal in the newborn.

*Pearl*: Pediatric ophthalmologists may perform an exam for retinopathy of prematurity and may not assess for myopia unless specifically asked to do so.

  - Echocardiogram
  - Abdominal US
  - Pass a nasal tube to detect choanal atresia.
  - Hygoglycemia and other endocrine abnormalities. Various hormone deficiencies (growth hormone, thyroid, ACTH) are more common in infants with oral clefts.
- In Pierre–Robin sequence, monitor for tachypnea, desaturation, or increased work of breathing.
  - Maintain the airway and reduce the work of breathing.
    - Avoid supine position. Feed in upright or forward leaning position. Babies prefer to sleep in prone or side positions.
    - Keep a laryngeal mask airway at the bedside. Intubation can be difficult.
    - Tachypnea and respiratory distress can limit growth even in the absence of desaturation.
  - As the mandible grows over time, respiratory compromise often resolves.
    - When respiratory distress is severe or unremitting, consider more invasive options, which should be rarely required: tongue–lip adhesion, mandibular distraction, tracheotomy.
  - Offer home monitoring for apnea in all but the mildest cases.

- Genetic testing
  - Microarray is appropriate in CP, especially when there are associated anomalies.
  - For suspected aneuploidy, chromosome analysis is the preferred first test.
  - The gene testing strategy (gene panel, exome) depends on the pattern of anomalies. Use gene testing to clarify the diagnosis, guide management decisions, and inform genetic counseling.
- Refer to multidisciplinary team for craniofacial anomalies for outpatient follow-up.
- Daily high dose preconceptional folic acid supplementation (4 mg/d) for the mother modestly reduces the recurrence risk in isolated CP.

# Further Reading

Burg ML, Chai Y, Yao CA, et al. (2016) Epidemiology, etiology, and treatment of isolated cleft palate. Front Physiol. 7:67. PMID 26973535

Côté A, Fanous A, Almajed A, Lacroix Y. (2015) Pierre Robin sequence: Review of diagnostic and treatment challenges. Int J Pediatr Otorhinolaryngol. 79:451–64. PMID 25704848

Dixon MJ, Marazita ML, Beaty TH, et al. (2011) Cleft lip and palate: Understanding genetic and environmental influences. Nat Rev Genet. 12:167–78. PMID 21331089

Izumi K, Konczal LL, Mitchel AL, et al. (2012) Underlying genetic diagnosis of Pierre Robin sequence: Retrospective chart review at two children's hospitals and a systematic literature review. J Pediatr. 160:645–50. PMID 22048048

Jackson A, Bromley R, Morrow J, et al. (2016) In utero exposure to valproate increases the risk of isolated cleft palate. Arch Dis Child Fetal Neonatal Ed. 101:F207–11. PMID 26408639

Rathé M, Rayyan M, Schoenaers J, et al. (2015) Pierre Robin sequence: Management of respiratory and feeding complications during the first year of life in a tertiary referral centre. Int J Pediatr Otorhinolaryngol. 79:1206–12. PMID 26092549

Shkoukani MA, Lawrence LA, Liebertz DJ, Svider PF. (2014) Cleft palate: A clinical review. Birth Defects Res C Embryo Today. 102:333–42. PMID 25504820

Yetman AT, Berhoukim RS, Ivy DD, et al. (2007) Importance of the clinical recognition of Loeys–Dietz syndrome in the neonatal period. Pediatrics. 119:e1199–202. PMID 17470566

# 13

# Craniosynostoses

## Clinical Consult

A newborn female with unilateral coronal craniosynostosis, ptosis, and facial asymmetry had a low anterior hairline and small ears with a prominent ear crus (Figure 13.1A). Her parents denied craniosynostosis in other relatives. Her family said that she looked like her mother and older sister, who were considered to be normal by relatives.

The genetic consultant suspected that the baby, her mother, and her sister were all affected with the same autosomal dominant disorder, **Saethre–Chotzen syndrome**. The mother and sister had a milder phenotype and had never had cranial surgery, but they shared the low anterior hairline, ptosis, and prominent ear cruses (Figure 13.1B). The same heterozygous pathogenic variant was found in *TWIST1* in the baby and her mother, confirming the diagnosis of Saethre–Chotzen syndrome in this family.

Saethre–Chotzen syndrome is a relatively common, highly variable craniosynostosis syndrome causing coronal craniosynsostosis, facial asymmetry, ptosis, small ear pinna with prominent ear crus, 2–3 finger syndactyly, and hallux valgus in some but not all individuals.

## Definition

- Craniosynostosis is premature fusion of one or more cranial sutures.
- Incidence 3–5/10,000 live births
- All cranial sutures are normally open in the newborn period.
  - The metopic suture is the first to fuse at 3–9 months.
- Premature closure of each suture represents a separate and distinct entity.
  - The head grows perpendicular to the direction of each suture, so each type of craniosynostosis affects the head shape in a unique way.
- Complications occur in both isolated and syndromic craniosynostosis.
  - Corneal exposure, strabismus (coronal craniosynostosis)
  - Increased intracranial pressure (ICP)

(A)

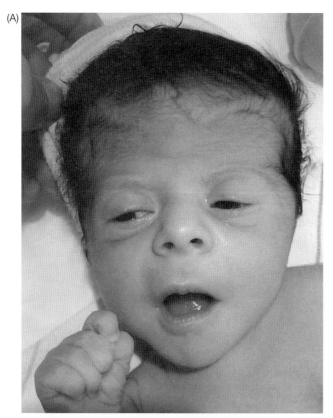

(B)

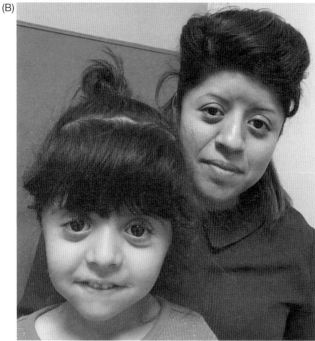

FIGURE 13.1 (A) This newborn female with unilateral coronal craniosynostosis, ptosis, and prominent eyes has Saethre–Chotzen syndrome. (B) This mother and child with Saethre–Chotzen syndrome have prominent eyes with infraorbital creases. Note the low anterior hairline in the mother and the ptosis in the child.

- Papilledema is a specific sign for raised ICP (98%), but it is not sensitive in young children. Under age 8 years, only 22% of children with raised ICP have papilledema.
  - Chiari I malformation (especially metopic craniosynostosis)

- Sleep apnea, obstructive and central types, common, especially with Chiari I (Addo, et al., 2013)
  - Foramen magnum decompression may be therapeutic.
- Isolated nonsyndromic craniosynostosis >85%
  - Risk factors for isolated, nonsyndromic craniosynostosis
    - Maternal smoking (OR 1.33)
    - Valproic acid exposure (metopic)
    - Twins*
    - Oligohydramnios and intrauterine head constraint
- Syndromic craniosynostosis
  - Associated with extracranial malformations and/or developmental delay
  - When the phenotype is mild, syndromic craniosynostosis may be mistaken for isolated craniosynostosis, which complicates diagnosis and counseling.
  - The most severe form is cloverleaf skull (Kleeblattschadel), most commonly seen in **thanatophoric dysplasia** and **Pfeiffer, Crouzon, and Apert syndromes**.
- Clinical diagnosis
  - Examination of the skull and face and palpation of all sutures may not be sufficient to establish the diagnosis.
  - Head ultrasound can be helpful.
  - Three-dimensional (3D) CT scan and plain radiographs may be more informative after the newborn period.
- Genetic factors
  - Monozygotic twins are concordant more often than dizygotic twins.
    - Sagittal craniosynostosis: MZ 30%: DZ 0%
    - Metopic craniosynostosis: MZ 43%: DZ 5%
  - Family history is positive in 6–8% of cases.
    - Familial cases are usually autosomal dominant with intrafamilial variability.
  - At least two dozen single genes have been identified.
    - The same genes can be associated with both syndromic and nonsyndromic craniosynostosis: *TWIST1, FGFR1-3, EFNA4, ALX4*.
      - Among patients with isolated, apparently nonsyndromic craniosynostosis, 10–15% have a pathogenic variant in a single gene.
    - Wilkie et al. (2010) identified a genetic diagnosis in 21%: pathogenic variants in single genes (86%), chromosome anomalies (15%), and one patient had both.

*Pearl*: The same genes are implicated in both premature fusion of cranial sutures and persistence of the fontanelles; the phenotype depends on whether the gene variant causes a gain-of-function or a loss-of-function. Delayed ossification of the skull, including parietal foramina, may be at the opposite expression of the same developmental process that causes craniosynostosis.

# Differential Diagnosis

- **Single suture, nonsyndromic craniosynostosis** (MIM 602849)

- o Can be sporadic or familial
- o Incidence of sporadic craniosynostosis of one suture: 1/1,700 to 1/2,500 live births
- **Sagittal craniosynostosis**: 50% of all craniosynostosis
  - o Incidence 1–2/5,000 live births
  - o 3.5 M:1 F; males predominate
    - ▪ Increased in twins
  - o Familial 2%
  - o Recurrence risk 2% when microarray is normal
  - o Clinical features: scaphocephaly or dolicocephaly—a long narrow skull with prominent occiput and frontal areas
    - ▪ Major malformations 22%, increased ICP ~10%
  - o Genetic testing: low detection rate
    - ▪ In 7%, there is both a heterozygous pathogenic variant in *SMAD6* and a common DNA variant near *BMP2*. Both genes impact bone development.
- **Coronal craniosynostosis**: 20–30% of all cases
  - o Incidence of unilateral coronal craniosynostosis 1/15,000 live births
  - o Bilateral: more likely syndromic
  - o 1 M:2 F; 60–75% female
  - o Familial 8%
  - o Recurrence risk 5% for unilateral coronal synostosis; ≥30–50% for bilateral
  - o Clinical features: when unilateral—anterior plagiocephaly, facial asymmetry, flattening of the forehead, depressed supraorbital ridge, shallow orbit with prominent eye (Figure 13.2)
    - ▪ Increased ICP ~40%, many are phenotypically mild
    - ▪ Coronal craniosynostosis can be seen with spina bifida.
    - ▪ Differentiate sporadic coronal craniosynostosis from mild presentations of Muenke and Saethre–Chotzen syndromes
  - o Genetic testing: *FGFR3, TCF12, FGFR2, TWIST1, EFN4*
  - o Among familial cases, ~75% have a recurrent pathogenic variant, P250R, in *FGFR3*; 17% of sporadic patients have this variant. This is the pathogenic variant responsible for Muenke syndrome.
    - ▪ Females with this variant have a higher rate of bilateral craniosynostosis.
- **Metopic craniosynostosis**: 15–20% of all cases
  - o Incidence 1/10,000 to 1/15,000 live births
    - ▪ Increased in twins
    - ▪ 3.3 M:1 F
  - o Familial 5–10%
  - o Recurrence risk 2–3% for isolated metopic craniosynostosis
  - o Syndromes account for 30% of trigonocephaly
    - ▪ Maternal use of valproic acid and maternal thyroid disease (usually Graves disease)
    - ▪ Cytogenetic anomalies: trisomy or deletion 9p; deletions of 7p, 11q24, or 22q11.2
  - o Clinical features: a narrow anterior cranial fossa, hypotelorism, pointed triangular-shaped forehead (trigonocephaly); anterior fontanelle closes prematurely 55%

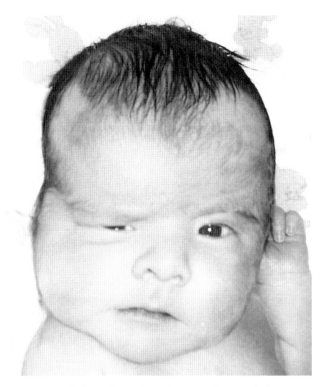

FIGURE 13.2 Unilateral coronal craniosynostosis causes facial asymmetry, which can make it easier to recognize than bilateral coronal suture closure. The left side is affected. The compensatory excess forward growth of the right forehead caused the orbital asymmetry.

- ▪ Chiari I malformation ~30%
- ▪ Of all single suture craniosynostoses, metopic craniosynostosis poses the highest risk of neurodevelopmental problems: 23–32%.
- ▪ Distinguish from a temporary metopic ridge—a normal variant seen in ~5% of infants that occurs when the metopic suture closes.
- **Lambdoid craniosynostosis**: 1–3% of all cases
  - o Most are unilateral.
  - o Demonstrate patency of the lambdoid suture by head US.
  - o Clinical features: when unilateral—causes posterior plagiocephaly and asymmetric flattening of the occiput
  - o Distinguish from positional plagiocephaly, which causes a skewed head shape.
    - ▪ Due to hypotonia, torticollis or preferred sleeping position
    - ▪ Treat with a helmet or molding band.
    - ▪ Deformational plagiocephaly is 100× more common that lambdoid craniosynostosis.
- **Multiple suture craniosynostosis**: 5% of all cases
  - o Two-suture fusion poses a higher chance of reoperation.
  - o Genetic testing: *FGFR2, ERF*
  - o The phenotype of *ERF*-related craniosynostosis involves multiple sutures in approximately half of affected individuals.
  - o Clinical features: increased risk for increased ICP and developmental delay with fusion of more than two sutures

- When coronal and sagittal sutures are both fused, 66% have ICP and 75% have Chiari I malformation on MRI.

*Pearl*: Multiple-suture fusion may occur with severe primary microcephaly; in these cases, the primary problem is failure of brain growth.

*Pearl*: Papilledema is present in ~25% of ICP. A normal fundoscopic exam does not rule out increased ICP.

- Syndromic craniosynostosis: <30% of all cases
  ○ Incidence: 1/15,000 live births
  ○ More than 180 syndromes
    - For a comprehensive review, see Raam and Muenke (2011).
    - Commonly due to pathogenic variants in *FGFR* genes, *TWIST1, ERF, EFNB1*
  ○ Chromosome anomalies occur in 6–28% of syndromic craniosynostosis.
    - Among children with syndromic and nonsyndromic craniosynostosis, Wilkie et al. (2010) found that 5% (13/244) had a chromosome anomaly. Some were only detectable on microarray.
      - All 13 were either syndromic or familial cases.
      - Among 92 nonsyndromic cases, none had clinically significant chromosome anomalies.
      - Almost all (11/13) of the chromosomally abnormal group had midline craniosynostosis (metopic or sagittal).
  ○ Clinical features: usually involve >1 suture and congenital anomalies, especially in limb, cardiac, CNS

# Common Syndromic Causes of Craniosynostosis

  ○ **Apert syndrome** (acrocephalosyndactyly, type 1, MIM 101200)
    - Autosomal dominant disorder due to recurrent gain-of-function heterozygous pathogenic variants in *FGFR2* (S252W and P253R in exon 7) in 98%
    - Most cases are sporadic, with de novo pathogenic variants.
      - Associated with advanced paternal age
      - De novo pathogenic variants arise exclusively in sperm.
    - Recurrence risk for siblings ~1% (Figure 13.3)
    - Clinical features: Bicoronal synostosis causes turribrachycephaly, but multiple sutures may be involved. Tall skull, malar and midface flattening with shallow orbits, proptosis, cleft palate (44%), choanal atresia, sleep apnea, hearing loss, ventriculomegaly. Cloverleaf skull is rare. Extensive syndactyly, often

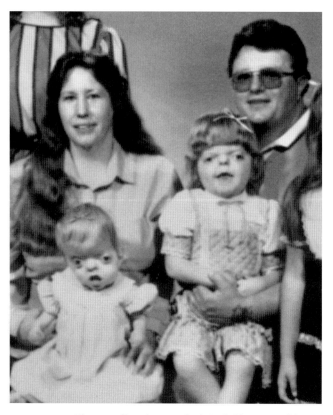

FIGURE 13.3  These unaffected parents had six children; two of their youngest had Apert syndrome. Increased paternal age and a selective growth advantage for spermatogonia with mutant *FGFR3* may increase the recurrence risk for Apert syndrome.

with fused phalanges, may involves all digits or the thumb may be separate. Radiohumeral fusion, cervical spine fusion
      - Cardiac and genitourinary anomalies occur in 10% each.
      - Tracheal anomalies: blind tracheal pouch, solid cartilaginous trachea
        - MRI of the trachea is indicated in lower respiratory compromise.
      - Variable intellectual disability (ID) is unrelated to the timing of corrective surgery.
        - Special education 44%
  ○ **Crouzon syndrome** (MIM 123500)
    - Autosomal dominant, due to gain-of-function heterozygous pathogenic variant in *FGFR2* (exons 7 and 8) or *FGFR3* (P250A) in 50%
    - Sporadic cases are associated with advanced paternal age.
    - Clinical features: usually bicoronal craniosynostosis and sometimes other sutures, frontal bossing, hypertelorism, strabismus, shallow orbits, exophthalmos, infraorbital creases, maxillary hypoplasia, prognathism
      - Beaked nose is typical in the older affected individual. Some have a flat midface but lack craniosynostosis.

- Mouth breathing and obstructive sleep apnea
- Hydrocephalus and papilledema are consequences of increased ICP.
- Patients with Muenke and Saethre–Chotzen syndromes have been misdiagnosed with Crouzon syndrome.
o **Muenke syndrome** (MIM 602849) is the most common syndromic form of craniosynostosis.
  - Incidence 1/30,000 births
  - Of all patients with craniosynostosis, 8% have Muenke syndrome.
  - Autosomal dominant trait, defined by the P250R variant in *FGFR3*: the single most common pathogenic variant that causes craniosynostosis, comprising up to 24% of all patients with a confirmed genetic cause (monogenic or chromosomal)
    - Any patient with unilateral or bilateral coronal craniosynostosis should be tested for this pathogenic variant.
    - 15–20% of individuals with this pathogenic variant, who do not have craniosynostosis, may still have other features of this syndrome, including developmental delay or deafness alone.
  - Advanced paternal age is a factor in sporadic cases.
  - Clinical features: variable unilateral or bilateral coronal suture synostosis, mild midface hypoplasia, macrocephaly, hypertelorism, down-slanting palpebral fissures, sensorineural hearing loss
    - The facial features can be easily mistaken for Saethre–Chotzen syndrome.
    - Brachydactyly, carpal and tarsal fusions
    - No syndactyly or deviation of the great toes
    - Low-frequency hearing loss 70%
  - Developmental delay 66%, ID 35%, attention deficit disorder 23%, seizures 20%
o **Pfeiffer syndrome** (MIM 101600)
  - Autosomal dominant trait; 70% have a gain-of-function heterozygous pathogenic variant in *FGFR1* (P252A), *FGFR2* (exons 7 and 8), or *FGFR3* (P250A)
  - Clinical features: variable craniosynostosis of coronal and sagittal sutures causes turribrachycephalymaxillary hypoplasia; proptosis; hypertelorism; choanal stenosis or atresia; tracheal anomalies; broad, radially deviated thumbs; broad great toes; short digits with soft tissue syndactyly; and radiohumeral synostosis (Figure 13.4).
    - Hydrocephalus and ID are common, but intelligence can be normal.
    - Chiari I malformation 50%
o **Saethre–Chotzen syndrome** (MIM 101400)
  - Autosomal dominant condition due, in 60%, to loss-of-function heterozygous pathogenic variant in *TWIST1* (a repressor of the FGFRs), gain-of-function variant in *FGFR3* (P250A), or in *TCF12* (20%)

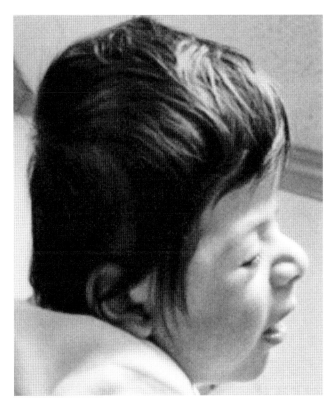

FIGURE 13.4  This infant with Pfeiffer syndrome has coronal craniosynostosis and broad great toes.

- Apparently, de novo *TWIST1* pathogenic variant can be due to parental germ line mosaicism. Recurrence risk for siblings is 2%.
- **Deletions or rearrangements at chromosome 7p21.1** may cause a similar phenotype.
  - Clinical features: Unilateral or bilateral coronal sutures are most commonly involved; facial asymmetry (especially with unilateral coronal involvement), low anterior hairline, hypertelorism, ptosis, small ear pinna, prominent ear crus, syndactyly of index and middle fingers, hallux valgus. Chiari I malformation 70%
    - Some do not have craniosynostosis.
    - Most have normal intelligence.
      - ID is more likely when *TWIST1* is deleted.

# Uncommon Syndromic Causes of Craniosynostosis

o **Carpenter syndrome** (MIM 201000)
  - Autosomal recessive trait, caused by biallelic pathogenic variants in *RAB23* or *MEGF8*
  - Clinical features: acrocephaly; variable craniosynostosis of the metopic, sagittal, coronal, and lambdoid sutures (Figure 13.5A); brachydactyly; syndactyly; postaxial,

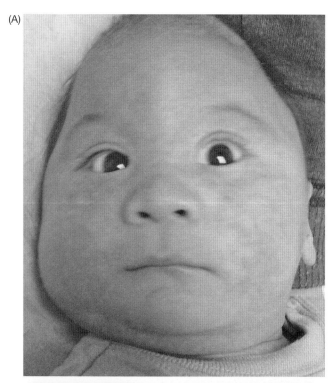

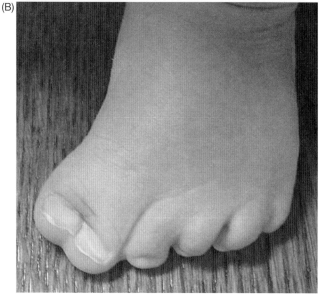

FIGURE 13.5 (A) This infant with acrocephaly due to metopic and coronal craniosynostosis has Carpenter syndrome. (B) Polysyndactyly typical of Carpenter syndrome.

central, and preaxial polydactyly (Figure 13.5B); cryptorchidism and large patellae
- Cardiac defects 50%
- Birth weight can be high, and later, obesity is part of the disorder.
- Mild learning problems to mild ID

o **Craniofrontonasal syndrome** (MIM 304110)
- X-linked dominant disorder, caused by a pathogenic variant in *EFNB1* in 80%
  - Heterozygous females are more severely affected than hemizygous males.
  - Recurrence risk is 10% for siblings of sporadically affected females.
    - High rate of gonadal mosaicism in parents
  - Clinical features in females: coronal craniosynostosis, craniofacial asymmetry, hypertelorism, frontonasal dysplasia with a broad bifid nasal tip
    - Syndactyly, grooved nails, thick wiry hair
    - Less common: pectus deformities, axillary pterygia, diaphragmatic hernia, arcuate uterus
  - Clinical features in males: hypertelorism, broad great toes, longitudinally grooved nails; no craniosynostosis
  - Cellular interference may explain the paradox of more severely affected females in an X-linked disorder.
    - X-inactivation in females causes two different cellular phenotypes, and effective cell–cell interaction does not occur between unlike cell types. This is the basis for the abnormal phenotype in females.
    - Males have only one cellular expression pattern, and their cells are still able to interact outside the *EFNB1* pathway. Their phenotype is mild unless they are mosaic for a pathogenic variant in *EFNB1*.

o **Curry–Jones syndrome** (MIM 601707)
- Autosomal disorder that is always mosaic, caused by a heterozygous de novo recurrent pathogenic variant in *SMO*
- Pathogenic variant is detectable in skin or tissue; not blood
- Clinical features: corpus callosum agenesis, unilateral craniosynostosis, facial asymmetry, microphthalmia and colobomas, polysyndactyly, ID 50% (Figure 13.6)
  - Skin: erythematous lesions resemble cutis aplasia. Later: atrophic linear scarring, streaky hyperpigmentation, freckling of soles of the feet and hands, skin trichoblastoma.
  - Severe gastrointestinal dysfunction
  - Smooth muscle hamartomas, medulloblastoma

o **Greig cephalopolysyndactyly syndrome** (MIM 175700)
- Autosomal dominant disorder, caused by a heterozygous pathogenic variant in *GLI3*
- Clinical features: metopic chraniosynostosis, trigonocephaly, preaxial and postaxial polysyndactyly (Figure 32.4)

o **Loeys–Dietz syndrome** (MIM 609192)
- Autosomal dominant disorder, caused by a heterozygous pathogenic variant, in 96%, in *TGFBR1*, *TGFBR2*, *SMAD3*, or *TGFB2*
  - ~25% have an affected parent.
  - Germline mosaicism can occur in a parent.
- Clinical features: triad of arterial tortuosity and aneurysms of the aorta and other arteries, hypertelorism, and bifid uvula or cleft palate
  - Craniosynostosis of any suture, usually sagittal, ~15%

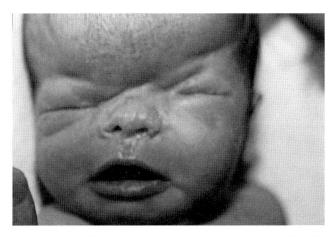

FIGURE 13.6 Infant with Curry–Jones syndrome. Note the unilateral craniosynostosis and the skin defects on the nose and philtrum.

- Skeletal: Marfanoid habitus is common in infancy; pectus deformities, cervical spine abnormality, scoliosis, joint laxity, arachnodactyly, pes planus, clubfoot.
- Aortic dissection has occurred in infants as young as 6-months-old.
  - Echocardiogram, MRA, and CT angiography are used to delineate arterial tortuosity.
  - Beta-blocker or Losartan therapy is warranted to reduce risks from arterial rupture.
○ **Shprintzen–Goldberg syndrome** (MIM 182212)
  ■ Autosomal dominant trait, caused by de novo pathogenic variant in *SKI*
  ■ A progressive disorder that may be difficult to diagnose in a newborn
  ■ Clinical features: craniosynostosis, prominent eyes, down-slanting palpebral fissures, hypertelorism, micrognathia (Figure 13.7); Marfanoid habitus, skeletal, connective tissue anomalies. Arachnodactyly, clubfeet, pectus, and scoliosis can be striking and severe.
    - Neurologic, cardiovascular anomalies
    - Phenotype overlaps that of Marfan and Loeys–Dietz syndromes, but it usually has significant ID.

# Other Causes of Craniosynostosis

○ Intrauterine factors
  ■ Breech head deformation sequence
    - Prominence of the occiput ("occipital shelf") and flat dome are common in breech presentation.
    - The head is molded by the uterine fundus.
    - It usually resolves spontaneously with time but can be associated with premature closure of the sutures.
  ■ Intrauterine constraint

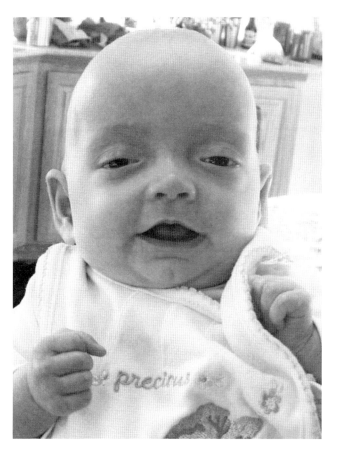

FIGURE 13.7 This baby with Shprintzen–Goldberg syndrome has hypertelorism with down-slanting palpebral fissures.
SOURCE: Courtesy of Carrie Rivas and the Shprintzen–Goldberg Syndrome Support Group.

- Uterine malformations (e.g., bicornuate uterus) can trap the fetal head and alter the fetal head shape.
- Early descent of the fetal head into the maternal pelvis
○ Teratogens*
  ■ **Fluconazole embryopathy**
    - First trimester therapy, with long-term high dose fluconazole (400–800 mg/day) for systemic or CNS fungal infection, can cause craniosynostosis.
    - Clinical features: multiple craniosynostoses, shallow orbits, hypertelorism, ptosis, digital anomalies, radioulnar or radiohumeral synostosis, skeletal anomalies, symphalangism.
  ■ **Maternal thyroid disorders**, fetal or neonatal hyperthyroidism
    - Transplacental passage of thyrotrophin receptor-stimulating antibodies (TRAb) from a mother with a current or past history of Graves disease can cause thyroid disease in the newborn with secondary accelerated bone maturation and premature fusion of the cranial sutures, often the metopic.
    - The thyrotoxic fetus
      - Occurs in 1/70 pregnancies complicated by maternal Graves disease

- Clinical features: craniosynostosis of one or multiple sutures, hydrops, tachycardia, poor growth, goiter
  - Secondary craniosynostosis can develop postnatally due to mechanical (e.g., position) or metabolic (e.g., hypophosphatemic rickets) factors.
  - **Methotrexate embryopathy**
    - Multiple craniosynostoses (usually coronal and/or lamboid) are a rare but established consequence of fetal methotrexate exposure.
      - Craniosynostosis may be secondary to microcephaly.
  - **Valproic acid embryopathy**
    - Adjusted OR 6.8 for craniosynostosis after first trimester exposure to valproic acid monotherapy
  - Craniosynostosis of postnatal onset
    - Microcephaly
      - Otherwise normal cranial sutures fuse prematurely in microcephalic infants because the normal forces associated with brain growth are absent while cranial bones grow at a normal rate.
      - Craniosynostosis in this situation is a *secondary* phenomenon.
      - Microcephaly with inadequate brain growth is the primary problem.
    - Positional plagiocephaly/torticollis
      - Increased pressure on one side of the head can cause secondary premature suture fusion.
      - Hypotonia, weakness or preferred sleeping or eating posture, can deform the head shape, initially causing asymmetric flattening of the occiput and, later, asymmetric prominence of the frontal region.
      - Infants with deformational plagiocephaly have lower developmental scores at 36 months and may be at risk for developmental delay.
      - Helmet treatment is more successful in the first months of life.
    - Prematurity
      - Dolicocephaly is common in premature infants whose heads are positioned only to the side.

# Evaluation and Management

- Take detailed pregnancy and family histories.
  - Document paternal age.
  - Ask about teratogenic exposures (valproic acid, methotrexate), history of maternal thyroid disease, uterine abnormalities, and pregnancy complications that cause intrauterine constraint, malpresentation, or limit fetal movement.
- Examine parents for unusual head shape, cranial asymmetry, ptosis, strabismus, hypertelorism, bifid uvula, prominent ear crus, syndactyly, broad deviated thumbs or great toes, and intellectual disability.

- Examine infant's head for asymmetry, position and size of the fontanelles, ridging of sutures, and movement across all of the sutures.
  - Posterior and bird's-eye views of the skull can reveal asymmetry (e.g., in the position of the ears when one is more anterior than the other).
- Evaluate for extracranial anomalies.
- Use imaging studies judiciously.
  - Head US can document suture patency and brain anatomy in the newborn period.
  - CT with 3D reconstruction, using both bone and soft tissue windows, is the investigation of choice for craniosynostosis, but its utility in the newborn should be weighed against the significant radiation dose.
    - 3D CT can usually be deferred to the craniofacial surgical team.
  - Skull radiographs are less sensitive than CT for diagnosing cranial suture patency.
  - MRI is ideal for visualizing brain anomalies but not for cranial sutures.
  - Consider early imaging with CT or MRI when two or more sutures are fused or when there is poor feeding, lethargy, or irritability in a baby with craniosynostosis of a single suture.
- Genetic testing
  - Begin with microarray for the following:
    - Familial craniosynostosis
    - Metopic craniosynostosis with or without trigonocephaly
    - Unexplained neurological impairment: poor feeding, hypotonia
    - Multiple congenital malformations that do not suggest a known syndrome
  - For isolated nonsyndromic coronal craniosynostosis, test for P250R variant in *FGFR3* as well as variants in *FGFR2*, *TWIST1*, and *TCF12*.
  - When multiple sutures are involved, consider *ERF*.
  - In the syndromic group, consider gene panels that include common recurrent pathogenic variants.
  - See genetic testing algorithm in Figure 3 of Johnson and Wilkie (2011).
- Anticipate common complications
  - Suspect increased ICP in multiple-suture craniosynostosis and when neurological exam is abnormal.
    - Do not be reassured by lack of papilledema.
  - For Chiari I malformation, order sleep study for respiratory insufficiency and apnea.
  - Manage obstructive or central sleep apnea prior to discharge, with CPAP, nasal stenting, choanal stenosis repair.
  - Treat for exposure keratitis when the baby does not close the eyelids during sleep.
  - Prevent iatrogenic dolicocephaly by frequently repositioning the head using gel-filled bags or blankets shaped into donuts under the occiput to redistribute pressure.

- Immediate surgical repair in the newborn period is rarely necessary.
- Refer patients with an unusual head shape, even if craniosynostosis has not been clearly established, for follow-up at a multidisciplinary craniofacial team clinic or a regional pediatric specialty surgical center within the first few months of life.
- Refer for genetic evaluation and counseling when craniosynostosis is familial, syndromic, or when multiple sutures are involved.

# Further Reading

Addo NK, Javadpour S, Kandasamy J, et al. (2013) Central sleep apnea and associated Chiari malformation in children with syndromic craniosynostosis: Treatment and outcome data from a supraregional national craniofacial center. J Neurosurg Pediatr. 11:296–301. PMID 23240845

Collett BR, Gray KE, Starr JR, et al. (2013) Development at age 36 months in children with deformational plagiocephaly. Pediatrics. 131:e109–15. PMID 23266929

Cunningham ML, Heike CL. (2007) Evaluation of the infant with an abnormal skull shape. Curr Opin Pediatr. 19:645–51. PMID 18025930

Eley KA, Johnson D, Wilkie AO, et al. (2012) Raised intracranial pressure is frequent in untreated nonsyndromic unicoronal synostosis and does not correlate with severity of phenotypic features. Plast Reconstr Surg. 130:690e–697e. PMID 2309662.

Johnson D, Wilkie AO. (2011) Craniosynostosis. Eur J Hum Genet. 19:369–76. PMID 21248745

Kruszka P, Addissie YA, Yarnell CM, et al. (2016) Muenke syndrome: An international multicenter natural history study. Am J Med Genet A. 170:918–29. PMID 26740388

Raam MS, Muenke M. (2011) Uncommon craniosynostosis syndromes: a review of thirteen conditions. In: Muenke M, Kress W, Collman H, Solomon BD editors. *Craniosynostoses: Molecular Genetics, Principles of Diagnosis and Treatment*. Monogr Hum Genet. Basel, Krager 19:119–42.

Twigg SR, Babbs C, van den Elzen ME, et al. (2013) Cellular interference in craniofrontonasal syndrome: Males mosaic for mutations in the X-linked *EFNB1* gene are more severely affected than true hemizygotes. Hum Mol Genet. 22:1654–62. PMID 23335590.

Twigg SR, Hufnagel RB, Miller KA, et al. (2016). A recurrent mosaic mutation in *SMO*, encoding the hedgehog signal transducer smoothened, is the major cause of Curry–Jones syndrome. Am J Hum Genet. 98:1256–65. PMID 27236920

Twigg SR, Wilkie AO (2015) A genetic–pathophysiological framework for craniosynostosis. Am J Hum Genet. 97:359–77. PMID 26340332

Wilkie AO, Byren JC, Hurst JA, et al. (2010) Prevalence and complications of single-gene and chromosomal disorders in craniosynostosis. Pediatrics. 126:e391–e400. PMID 20643727

# Part IV

# Central Nervous System

# 14

# Macrocephaly and Megalencephaly

## Clinical Consult

A 2-month-old baby with macrocephaly was referred for outpatient genetics consultation. Prenatal diagnosis of macrocephaly prompted elective cesarean section at 38 weeks' gestation. Head circumference (HC) was 39 cm at birth, whereas other growth parameters were normal. She had frontal bossing, hypertelorism, and no other notable dysmorphic features (Figure 14.1). Her father was also macrocephalic, raising the question of familial macrocephaly. Skin lesions started in his teens, and he reported his dermatologist removes multiple basal cell nevi every 6 months. Focused questioning revealed a history of jaw cysts and mild learning problems. On exam, he had palmar and plantar pits. Their physical features and history established the clinical diagnosis of **Basal cell nevus syndrome** (Gorlin syndrome) in father and baby. The parents were counseled to use sunscreen daily and to monitor HC and development. The family was given a 50% recurrence risk for future children. Eight months later, this child presented with an increasing HC and bulging fontanel. A CT scan revealed a probable medulloblastoma, a known rare complication in this syndrome. Establishing this diagnosis was important because radiation therapy was avoided.

## Definition

- Macrocephaly (MAC) is defined as a head circumference (HC) > +2 SD for gestational age and sex, equivalent to >97th percentile. Hydrocephalus* is discussed in detail in another chapter.
  - Relative macrocephaly is a HC that, although normal for age and sex, is disproportionately large compared to other growth parameters.
- Megalencephaly (MEG) refers to enlarged brain parenchyma, with or without cortical malformations or asymmetry. Patients with MEG usually also have MAC.
  - The medical literature does not always distinguish MAC and MEG.
  - Cranial imaging differentiates between brain overgrowth and other causes of MAC.
- Etiologies

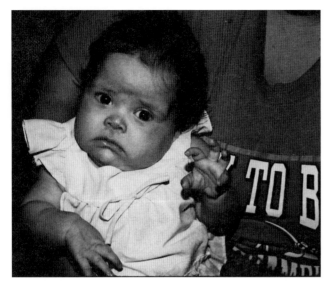

FIGURE 14.1  Basal cell nevus syndrome (Gorlin syndrome in an infant with macrocephaly. Her father had multiple basal cell nevi, allowing this diagnosis.

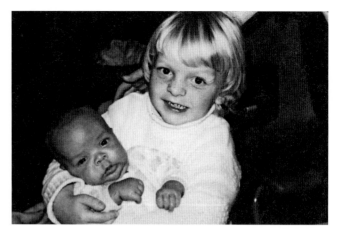

FIGURE 14.2  Familial macrocephaly Child with macrocephaly and his older sibling, also with macrocephaly. Father is also macrocephalic, consistent with autosomal dominant inheritance.

- o **MAC without MEG**
  - ■ Ventriculomegaly, hydrocephalus, benign enlargement of subarachnoid spaces, intracranial hemorrhage, arteriovenous malformations (AVMs), increased intracranial pressure
- o **MAC with MEG**
  - ■ RAS pathway disorders, generally caused by germline variants (rarely mosaic) such as **Noonan*** and **Costello syndromes**
  - ■ *P13K–AKT–mTOR* pathway variant disorders are generally somatic and mosaic, e.g. **Proteus syndrome**
  - ■ *PTEN*-related disorders e.g. **Cowden syndrome**
  - ■ Disorders of chromatin remodeling including **Sotos** and **Weaver syndromes**

## Differential Diagnosis

- **Familial macrocephaly** (MIM 153470)
  - o Most common cause of MAC in healthy infants
    - ■ 40% of macrocephalic infants who appear otherwise normal have a parent with MAC.
    - ■ HC stabilizes by ~6 months (Figure 14.2).
  - o Enlarged subarachnoid spaces are the most common finding on cranial imaging.
  - o More boys and their fathers are affected.
  - o Development is usually normal.
    - ■ Small increased risk for developmental issues
    - ■ Autism ~5%

*Pearl*: In a series of autistic children macrocephaly is a consistent frequent finding (~15-30%) even in the absence of any known genetic etiology. Often the macrocephaly is not present at birth.

- **Hydrocephalus**
  - o Associated CNS malformation in ~50%: Chiari malformation, Dandy–Walker malformation, aqueductal stenosis
  - o Many nonsyndromic (hemorrhage, tumor) and syndromic causes (**X-linked hydrocephalus** MIM 307000)
- **Metabolic disorders**
  - o MAC/MEG is a common feature but is not always present in the neonatal period.
  - o Lysosomal storage diseases
    - ■ Autosomal recessive disorders: **Tay–Sachs** (MIM 277800), **Sandhoff disease** (MIM 268800), **Hurler** (MIM 607014) and **Hunter** syndromes (MIM 309900)
  - o Metabolic encephalopathies
    - ■ Autosomal recessive disorders: **Alexander disease** (MIM 203450) and **Canavan disease** (MIM 271900).
    - ■ **Megalencephalic leukoencephalopathy** (MIM 604004): impressive neonatal MAC, severe white matter disease, with relatively mild neonatal symptoms

*Pearl*: In **Glutaric aciduria I**, a neurodegenerative disorder, a large head is the only presenting sign in most affected neonates.

- o Organic acid disorders
  - ■ **Glutaric aciduria I** (MIM 231670)
    - • Autosomal recessive disorder, due to biallelic variants in *GCDH*. Enzyme defect in glutaryl-CoA dehydrogenase
    - • Clinical features: MAC/MEG, progressive dystonic movements from 6 to 18 months. Encephalopathic crises associated with infection. Increased risk for subdural hemorrhage.
    - • Newborn screening identifies elevated glutaric acid in most cases. Diagnose with urine organic acid analysis or plasma acylcarnitine profile.

- **D-2-hydroxyglutaric aciduria** (MIM 600721)
  - Autosomal recessive disorder, due to variants in *D2HDGH*
  - Clinical features: hypotonia, MAC, ID, encephalopathy, seizures, cardiomyopathy
    - Milder form has later onset
- Peroxisomal disorders
  - **Zellweger syndrome spectrum** (MIM 214100)
    - Autosomal recessive disorders, caused by biallelic variants in several peroxin (PEX) genes
      - Overlapping clinical and molecular phenotypes from neonatal **adrenoleukodystrophy** (MIM 602136) to classic **Zellweger** (MIM 214100) and **infantile Refsum disease** (MIM 601539)
    - Clinical features: MAC, large fontanels, dysmorphic face, high forehead, hypertelorism (see Figure 1.4)
      - Hypotonia, hepatomegaly, liver and renal dysfunction, cataracts, epiphyseal stippling
      - Elevated plasma very long-chain fatty acids
- **Chromosome disorders**
  - Microdeletions and microduplications: 1q21.1, 5q35.5, 16p11.2; **chromosome 14 maternal uniparental disomy** (MIM 608149)
- **Syndromic MAC with variable overgrowth**
  - Hemimegalencephaly: one side of brain larger than the other often with cortical dysplasia; frequent seizures, ID. May be isolated or syndromic (below)
    - **Linear nevus sebaceous syndrome** (MIM 162900)
      - Usually large congenital nevus with multiple and variable effects on CNS, skeletal development and other organs. Caused by somatic mosaic variants in *HRAS, KRAS,* and *NRAS*
    - **Tuberous sclerosis** (MIM 191900)
      - Multisystem disorder affecting CNS, heart, skin, kidneys, lungs, and eyes caused by variants in *TSC1* and *TSC2*
    - **Curry–Jones syndrome** (MIM 601707)
      - Cerebral hemisphere overgrowth, contralateral cortical dysplasia, dilated ventricles, early onset intractable seizures, infantile spasms. Multi-system disorder caused by mosaic de novo variants in *SMO*
  - **Bannayan–Riley–Ruvalcaba syndrome** (BRRS, MIM 153480) (also called Riley–Smith syndrome or Ruvalcaba–Myhre–Smith syndrome)
    - Autosomal dominant multiple hamartoma syndrome, caused by heterozygous variants in *PTEN,* in 60%
    - Clinical features: MAC, BW and length >97%, large phallus and testes. MAC may be progressive
      - GI: ileal and colonic hamartomatous polyps, intussusception
      - Skin: hemangiomas, café-au-lait spots, lipomas, penile freckling (later)
      - CNS: hypotonia, thick corpus callosum

- Later: delay, ID, autism
  - Increased tumor risk merits surveillance in childhood.
- **Cowden syndrome** (MIM 158350), caused by variants in *PTEN* in ~80%, has an overlapping phenotype. Most clinical findings are of adult onset.

*Pearl*: A variable percentage of autistic children with MAC have *PTEN* mutations.

- **Neurofibromatosis, type 1** (NF1, MIM 162200)
  - Autosomal dominant disorder, due to pathogenic variants in *NF1*
  - Clinical features: HC > +2 SD in ~25%. Pale café-au-lait spots usually become obvious in the first few months.
    - Rarely diagnosed at birth, except in severely affected newborns with a large deletion that includes *NF1*
  - Other autosomal dominant disorders affecting the same gene pathway (RASopathies) can have overlapping phenotypes.
    - **Legius syndrome** (MIM 611431) caused by variants in *SPRED1*
      - Multiple café au lait macules without neurofibromas; otherwise similar to NF1
    - Noonan*, CFC, and Costello syndromes due to variants in multiple RAS pathway genes
- *PIK3CA*-related overgrowth syndromes (PROS)
  - Congenital lipomatous overgrowth, vascular malformations, epidermal nevi, skeletal/spinal **anomalies** (CLOVES, MIM 612918), **megalencephaly capillary malformation polymicrogyria syndrome** (MCAP, MIM 602501) (Figure 14.3), **megalencephaly-polymicrogyria–polydactyly–hydrocephalus** syndrome (MPPH, MIM 603387) are distinct but overlapping conditions in this spectrum
  - Usually sporadic, mosaic overgrowth disorders, caused by gain-of-function heterozygous variants in *PIK3CA* or *PIK3R2*.
    - Rarely, a *PIK3CA* germline variant causes isolated MEG (Figure 14.4) with a fairly good prognosis.
  - Complex segmental **overgrowth** with vascular malformations.
- **Proteus syndrome** (MIM 176920)
  - Sporadic disorder, due to mosaic, activating mutation in *AKT1*
  - Clinical features: Progressive asymmetric, disproportionate overgrowth, cerebriform connective tissue nevi, exostoses, lipomas, hemangiomas
    - MAC is of prenatal onset and may be the only finding in the newborn, HC > +4–5 SD; other growth parameters are only mildly increased at birth.
    - Vascular stasis increases risk for deep vein thrombosis (DVT).

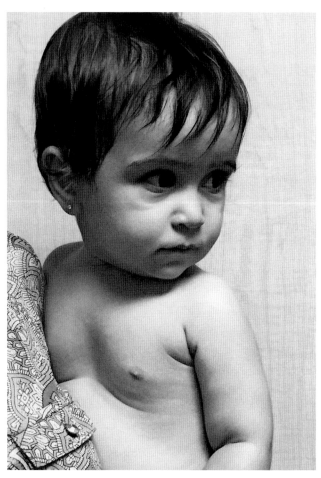

FIGURE 14.3 Germline mutation in *PIK3CA* in a child with isolated macrocephaly.

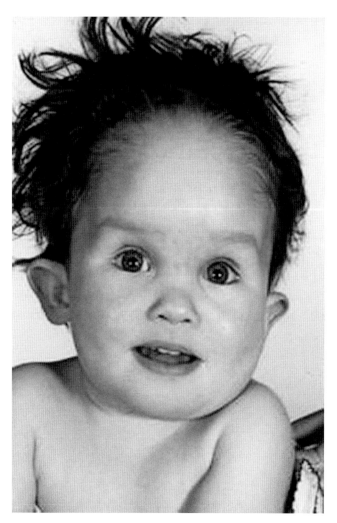

FIGURE 14.4 FG syndrome in infant with hypotonia, macrocephaly, high forehead and small ears. Note frontal upsweep to hair.

- **Syndromes with relative MAC and IUGR**
  - **Russell–Silver syndrome** (Silver–Russell syndrome, MIM 180860)
    - Usually sporadic disorder, due to epigenetic alterations, uniparental disomy, or mutation in growth-related genes, including *CDKN1C*
    - Clinical features: IUGR, short stature, failure to thrive, relative macrocephaly, limb asymmetry, clinodactyly
  - **Wiedemann–Rautenstrauch syndrome** (neonatal progeriod syndrome, MIM 264090)
    - Autosomal recessive neonatal progeriod disorder; no known responsible gene
    - Clinical features: MAC, pseudohydrocephalus, paucity of subcutaneous fat, prominent veins, short stature, failure to thrive
      - Early lethality is common.
- **Syndromic MAC—other causes**
  - **Simpson–Golabi–Behmel syndrome, types 1 and 2** (MIM 312870; 300209)
    - X-linked recessive disorders, due to hemizygous variants in *GPC3, OFD1,* or *PIGA*

- Clinical features: MAC, prenatal and postnatal over-growth, dysmorphic coarse facial features, submucous cleft palate, intestinal malrotation, coccygeal skin tag and bony appendage
  - Limbs: hypoplastic index fingernails, postaxial polydactyly, bilateral syndactyly of fingers 2 and 3
  - May have early lethality
  - **Sotos syndrome** (MIM 117550)
    - Autosomal dominant disorder, due to heterozygous variant or deletion of *NSD1*
      - **Malan syndrome** (Sotos 2, MIM 614753), caused by heterozygous variants in *NFIX*, has a similar phenotype.
    - Clinical features: macrosomia usual at birth with rapid somatic growth and advanced bone age, MAC, tall prominent forehead and jaw
      - MAC usually persists; other growth parameters normalize

- o **Weaver syndrome** (MIM 277590)
  - ■ Autosomal dominant disorder, due to heterozygous variants in *EXH2*
    - ● Features overlap with **Sotos syndrome**
  - ■ Clinical features: pre- and postnatal overgrowth, MAC, dysmorphic features, round face, thin deep-set nails, limited elbow and knee extension, camptodactyly, loose skin
- o **Basal cell nevus syndrome** (Gorlin syndrome, MIM 109400); see Clinical Consult
  - ■ Autosomal dominant disorder, due to mutation in *PTCH1, PTCH2*, or *SUFU*
  - ■ Clinical features: MAC, high prominent forehead, absent corpus callosum, bifid ribs, skeletal anomalies, polydactyly, cardiac fibroma
    - ● Later: malignant basal cell nevi as young as 2 years
    - ● Cancer risk: medulloblastoma 5–10%
    - ● Odontogenic jaw keratocysts in first decade
- o **FG syndrome** (Opitz–Kaveggia syndrome, MIM 305450)
  - ■ X-linked recessive disorder, caused by distinct variant in *MED12*
    - ● An allelic disorder, **Lujan syndrome** (Lujan Fryns, MIM 309520), due to a *MED12* variant; causes MAC, hypotonia, Marfanoid features, and CNS and cardiac anomalies
  - ■ Clinical features: relative or absolute MAC, hypotonia, failure to thrive, constipation, anal stenosis
    - ● High forehead, frontal upsweep of hair, long myopathic face, small ears (Figure 14.4)
  - ■ Unrelated disorders with shared features of macrocephaly, hypotonia, dysmorphic facies, and constipation in males with ID have been designated as subtypes of FG syndrome, causing diagnostic confusion. These are clinically and molecularly distinct from FG syndrome.
    - ● **FG syndrome 2** (MIM 300321)
      - ● X-linked disorder, due to hemizygous variant in *FLNA*; causes CNS anomalies and GI dysmotility
    - ● **FG syndrome 4** (MIM 300422)
      - ● X-linked disorder, due to hemizygous variant in *CASK*; causes hypotonia, relative macrocephaly (or microcephaly), constipation, and dysmorphic features
- o **Skeletal dysplasias\* and Craniosynostosis\***
  - ■ **Achondroplasia\*, Campomelic dysplasia** and **Short Rib Polydactyly syndromes** and other skeletal dysplasias cause relative MAC
  - ■ **Muenke syndrome** (MIM 602849), **Cole Carpenter syndrome** (MIM 112240) and other craniosynostosis syndromes may have MAC
- o **Previously uncharacterized macrocephaly syndromes**
  - ■ Variants in *ASXL2, CHD4, DICER1, DNMT3A, HERC1, MTOR, PAK3, TCF20*, and others have been delineated by exome sequencing.

# Evaluation and Management

- Document family and pregnancy histories.
- Measure parental head circumferences.
  - o Measure head circumference and calculate standard deviation (see https://simulconsult.com/resources/measurement.html?type=head)
- Evaluate for other anomalies and cardinal signs especially body symmetry, skin abnormalities.
- Imaging studies
  - o Brain MRI: non-sedated fast MRI of brain in newborn period can avoid general anesthesia later.
  - o Skeletal radiographs: for limb or trunk shortening
- Genetic testing should be guided by the clinical presentation.
  - o Chromosome microarray is a preferred first-line test.
  - o Urine organic acids, plasma amino acids, plasma very long-chain fatty acids, acylcarnitine profile, lysosomal enzymes when metabolic or storage disorders are suspected
  - o Single gene analysis, gene panel, or exome sequencing testing as indicated by presentation and initial testing results
    - ■ Consider *PTEN* testing in isolated MAC, especially HC > +3 SD.
    - ■ Several commercial genetic testing companies offer macrocephaly/overgrowth panels
    - ■ Exome sequencing test is useful in familial MAC with ID and unexplained or complex phenotypes
    - ■ Mosaic gene mutations in disorders with segmental overgrowth may not be detected in blood, and may require biopsy (usually skin) of affected tissue
- Anticipate common complications: feeding problems, and seizures. Monitor HC and SD.
- Careful long-term follow-up is needed as many phenotypes evolve.
- Recent use of a *PIK3CA* inhibitor shows early therapeutic promise in the PROS syndromes

# Further Reading

Busa T, Milh M, Degardin N, et al. (2015) Clinical presentation of PTEN mutations in childhood in the absence of family history of Cowden syndrome. Eur J Paediatr Neurol. 19:188–92. PMID 2554989

Cottereau E, Mortemousque I, Moizard MP, et al. (2013) Phenotypic spectrum of Simpson–Golabi–Behmel syndrome in a series of 42 cases with a mutation in GPC3 and review of the literature. Am J Med Genet C Semin Med Genet. 163C:92–105. PMID 23606591

Jansen LA, Mirzaa GM, Ishak GE, et al. (2015) PI3K/AKT pathway mutations cause a spectrum of brain malformations from megalencephaly to focal cortical dysplasia. Brain. 138:1613–28. PMID 25722288

Lyons MJ. (2016) *MED12*-related disorders. In: Pagon RA, Adam MP, Ardinger HH, et al. editors. GeneReviews [Internet]. Seattle, WA: University of Washington, Seattle; 1993–2016. PMID 20301719

Mirzaa GM, Poduri A. (2014) Megalencephaly and hemimegalencephaly: Breakthroughs in molecular etiology. Am J Med Genet C Semin Med Genet. 166C:156–72. PMID 24888963

Pavone P, Praticò AD, Rizzo R, et al. (2017) A clinical review on megalencephaly: A large brain as a possible sign of cerebral impairment. Medicine (Baltimore). 96:e6814. PMID 28658095

Venot Q, Blanc T, Rabia SH, et al. (2018) Targeted therapy in patients with PIK3CA-related overgrowth syndrome. Nature. 558(7711):540–546. PMID 29899452

# 15

# Microcephaly

## Clinical Consult

A term baby girl presented with severe microcephaly. Her head circumference was 27 cm (*z* score –8 SD); and she had a sloping, posteriorly recessed forehead (Figure 15.1). There were no other apparent birth defects. The mother was well during gestation, and the family had not traveled outside the United States. A small fetal head was first noted on ultrasound at 24 weeks' gestation, followed by progressive fall off. Her other growth parameters were normal. A brain MRI showed a simplified gyral pattern but no other structural abnormalities. The baby's status deteriorated, and she died at 1 week of age. A microarray was normal. DNA was banked. The likelihood of autosomal recessive inheritance was discussed with the family.

Three years later, the parents had another pregnancy followed closely with fetal ultrasound. At 22 weeks' gestation, the fetal head circumference fell below the third percentile. Fetal MRI confirmed recurrence of microcephaly. The couple chose to discontinue the pregnancy. Exome sequencing failed to reveal the cause of the severe **autosomal recessive primary microcephaly** in this family. Many new genes responsible for primary microcephaly are being described. If the parents desire more children, past negative exome results should be reanalyzed and referral to the Undiagnosed Disease Network considered. https://undiagnosed.hms.harvard.edu/

## Definition

- Microcephaly is defined as a head circumference (HC) > –2 SD for sex and gestational age.
- This discussion is limited to microcephaly that presents in the newborn period. Syndromes associated with a later onset or "acquired" microcephaly are not discussed here.
- Incidence 0.5%
  - 25,000/year in the United States
  - Severe microcephaly, > –3 SD, affects 0.14% of newborns.
- Etiology highly heterogeneous
  - Proportionate microcephaly: other growth parameters also small
    - Prognosis for intellectual development may be more favorable.

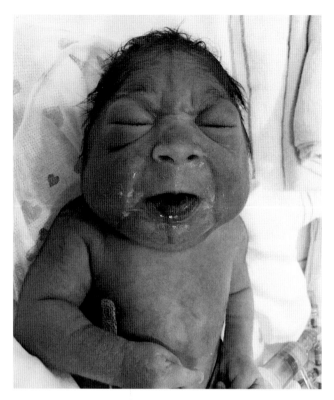

FIGURE 15.1   Neonate with severe prenatal-onset autosomal recessive microcephaly genetic cause unknown.

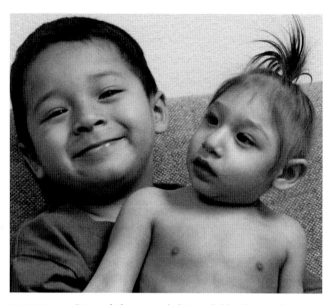

FIGURE 15.2   Primordial microcephaly in a child with severely reduced head and body size. Cause unknown despite exome sequencing. Note normal sized younger sib.

   o Syndromic microcephaly: associated with anomalies in other organ systems
      ■ Often due to a chromosomal or monogenic disorder

*Pearl*: Express head circumference in terms of standard deviations (SD), rather than percentiles. The SD is an important factor in forming the differential diagnosis. https://simulconsult.com/resources/measurement. html?type=head

## Differential Diagnosis

• **Autosomal recessive primary microcephaly**
   o A heterogeneous group of disorders, causing significant congenital microcephaly (MCPH 1–15, MIM 251200 and others)
      ■ HC $z$ score usually –4 to –12 SD below the mean for gestational age
   o Evident by 32 weeks' gestation
   o Prevalence 1/1,000,000 (Caucasians)
      ■ More common in Asians and Middle Eastern groups (e.g., northern Pakistan)
      ■ Consanguinity is common.

   o More than 15 genes are currently known (e.g. ASPM, CNPJ, *ANKLE2*), but half or more of affected patients from North America or Western Europe have no identifiable gene mutations (Figure 15.2).
      ■ Most genes impair cell division and cell cycle regulation.
      ■ Variants affect neuronal precursor cells, reducing the number of neurons produced in fetal life.
      ■ Spontaneous chromosome breakage and abnormal chromosome morphology may be seen.
   o Clinical features: simplified gyral patterning and small size on brain MRI; structural CNS defects uncommon; no visceral anomalies
      ■ Severe outcome in many: poor feeding, failure to thrive, ID, seizures, spastic quadriplegia, early death
      ■ Some have better prognosis: ambulation possible, body size small
      ■ Brain MRI is important for clinical categorization
• **Syndromes of primordial microcephaly with DWARFISM**
   o **Majewski osteoplastic dysplasia II** (MOPD II, MIM 210720)
      ■ Autosomal recessive disorder, caused by biallelic variants in *PCNT*
      ■ Clinical features: severe IUGR, microcephaly (see Figures 2.1 and 2.2) Distinctive facial features: prominent nose and eyes, high squeaky voice
         • Elements of a primary skeletal dysplasia with mesomelic shortening of the forearms and legs in early life
         • High frequency of Moyamoya leads to stroke.
         • Mild ID usual

○ **Seckel syndrome** (MIM 210600)
  ■ Heterogeneous group of autosomal recessive disorders
    • Eight subtypes; biallelic variants in *ATR* and seven other genes at present
  ■ Clinical features: IUGR, microcephaly, short stature, receding forehead, prominent beaked nose, micrognathia, intellectual disability
    • Hematologic abnormalities with chromosome breakage in 15–25%
    • Skeletal survey in the first years of life can distinguish between Seckel and MOPD II syndromes.
○ **Meier–Gorlin syndrome** (ear, patella, short stature syndrome, MIM 224690)
  ■ Autosomal recessive disorders due to mutations in *ORC1, ORC4, ORC6, CDT1, CDC6* and others. At least seven subtypes exist.
    • Biallelic variants in *CDC45* cause craniosynostosis.
    • One form is autosomal dominant: *GMNN*.
  ■ Clinical features: classic triad in 82%: severe IUGR, bilateral microtia, patellar aplasia/hypoplasia
    • Microcephaly is not present in all patients.
    • Additional findings: micrognathia, small mouth, full lips, breast underdevelopment, genital hypoplasia 42%, feeding problems, congenital pulmonary emphysema (see Figure 2.4)
    • Intellect is usually normal.
• **Chromosomal abnormalities associated with microcephaly**
○ Aneuploidy
  ■ **Trisomy 18***
  ■ **Down syndrome***: Mean HC is –2 SD less than that of the general newborn population.
○ Microdeletions
  ■ **4p-* (Wolf–Hirschhorn syndrome)**
    • Microcephaly 90%
  ■ **5p-* (cri du chat)**
    • Microcephaly is a hallmark of this disorder.
  ■ 7q11.23 deletion causes **Williams syndrome***.
  ■ 17q21.31 includes the locus for the *EFTUD2* gene responsible for **mandibulofacial dysostosis with microcephaly** syndrome (MIM 160536) (see Figure 12.4).
    • Clinical features: first and second branchial arch anomalies resemble oculo-auriculo-vertebral syndrome, hearing loss, microcephaly in most—may normalize in later life
    • Esophageal atresia ~27%
  ■ **Chromosome 22q11.2 deletion***: HC < second percentile in 25–50% of affected newborns.
• **Single gene disorders with isolated microcephaly, without major CNS defects**
○ Microcephaly can occur as an autosomal dominant trait without intellectual disability (MIM 156580).

○ **Lethal neonatal rigidity and multifocal seizure syndrome** (MIM 614498)
  ■ Autosomal recessive disorder, caused by mutations in *BRAT1*
  ■ Clinical features: progressive microcephaly, dysmorphic features, hypertonia, intractable neonatal seizures with suppression-burst pattern on electroencephalogram (Otahara syndrome)
• **Single gene disorders with major structural CNS malformations**
○ **Congenital disorders of glycosylation** (MIM 212065)
  ■ A large group of autosomal recessive disorders that limit glycosylation of proteins: more than 111 types
  ■ Clinical features: microcephaly with cerebellar abnormalities, liver disease, hypotonia, abnormal eye movements, dysmorphic features, inverted nipples, abnormal fat distribution, feeding problems
    • In order of decreasing frequency: abnormal coagulation, increased thyroid-stimulating hormone, cardiomyopathy
    • Can present as severe neonatal encephalopathy
  ■ Laboratory studies: Transferrin glycosylation products are abnormal on isoelectric focusing (electrophoresis).
    • Screening for both N- and O-glycosylation defects in a qualified reference laboratory refines the diagnosis. Exome sequencing may speed diagnosis.
○ **Pontocerebellar hypoplasia** (MIM 607596)
  ■ A group of autosomal recessive disorders, caused by multiple genes including *VRK1* and *TSEN54*
  ■ Clinical features: severe hypoplasia of the cerebellum and pons, evolving loss of cerebral cortex and basal ganglia, severe developmental delay, respiratory and feeding issues, seizures, visual limitations. Rarely, sex reversal
    • Most do not survive beyond a few years.
○ **Microcephaly with lobar holoprosencephaly** (MIM 612703)
  ■ Autosomal recessive disorder, caused by biallelic variants in *STIL*
○ **Pyruvate dehydrogenase complex deficiency**
  ■ The mitochondrial pyruvate dehydrogenase complex is made up of enzymatic subunits (E1-alpha, E1-beta, E2, E3, E3 binding protein) coded by at least six nuclear genes: *PDHA1, PDHB, DLAT, DLD, PDHX, PDP1*. The following are the two most common causes of PDC deficiency:
  ■ **Pyruvate dehydrogenase E1-alpha deficiency** (MIM 312170)
    • X-linked recessive disorder, caused by pathogenic variants in *PDHA1*; most common cause of PDC deficiency
    • Carrier mothers may be symptomatic with intermittent weakness or dystonia precipitated by exercise.

- Clinical features: severe microcephaly, absent corpus callosum and other structural CNS anomalies, neonatal encephalopathy, hypotonia, lethargy, seizures and profound ID
- Laboratory testing
  - Biochemical studies: elevated lactate in blood and CSF, may occasionally be normal. Enzymatic assays and functional studies confirm the diagnosis
- Therapy: Some patients respond to vitamin $B_1$, thiamine.
- **Pyruvate dehydrogenase E3-binding protein deficiency** (MIM 245349)
  - Autosomal recessive disorder, caused by biallelic variants in *PDHX*
  - Clinical features: ventriculomegaly, dysgenesis of corpus callosum and other CNS anomalies, neonatal lactic acidosis, hypotonia, microcephaly ~22%, progressive neurological dysfunction, seizures, death during childhood

*Pearl*: The most common cause of fused sutures in microcephaly is failure of growth of the underlying brain. Infants with primary craniosynostosis almost always have a normal head circumference.

- **Microcephaly syndromes associated with non-CNS anomalies**
  - **Cornelia de Lange syndrome\*** (MIM 122470)
    - Both autosomal and X-linked forms exist.
    - Five cohesin genes are known to date, most common being *NIPBL*
  - **Neu–Laxova syndrome** (MIM 256520)
    - Autosomal recessive defects in the serine biosynthetic pathway cause this characteristic multiple anomaly lethal syndrome.
      - Severe brain changes and cataracts distinguish this from **Harlequin ichthyosis** (MIM 242500).
    - Clinical features: profound microcephaly with lissencephaly, severe hydrops, dramatic swelling of hands and feet, severe ichthyotic skin changes, cataracts (see Figure 5.4)
  - **Dubowitz syndrome** (MIM 223370)
    - Autosomal recessive; responsible gene unknown. Many "look alike" disorders.
    - Clinical features: pre- and postnatal growth deficiency, severe eczema of face and flexural areas, unusual face somewhat similar to that of fetal alcohol spectrum disorder\* (Figure 15.3)
      - Recurrent infections suggest immunodeficiency.
  - **Smith–Lemli–Opitz syndrome\*** (MIM 270400)
    - Autosomal recessive multiple malformation syndrome, caused by defect in cholesterol biosynthesis pathway
    - Clinical features: low birth weight, microcephaly, characteristic face and variable clinical course

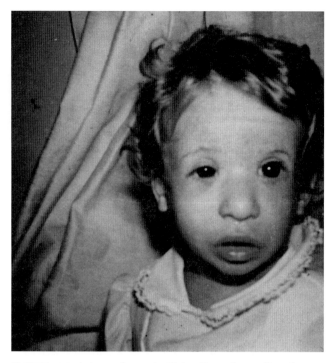

FIGURE 15.3 Autosomal recessive Dubowitz syndrome. One of sibs with severe microcephaly, ptosis, and eczema, all classical characteristic features.

- **Microcephaly with or without chorioretinopathy, lymphedema, or mental retardation** (MIM 152950)
  - Autosomal dominant disorder, caused by heterozygous variants in *KIF11*
  - Clinical features: congenital microcephaly, chorioretinopathy, also retinal folds, microphthalmia, lymphedema of dorsa of the feet
- **Microcephaly with chorioretinopathy** (MIM 251270)
  - Autosomal recessive disorder, caused by biallelic variants in *TUBGCP6*
- **Microcephaly capillary malformation syndrome** (MIC-CAP, MIM 614261)
  - Autosomal recessive disorder caused by biallelic variants in *STAMBP*
  - Clinical features: severe progressive microcephaly, refractory epilepsy, profound developmental delay, multiple small capillary malformations over the body
    - Variable dysmorphic facial features, distal limb abnormalities with nail hypoplasia, mild cardiac defects

- **MICROCEPHALY DUE TO TERATOGENS**
  - **Fetal alcohol spectrum disorder\***
    - Reduction in head circumference in severely affected infants
  - **TORCH infections**, especially CMV, rubella
  - **Zika virus infection**

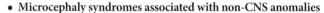

(A)

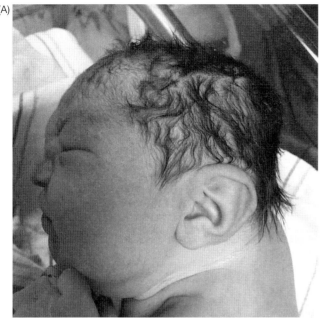

(B)

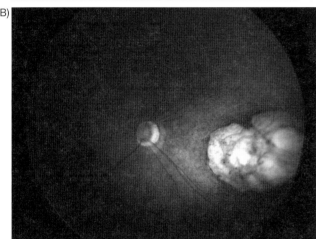

FIGURE 15.4 (A) Congenital Zika infection in an infant with severe microcephaly with redundant frontal scalp skin and occipital prominence. (B) Optic atrophy and macular abnormalities in congenital Zika infection. SOURCE: Courtesy of Derick Holt, MD. Eye-Q Vision Care- Fresno, California.

- Maternal infection with Zika virus associated with disruptive CNS abnormalities, including congenital microcephaly. Mean HC at birth 29 cm
- Prenatal findings
  - Microcephaly on fetal US in the third trimester
  - Fall off in fetal HC in the mid- to late second trimester
- Clinical features: variable microcephaly, redundant scalp folds and body folds (Figure 15.4A), severe optic nerve and macular abnormalities (Figure 15.4B), joint contractures ~11%, seizures, spasticity
  - Cranial imaging: ventriculomegaly, gyral abnormalities, enlarged cisterna magna, intracranial calcifications

- Follow CDC and WHO guidelines for diagnostic testing and reporting: http://www.cdc.gov/zika/index.html.
  - **Maternal HIV**
    - Head circumference is lower in offspring of untreated HIV-positive mothers than in offspring of unaffected mothers; some are microcephalic with ID.
    - There is no clear evidence for microcephaly in offspring of HIV-positive mothers treated with antiretroviral medications.
  - **Maternal phenylketonuria**
    - Consider when there is more than one affected sib with microcephaly, especially in the presence of cardiac defects.
      - Diagnose with history of no dietary control: confirm with maternal serum phenylalanine level.
  - **Maternal hyperthermia**
    - May cause microcephaly when hyperthermia is severe and untreated, usually in late first and early second trimester
  - **Maternal methylmercury toxicity**
    - Methylmercury is neurotoxic at high levels.
    - Low to moderate consumption of fish is not associated with adverse outcomes.
- **MICROCEPHALY DUE TO CNS DISRUPTIVE EVENTS IN PREGNANCY**
  - IUFD of MZ co-twin
  - In utero vascular events cause hydranencephaly and schizencephaly. Porencephaly is due to early third trimester middle cerebral artery infarction.
    - Causes may include congenital infection such as CMV or Zika virus or rarely maternal trauma.
  - Autosomal dominant variants in *COL4A1* and *COL4A2* cause small vessel disease that can result in hydrocephaly, porencephaly, or microcephaly, as well as stroke and seizures.
  - Other rare autosomal recessive disorders are reported with severe microcephaly and a clinical appearance of brain disruption.

## Evaluation and Testing

- Obtain detailed pregnancy history: trauma, twins, fetal US head measurements/anomalies.
- Document teratogenic exposures: alcohol, methylmercury, hyperthermia, rash, illnesses, travel to Zika endemic areas.
- Document family history: consanguinity, other affected infants, maternal PKU.
- Measure head twice around largest circumference and graph per gestational age; calculate standard deviation. https://simulconsult.com/resources/measurement.html?type=head Evaluate fontanels and sutures.
- Measure parental head circumferences.

- Document perinatal asphyxia or lack of it with blood gases, signs of multi-organ failure, Apgar scores.
  - Order placental histology when there is IUGR or history of twins.

Evaluate dysmorphic features, eye findings, and other congenital anomalies.

- Perform cranial imaging to identify structural CNS malformations, disruptive lesions, and migrational abnormalities.
  - Brain MRI: preferred for structural CNS anomalies
  - Head ultrasound: limited value, especially if the fontanelles are closed or small
  - Head CT: useful for calcifications
- Laboratory studies
  - Chromosome microarray
  - Viral studies
    - TORCH and LCMV titers and urine for CMV, include TORCH titers on mother
    - Zika virus testing in mother and neonate
  - Metabolic testing
    - With hypotonia and cerebellar hypoplasia, test for the congenital disorders of glycosylation, especially Congenital Disorder of Glycosylation type II.
      - Order both N- and O-glycosylation testing and/or exome sequencing.
    - Quantitative urine organic acids and plasma lactate
    - 7-Dehydrocholesterol level, if Smith–Lemli–Opitz syndrome suspected
    - Maternal phenylalanine, if siblings also have microcephaly and/or congenital heart defects
    - Methylmercury level, if exposure is suggestive
  - Molecular testing
    - Single gene testing for specific syndromes when clinical diagnosis is clear
    - Primary autosomal recessive microcephaly gene panel should be considered if brain MRI is consistent: small brain with simplified gyral patterning.
    - Exome sequencing test for syndromic, complex, and atypical microcephaly phenotypes
    - See Genetic Testing Registry website for availability of specific gene testing: http://www.ncbi.nlm.nih.gov/gtr

- If financial constraints or unsure as to best test, bank DNA for future testing; early death may preclude later testing.
  - Collect blood in EDTA (lavender top) tube; send for DNA extraction.
- Obtain photographs and autopsy (including brain and eyes) in the event of demise.
  - Where available, utilize regional pediatric neuropathology service.

*Pearl*: In an emergency, collect blood on newborn screening filter paper; place in zippered plastic bag; freeze for later use.

# Further Reading

Ashwal S, Michelson D, Plawner L, Dobyns WB; Quality Standards Subcommittee of the American Academy of Neurology and the Practice Committee of the Child Neurology Society. (2009) Practice parameter: Evaluation of the child with microcephaly (an evidence-based review): Report of the Quality Standards Subcommittee of the American Academy of Neurology and the Practice Committee of the Child Neurology Society. Neurology. 73:887–97. PMID 19752457

de Munnik SA, Hoefsloot EH, Roukema J, et al. (2015) Meier–Gorlin syndrome. Orphanet J Rare Dis. 10:114. PMID 26381604

DeBrosse SD, Okajima K, Zhang S, et al. (2012) Spectrum of neurological and survival outcomes in pyruvate dehydrogenase complex (PDC) deficiency: Lack of correlation with genotype. Mol Genet Metab. 107:394–402. PMID 23021068

Del Campo M, Ribeiro EM, et al.; Zika Embryopathy Task Force-Brazilian Society of Medical Genetics ZETF-SBGM. (2017) The phenotypic spectrum of congenital Zika syndrome. Am J Med Genet A. 173:841–57. PMID 28328129

Faheem M, Naseer MI, Rasool M, et al. (2015) Molecular genetics of human primary microcephaly: An overview. BMC Med Genomics. 8(Suppl. 1):S4. PMID 25951892

Khetarpal P, Das S, Panigrahi I, Munshi A. (2015) Primordial dwarfism: Overview of clinical and genetic aspects. Mol Genet Genomics. 291:1–15. PMID 26323792

Namavar Y, Barth PG, Poll-The B, Baas F. (2011) Classification, diagnosis and potential mechanisms in pontocerebellar hypoplasia. Orphanet J Rare Dis. 6:50. PMID 21749694

Naveed M, Kazmi SK, Amin M, et al (2018) Comprehensive review on the molecular genetics of autosomal recessive primary microcephaly (MCPH). Genet Res (Camb). 100:e7. PMID 30086807

# 16

# Cerebellar Anomalies

## Clinical Consult

A newborn male, with congenital hydrocephalus and hypotonia, fed poorly. He had mildly dysmorphic facial features, a large brachycephalic head, broad forehead, hypertelorism, midface hypoplasia, thin lips, and low-set ears. The genetics consultant noted biparietal scalp alopecia (Figure 16.1A). A brain MRI revealed absence of the cerebellar vermis, continuity of the cerebellar hemispheres across the midline, rhombencephalosynapsis (Figure 16.1B), and aqueductal stenosis. The diagnosis of **Gomez–Lopez–Hernandez syndrome** was made on clinical grounds because no responsible gene has been identified. This is a rare, under-recognized condition that should be considered whenever the cardinal sign, rhomboencephalosynapsis, is present. Biparietal alopecia and reduced corneal sensitivity are specific and useful signs.

## Definition

- Congenital cerebellar disorders in the newborn include dysgenesis, hypoplasia, and malformation of the cerebellar hemispheres and/or vermis and Dandy–Walker malformation (DWM). Brainstem anomalies are common.
  - Neurodegenerative cerebellar disorders and spinocerebellar ataxias are not included here.
  - For extensive reviews of pediatric cerebellar disorders, see Poretti et al. (2014) and Klein et al. (2016).
- Incidence 1/4,000–5,000 live births
- Nonspecific features of cerebellar dysgenesis in the newborn
  - Hypotonia,* spasticity
  - Apnea, tachypnea, episodic panting
  - Abnormal eye movements, oculomotor apraxia, ptosis, visual inattentiveness, nystagmus
  - Feeding problems, aspiration
  - Seizures
- Cerebellar lesions can be isolated, associated with other brain malformations, or syndromic.
  - Neuroimaging is essential.
- **Isolated Dandy–Walker malformation** (DWM, MIM 220200)

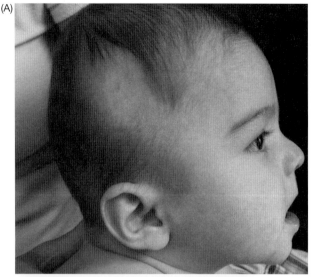

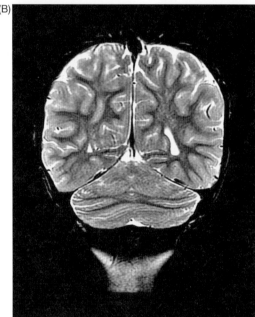

FIGURE 16.1 (A) This boy with Gomez–Lopez–Hernandez syndrome has parietal alopecia, which is a cardinal sign of this disorder. Note the low-set ears. (B) This brain MRI shows absence of the cerebellar vermis and rhomboencephaloosynapsis in Gomez-Lopez-Hernandez syndrome.

o Incidence ~1/10,000 (United Kingdom)
o Usually sporadic
  ▪ Low recurrence risk: 1–5%
o Etiology
  ▪ Chromosome anomalies: ~50%
  ▪ Monogenic in a small proportion: *FOXC1, ZIC1, ZIC4*
o Clinical features: hypoplasia or aplasia of the cerebellar vermis, malposition (elevation) of cerebellum, enlarged posterior fossa and cystic dilatation of the fourth ventricle. Cerebral hemisphere hypoplasia, hydrocephaly and other brain malformations in 30–50%

  ▪ Corpus callosum agenesis
  ▪ Encephalocele
  ▪ CNS migration anomalies
  ▪ ID in ~50%
• Etiology
  o Nongenetic: prematurity, hypoxic–ischemic injury, vascular events (hemorrhage), CMV, herpes infection, teratogenic

*Pearl:* Isolated unilateral cerebellar hypoplasia is often caused by an in utero cerebellar hemorrhage or other vascular disruption. It has a low recurrence risk.

  o Genetic: chromosome anomalies, metabolic and malformation syndromes, sporadic somatic mutations
• Chromosome anomalies
  o Aneuploidy: **Down syndrome,\* trisomies 9, 13,\* 18\***
  o Deletions: 1p36, 3q, 5p\* (cri du chat syndrome), 6p25 (with optic disc colobomas), 13q
  o Duplications: 3q, 17p13.3, Xq28
• Teratogens\*
  o Prenatal exposures: **alcohol,\* cocaine, retinoic acid, misoprostol, valproic acid, other anticonvulsant medications**
  o Congenital infections: **herpes, CMV, Zika virus**

## Differential Diagnosis

• **SYNDROMES WITH UNILATERAL CEREBELLAR HYPOPLASIA**
  o **Familial porencephaly** (MIM 175780)
    ▪ Autosomal dominant trait, caused by heterozygous pathogenic variant in *COL4A1, COL4A2*
    ▪ Clinical features: usually unilateral porencephaly, cerebellar hypoplasia, or atrophy, due to vascular occlusion, hemiplegia, seizures
  o **Osteogenesis imperfecta XV** (MIM 615220)
    ▪ Autosomal recessive disorder, due to biallelic *WNT1* pathogenic variants
    ▪ Variable ID, often severe; extreme short stature
  o **PHACE association** (*p*osterior fossa brain malformations, *h*emangioma of the head or neck, *a*rterial defects of the head or neck, *c*ardiac defects, and *e*ye anomalies, MIM 606519)
    ▪ Sporadic, likely somatic mutation
      • No causative gene
    ▪ 1 M:8 F; female preponderance (Figure 41.4)
    ▪ Clinical features: posterior fossa anomalies, usually unilateral cortical dysgenesis, arachnoid cyst, hemangiomas of the head and neck, sternal anomalies, coloboma, glaucoma, microphthalmia, optic nerve hypoplasia, cardiac defects

- **SYNDROMES WITH DWM**
  - **Cranio-cerebello-cardiac syndrome** (3C syndrome, Ritscher–Schinzel syndrome, MIM 220210)
    - Genetically heterogeneous
      - Biallelic pathogenic variants in *KIAA0196* among Canadian First Nations; other genes unknown
      - Microdeletion 6p25 may produce a similar phenotype.
    - Clinical features: cerebellar hypoplasia, vermis hypoplasia, DWM, macrocephaly, brachycephaly, prominent forehead, hypertelorism, down-slanting palpebral fissures, coloboma, cleft palate, cardiac defects (especially septal defects) (Figure 16.2)
  - **Meckel syndrome** (Meckel–Gruber syndrome, MIM 249000)
    - Lethal autosomal recessive ciliopathies, caused by pathogenic variants in *MKS1* and other genes
    - Clinical features: DWM; hydrocephalus; holoprosencephaly; occipital encephalocele 60–80%; large, cystic, dysplastic kidneys >95%; hepatic portal fibrosis; post-axial polydactyly 80%; bowed long bones; cardiac defects (Figure 26.2)
  - **Walker–Warburg syndrome** (muscle–eye–brain disease, Fukuyama muscular dystrophy, MIM 236670) and other muscular dystrophy α-dystroglycanopathies
    - Autosomal recessive disorders with variable muscle, eye, and brain anomalies; many responsible genes: *POMT1, POMT2, POMGNT1, FKTN, FKRP, LARGE, ISPD, GTDC2*
    - Clinical features: hydrocephalus, DWM, dysplastic, cystic, cobblestone-type lissencephaly, corpus callosum anomalies, seizures, microphthalmia, optic nerve hypoplasia, retinal dysplasia, cataract, coloboma, hypotonia
      - Creatine kinase markedly elevated

- **METABOLIC DISORDERS WITH CEREBELLAR ANOMALIES**
  - **Adenylosuccinase deficiency** (MIM 103050)
    - Autosomal recessive disorder, due to biallelic pathogenic variants in *ADSL*, causes an enzymatic defect in de novo purine synthesis
    - Clinical features: fatal neonatal encephalopathy, lack of spontaneous movement, intractable seizures, respiratory failure
      - Succinylpurines (SAICAr, S-Ado) in CSF, plasma, urine
  - **Congenital disorder of glycosylation, type 1a** (MIM 212065)
    - Autosomal recessive carbohydrate-deficient glycoprotein disorders. CDGIa, the most severe form, with a neonatal onset, is caused by biallelic pathogenic variants in *PMM2*.
    - Clinical features: olivopontocerebellar atrophy, encephalopathy, hypotonia, retinal degeneration, strabismus, roving eye movements, inverted nipples, decreased or abnormal fat distribution, cardiomyopathy, hydrops, coagulopathy, hepatopathy, stroke-like episodes, seizures, failure to thrive, poor feeding
      - Abnormal transferrin electrophoresis
  - **Carnitine palmitoyltransferase II deficiency** (CPT2, MIM 600649)
    - Autosomal recessive fatty acid oxidation disorder, caused by biallelic pathogenic variants in *CPT2*
    - Clinical features: lethargy, respiratory arrest, seizures
      - Arrhythmia following febrile illness
      - Elevated acylcarnitines, elevated liver enzymes, low plasma carnitine
  - **Smith–Lemli–Opitz syndrome*** (MIM 270400)
    - Autosomal recessive malformation syndrome, due to pathogenic variants in *DHCR7*, causes impaired cholesterol biosynthesis

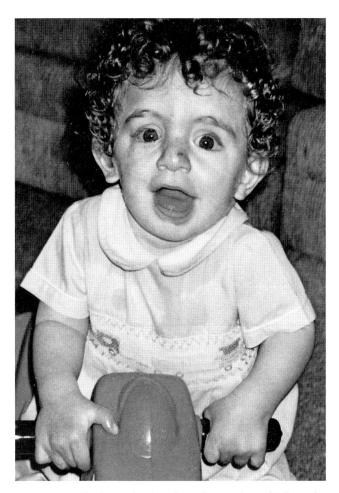

FIGURE 16.2 This boy with 3C syndrome has tetralogy of Fallot and Dandy Walker malformation, cardinal signs of this disorder. Note macrocephaly, brachycephaly, wide forehead, and down-slanting palpebral fissures.

- Clinical features: hypotonia, cleft palate, polydactyly, CNS and cardiac anomalies, ambiguous genitalia in males (Figure 27.3)
  - Elevated 7-dehydrocholesterol
- o **Zellweger syndrome** (cerebrohepatorenal syndrome, MIM 214100)
  - Prototypic autosomal recessive peroxisomal biogenesis disorder, caused by biallelic pathogenic variants in *PEX* genes
  - Clinical features: weak suck, hypotonia, CNS and cardiac anomalies, hepatomegaly, renal cysts; features overlap neonatal adrenoleukodystrophy and infantile Refsum disease; early lethality (Figure 1.4)
    - Elevated very long-chain fatty acids
- o Other metabolic disorders: **copper metabolism disease** (*SLC33A1*; MIM 614482), mitochondrial disorders (Leigh disease, **pyruvate dehydrogenase deficiency**, MIM 256000), **molybdenum cofactor deficiency** and **isolated sulfite oxidase deficiency** (MIM 252150), **mucopolysaccharidoses** (types I and II), **nonketotic hyperglycinemia** (MIM 605899)

*Pearl*: Pathogenic variants in more than 15 X-linked genes have been implicated in cerebellar hypoplasia.

- • **X-LINKED CEREBELLAR DISORDERS**
  - o **Microcephaly with pontine and cerebellar hypoplasia** (MIM 300749)
    - Heterozygous pathogenic variant or deletion in *CASK*, primarily affects females
    - Clinical features: pontocerebellar hypoplasia, dilated fourth ventricle, microcephaly, hypotonia, seizures, broad nasal bridge, large ears, micrognathia, hypertelorism, sensorineural hearing loss
  - o **Opitz G/BBB syndrome** (MIM 300000)
    - Pathogenic variant in *MID1*
    - Clinical features: hypertelorism, cleft lip/palate, esophageal abnormality, imperforate anus, hypospadias
  - o **Oral-facial-digital syndrome, type 1** (MIM 311200)
    - X-linked dominant ciliopathy, caused by heterozygous pathogenic variant in *OFD1*; lethal in males
    - Clinical features: CNS 40%, alopecia, milia on the face, midline cleft lip/palate (Figure 11.6), multiple hyperplastic oral frenulae, cleft alveolar ridge, lobulated tongue, polydactyly, syndactyly, polycystic kidneys
  - o **X-linked intellectual disability with cerebellar hypoplasia** (MIM 300486)
    - Pathogenic variant or deletion of *OPHN1* at Xq12; females can be mildly symptomatic
    - Clinical features: cerebellar hypoplasia, posterior vermis agenesis, dilated cerebral ventricles, hypotonia, strabismus, early onset seizures, ID

- • **OTHER CEREBELLAR SYNDROMES**
  - o **COACH syndrome** (MIM 216360)
    - Autosomal recessive ciliopathy, associated with pathogenic variants in *TMEM67, CC2D2A, RPGRIP1L*
    - Clinical features: cerebellar vermis hypo/aplasia, congenital ataxia, coloboma, hepatic fibrosis
  - o **Gomez–Lopez–Hernandez syndrome** (cerebello–trigeminal–dermal dysplasia, MIM 601853; see Clinical Consult)
    - Sporadic condition; no identified genetic cause
    - Clinical features: rhomboencephalosynapsis (fusion of the cerebellar hemispheres), absent cerebellar vermis, agenesis of septum pellucidum, hydrocephalus, hypotonia, dysmorphic features, biparietal scalp alopecia, trigeminal anesthesia (corneal opacities are secondary to diminished sensation), head shaking and figure-eight head movements, occasional VATER/VACTERL spectrum anomalies (Figure 16.1)
  - o **Joubert syndrome** (MIM 213300)
    - Autosomal recessive ciliary defects, caused by biallelic pathogenic variants in >20 genes
    - MRI features: cerebellar vermis hypoplasia/dysplasia, polymicrogyria, agenesis of the corpus callosum
      - Molar tooth sign on brain MRI (Figure 16.3) is diagnostic: elongated superior cerebellar peduncles and

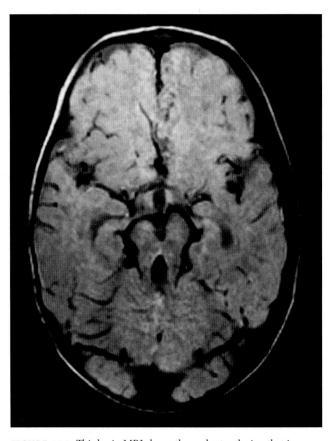

FIGURE 16.3 This brain MRI shows the molar tooth sign that is characteristic of Joubert syndrome.
SOURCE: Courtesy of Dr. Ghayda Mirzaa, University of Washington, Seattle, WA.

abnormally deep interpeduncular fossa. Note that a molar tooth sign can be seen in other related ciliopathy syndromes: COACH syndrome (MIM 216360), Senior-Loken syndrome (MIM 266900), Varadi-Papp syndrome (Oro-facial-digital syndrome, type VI, MIM 277170).

- ■ Clinical features: encephalocele, oculomotor apraxia, retinal dystrophy, coloboma, alternating episodes of apnea and hyperventilation, cystic kidneys, nephronophthisis, polydactyly, hypotonia.

- ○ **Pancreatic and cerebellar agenesis** (MIM 609069)
  - ■ Autosomal recessive trait, caused by biallelic pathogenic variants in *PTF1A*
  - ■ Clinical features: hypoplasia or agenesis of cerebellum and/or vermis, optic nerve hypoplasia, flexion contractures, talipes equinovarus, severe IUGR, triangular face, small chin. Agenesis of the pancreas causes neonatal diabetes mellitus and meconium ileus.

- ○ **Pontocerebellar hypoplasias** (PCH, MIM 607596)
  - ■ Severe autosomal recessive neurodegenerative disorders of the brainstem and cerebellum
    - • Heterogeneous—10 major types
      - • Homozygous recurrent pathogenic variant in *TSEN54*, p.A307S, occurs in >50%, causing a flat "dragonfly" cerebellum with preserved vermis on MRI coronal views.
      - • Type 1, PCH1B (MIM 614678), with anterior horn cell disease and joint contractures, is caused by pathogenic variants in *EXOSC3*.
      - • No molecular diagnosis in 35–40%
  - ■ Clinical features: hypoplasia and dysplasia of cerebellum and pons, hypotonia, weakness, spasticity, clonus, contractures, extrapyramidal dyskinesia, chorea, dystonia, microcephaly, progressive cortical atrophy, optic atrophy, seizures, poor feeding

## Evaluation and Management

- • Obtain pregnancy history: illness, medication use, teratogens, toxins, trauma.
- • Document family history: consanguinity, X-linked inheritance pattern.
- • Evaluate for distinctive features to narrow differential diagnosis (e.g., biparietal alopecia).
  - ○ Ophthalmology evaluation, echocardiogram, and abdominal US
  - ○ Hearing assessment as soon as practical
- • Brain MRI: Neuroimaging is key.

- ○ Request sufficient cuts to identify or rule out molar tooth sign. When a molar tooth sign is present, consider Joubert syndrome or a related ciliopathy.
- • Perform gene testing as indicated by the differential diagnosis.
  - ○ Chromosome microarray
  - ○ Gene panels or genomic testing may be the most cost-effective strategies, but careful phenotyping is essential to chose the appropriate test.
- • Other laboratory studies
  - ○ Very long-chain fatty acids (peroxisomal disorders), creatine kinase, liver enzymes, carnitine, isoelectric focusing of transferrin, lactate, pyruvate, acylcarnitine panel, 7-dehydrocholesterol, plasma amino acids (quantitative; for glycine), and urine organic acids (quantitative)
  - ○ Creatine kinase is elevated in Walker–Warburg syndrome, cobblestone-type lissencephaly
  - ○ Elevated glucose and absent insulin levels suggest *PTF1A*-related cerebellar and pancreatic agenesis.

## Further Reading

Cotes C, Bonfante E, Lazor J, et al. (2015) Congenital basis of posterior fossa anomalies. Neuroradiol J. 28:238–53. PMID 26246090

Doherty D, Millen KJ, Barkovich AJ. (2013) Midbrain–hindbrain malformations: Advances in clinical diagnosis, imaging, and genetics. Lancet Neurol. 12:381–393. PMID 23518331

Elliott AM, Simard LR, Coghlan G, et al. (2013) A novel mutation in KIAA0196: Identification of a gene involved in Ritscher–Schinzel/3C syndrome in a First Nations cohort. J Med Genet. 50:819–22. PMID 24065355

Klein JL, Lemmon ME, Northington FJ, et al. (2016) Clinical and neuroimaging features as diagnostic guides in neonatal neurology diseases with cerebellar involvement. Cerebellum Ataxias. 3:1. PMID 26770813

Namavar Y, Barth PG, Poll-The BT, Baas F. (2011) Classification, diagnosis and potential mechanisms in pontocerebellar hypoplasia. Orphanet J Rare Dis. 6:50. PMID 21749694

Poretti A, Boltshauser E, Doherty D (2014) Cerebellar hypoplasia: Differential diagnosis and diagnostic approach. Am J Med Genet C Semin Med Genet. 166C:211–26. PMID 24839100

Rudnik-Schöneborn S, Barth PG, Zerres K. (2014) Pontocerebellar hypoplasia. Am J Med Genet C Semin Med Genet. 166C:173–83. PMID 24924738

Scott K, Gadomski T, Kozicz T, Morava E. (2014) Congenital disorders of glycosylation: New defects and still counting. J Inherit Metab Dis. 37:609–617. PMID 24831587

Tully HM, Dempsey JC, Ishak GE, et al. (2012) Beyond Gómez–López–Hernández syndrome: Recurring phenotypic themes in rhombencephalosynapsis. Am J Med Genet A. 158A:2393–406. PMID 22965664

Zanni G, Bertini ES. (2011) X-linked disorders with cerebellar dysgenesis. Orphanet J Rare Dis. 6:24. PMID 21569638

# 17

# Holoprosencephaly

## Clinical Consult

A genetics consultation was requested on a four month old female infant to appease a nurse who suspected Down syndrome. The patient had been admitted for dehydration and hypernatremia without a history of vomiting or diarrhea. As a term female infant, she had been admitted briefly to the NICU for mild respiratory distress and hypernatremia. She responded to IV hydration and was discharged on day 3. At 4 months of age, she had her first upper respiratory tract infection and slept through her usual nighttime feedings. When she was lethargic the next morning, her mother took her to the emergency department. Her urine output never diminished, and her mother recalled that she had several wet diapers while she was evaluated there . . .

The geneticist noted microcephaly, hypotelorism, and a flat midface (Figure 17.1). When the geneticist held her glasses under the baby's nose, there was condensation from only one nostril. She could not pass a number 6 French nasogastric tube on the obstructed side. All urine samples were dilute (specific gravity <1.005), even when fluids were restricted for several hours. Her findings suggested diabetes insipidus (DI), which can cause dehydration and recurrent hypernatremia. **Lobar holoprosencephaly** (HPE) was diagnosed on brain MRI.

Even mild unexplained hypernatremia in the newborn should be investigated. In this patient, it was the first sign of DI and HPE. Her oral intake was sufficient to maintain hydration until she fell behind on her feedings with her first cold. The facial phenotype associated with lobar HPE may be mild. In this case, her nurse recognized subtle dysmorphic facial features and appropriately raised concern.

*Pearl*: Choanal atresia and congenital nasal pyriform aperture stenosis are often seen in holoprosencephaly.

## Definition

- Holoprosencephaly (HPE, MIM 236100) is caused by failure of the prosencephalon to divide into two hemispheres between days 18 and 28 of gestation.
- Incidence 1/10,000 live births
  - Occurs in 1/250 conceptions, but most do not survive

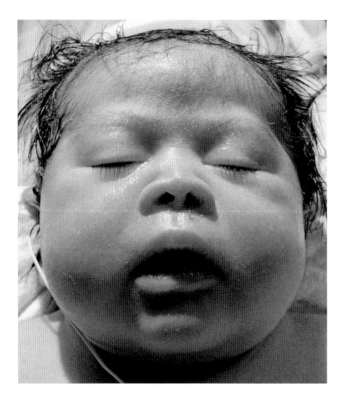

FIGURE 17.1 Hypotelorism and frontal bossing in an infant with lobar holoprosencephaly. Note the smooth upper lip that lacks the cupid's bow shape.

- 2 M:3 F, females predominate
- A specific genetic cause can be found in 80–90%.
- A multiple-hit model is widely accepted: a combination of environmental factors and pathogenic variants in the major and minor HPE genes causes the disorder, accounting for the range of severity even within the same family.
- Recurrence risk for sporadic case: 13–14%
  o Higher risk when family history is positive for HPE or related findings
- In familial HPE, incomplete penetrance and variable expressivity are common.
  o Up to one-third of gene carriers are clinically unaffected.
- The diagnosis is established with brain imaging, preferably MRI.
- Anatomic types are listed from most to least severe:
  o Alobar: monoventricle, no separation of the thalami
    ■ Most severe; two-thirds of all cases
    ■ Cebocephaly: hypotelorism, single-nostril nose
    ■ Ethmocephaly: hypotelorism, with proboscis
    ■ Cyclopia: single or fused eyes
    ■ Other variants, difficult to classify, occur.
  o Semilobar: frontal and parietal lobes fused hemispheres divided posteriorly but not anteriorly
  o Lobar: hemispheres fused ventrally, splenium and corpus callosum present
  o Middle interhemispheric variant: absent body of the corpus callosum

o Microforms exist in patients as well as relatives who do not have gross brain malformations: small HC, hypotelorism, anosmia, solitary median maxillary central incisor (SMMCI) (Figure 17.2), absent midline maxillary frenulum.

*Pearl*: When HPE is suspected but MRI brain images are normal, review the images for maxillary tooth buds to detect SMMCI. This microform of HPE is often overlooked by radiologists. Examine parents for SMMCI and other microforms to identify families with autosomal dominant HPE.

- Associated brain anomalies
  o Microcephaly ~50%
  o Hydrocephalus
  o Absent corpus callosum
  o Absent ophthalmic, olfactory tracts
  o Absent septum pellucidum
  o Pituitary dysfunction, DI
- Craniofacial anomalies 80%
  o "The face predicts the brain."
    ■ Severe facial features predict severe CNS malformation in ~80%.
  o Eye spacing and anomalies: hypotelorism (may be the only eye feature in mild cases); coloboma, microphthalmia (may be severe), cyclopia and proboscis
  o Nasal airway obstruction: choanal atresia or congenital pyriform aperture stenosis
  o Nasal depression: absent or hypoplastic columella or premaxilla, absent ethmoid bone

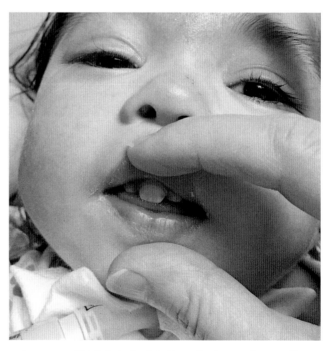

FIGURE 17.2 This infant of a diabetic mother has a solitary median maxillary central incisor. Maternal diabetes is a major risk factor for holoprosencephaly and its microforms.

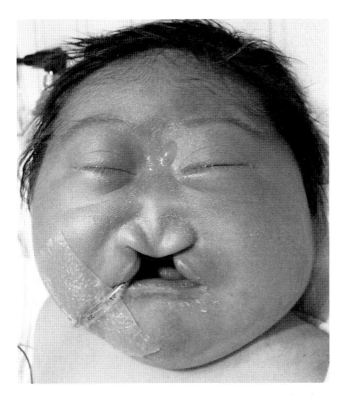

FIGURE 17.3 The premaxilla and nasal septum, which are induced by midline structures in the brain, are absent in this infant with microcephaly and holoprosencephaly.

- Oral cavity
  - Median or typical cleft lip
  - Agenesis or hypoplasia of premaxilla (Figure 17.3)
  - SMMCI
  - Absent midline upper maxillary frenulum

*Pearl*: An absent midline upper (maxillary) frenulum is a reliable sign in both severe and mild forms of HPE.

- Sequelae: developmental delay, pituitary dysfunction, seizures
- Prognosis varies with the severity of the lesion and the etiology.
  - Alobar form: Survival beyond infancy is rare.
  - Lobar form: >40% of survivors ambulate, speak, and use their hands.
  - Abnormal chromosomes: Only 2% survive >1 year.
  - Normal chromosomes: 30–50% survive >1 year.

# Differential Diagnosis

- Nonsyndromic, isolated HPE
  - Single gene variants account for ~25% of HPE.
    - Point mutations are more likely in live-borns; microdeletions are more likely in fetuses.

- Most are autosomal dominant with incomplete penetrance.
  - Five major genes cause ~25% of isolated HPE; most pathogenic variants are de novo.
    - *SHH* ~6%
      - Often with SMMCI and microforms
      - In autosomal dominant HPE families, pathogenic variants in *SHH* are the most common: 37%.
    - *ZIC2* ~5%
      - Face is less severely affected, often semilobar HPE
      - 70% de novo
    - *GLI2* ~3%
      - SMMCI and other microforms are more common than full HPE; hypopituitarism.
    - *SIX3* ~3%
      - Associated with alobar HPE
    - *FGF8* ~2%
      - Semilobar HPE and microforms
    - Many other genes are less commonly involved: *TGIF* 1%, and *DISP1, FAST1, FOXH1, HPE6, NODAL, PTCH1, STIL, TDGF, TMEM1*.
- Chromosome anomalies are the most common cause of HPE: 30–50% of live-born.
  - Aneuploidy and balanced translocations or inversions
    - **Trisomy 13** over half of chromosome anomalies in HPE
    - **Trisomy 18**
    - **Klinefelter syndrome** (47,XXY)
    - **Triploidy** (69,XXX, 69,XXY)
    - Translocations, inversions, deletions
  - Microarray abnormalities (copy number variants, CNV)
    - CNV: 20–25%
    - ≥12 chromosome regions are associated with HPE.
      - Del 1q41, del 2p21, dup 3p24-ter, dup 5q35.1, del 7q36.3 (*SHH*), del 8p, del 13q (*ZIC2*), del 18p (*TGIF*), ring 18, del 21q22.3, del 22q11.2
- Teratogenic agents 10–15% of HPE
  - Maternal disorders
    - **Maternal diabetes mellitus** in the first trimester
      - Risk for HPE in the infant of a diabetic mother is 1–2%, 100× the general population risk.
      - The most likely cause of HPE when chromosomal analysis is normal
    - Maternal infections: rare—CMV, toxoplasma, rubella
  - **Fetal alcohol spectrum disorder**: HPE is rare with heavy and early exposure (OR 2.0; Croen et al., 2000).
  - Tobacco: Cigarette smoking increases risk for HPE (OR 4.1).
    - Higher risk when cigarette smoking occurs with alcohol consumption (OR 5.4; Croen et al., 2000)
  - Retinoic acid (isotretinoin) and vitamin A derivatives: HPE is rare.
  - Cholesterol-lowering statins: Human data are inconclusive, and risk is low.

(A)

(B)

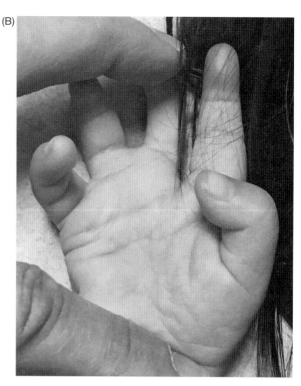

FIGURE 17.4 (A) This girl with Hartsfield syndrome has holoprosencephaly with digital anomalies. Note her tall forehead, frontal upsweep of hair and poorly defined cupid's bow of the upper lip. (B) There is a mild cleft in her right hand between her index and middle fingers and partial syndactyly of the middle and ring fingers.

- Monogenic syndromes cause ~25% of HPE.
  - Approximately 25 multiple congenital anomaly syndromes include HPE.
  - **Hartsfield syndrome** (MIM 615465)
    - Autosomal dominant disorder caused by heterozygous pathogenic variant in *FGFR1*
    - Clinical features: HPE, microcephaly, hypertelorism, cleft lip and palate, ectrodactyly, absent digits, syndactyly (Figure 17.4)
  - **Holoprosencephaly polydactyly syndrome** (pseudotrisomy 13 syndrome, MIM 264480)
    - Lethal rare, heterogeneous condition, more common in fetuses
    - Autosomal recessive disorder, likely a ciliopathy
      - Pathogenic variants in *RPGRIP1L*, a gene associated with primary cilia, were found in two fetuses from one family (CJC, unpublished results).
    - Clinical features: similar to **Meckel syndrome** but kidneys are normal; HPE, posterior encephalocele, exencephaly, postaxial polydactyly, anomalies of eyes, heart, genitalia (Figure 17.5)
  - **Meckel syndrome** (Meckel–Gruber syndrome, MIM 249000)
    - Autosomal recessive ciliopathy, usually lethal in newborns
    - Overlaps with other ciliopathy syndromes, including **Joubert syndrome**

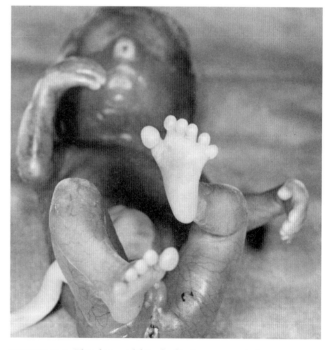

FIGURE 17.5 This deceased fetus had holoprosencephaly, cebocephaly, microphthalmia, omphalocele, and postaxial polydactyly of the left hand and foot. Chromosome analysis was normal, 46,XY. His consanguineous parents had a prior pregnancy with a similarly affected male fetus.
SOURCE: Reprinted with permission from the Journal of Medical Genetics (J Med Genet 1990;27:50–52).

- Biallelic pathogenic variants in *MKS1* cause Meckel type 1; approximately 12 genes are implicated in other Meckel syndrome subtypes.
- Clinical features: not all classic features need be present, enlarged cystic kidneys, CNS anomalies, occipital encephalocele, hydrocephalus, Dandy–Walker anomaly, postaxial polydactyly, fibrotic liver.
  - **Pallister–Hall syndrome** (MIM 146510)
    - Autosomal dominant disorder, caused by heterozygous pathogenic variant in *GLI3*
    - Most are sporadic; an occasional parent is affected.
    - Clinical features: IUGR, hypothalamic hamartoma, multiple frenulae, central and postaxial polydactyly, nail dysplasia, renal agenesis, imperforate anus, cardiac defects. HPE has been reported in only a few patients.
  - **Smith–Lemli–Opitz syndrome\*** (SLOS, MIM 270400)
    - Autosomal recessive trait, caused by biallelic pathogenic variants in *DHCR7*; affects cholesterol biosynthesis
    - Clinical features: ptosis, cleft palate, cardiac, thumb anomalies, atypical genitalia in males, hypotonia. HPE phenotype ranges from mild to severe.
    - Elevated serum 7-dehydrocholesterol is a diagnostic and reliable finding.

## Evaluation and Management

- Take a pregnancy history: maternal diabetes mellitus, teratogens.
- Document family history: consanguinity, microcephaly, infant death, intellectual disability, multiple congenital anomalies.
- Examine parents for microforms: microcephaly, hypotelorism, anosmia, SMMCI, absent upper maxillary frenulum.
- Prenatal diagnosis can be challenging; false positives occur with ultrasound imaging alone, confirm with postnatal brain MRI.
- Examine patient for associated anomalies: coloboma, choanal atresia, cleft palate, diabetes insipidus or other endocrinopathies, heart defects, renal cysts, limb anomalies, scalp defect, hearing deficits.
- EEG and brain imaging, MRI preferred. Check for SMMCI.
- Order 7-dehydrocholesterol when SLOS is suspected.
- Genetic testing
  - Chromosome microarray is preferred first test.
  - Chromosome analysis is preferred when aneuploidy, such as trisomy 13 or 18, is suspected.

*Pearl*: Approximately 2% of patients with HPE have both a chromosome anomaly and a pathogenic variant/deletion in a single gene. Both chromosome and genetic testing are recommended in all patients with HPE.

- Select a gene panel that is appropriate to the phenotype.
  - *GLI2* is more common in HPE with pituitary anomalies.
  - *SIX3* and *SHH* are more common in HPE with colobomas.
  - *SHH* and *ZIC2* are more common in HPE with GU defects.
  - Consider participation in a NIH-sponsored research protocol for common and more extensive genomic testing (https://clinicaltrials.gov/ct2/show/NCT00088426).
  - When a pathogenic variant or CNV is detected, test parents to determine if it is familial or de novo.
- Offer genetic consultation and counseling.
- Acknowledge widely variable outcomes when discussing prognosis.
  - Development and long-term survival differ by severity of HPE.
- Inform families about support groups: Families for HoPE (https://familiesforhope.org).

## Further Reading

Croen LA, Shaw GM, Lammer EJ. (2000) Risk factors for cytogenetically normal holoprosencephaly in California: A population-based case–control study. Am J Med Genet. 90:320–5. PMID 10710231

Dubourg C, Carré W, Hamdi-Rozé H. (2016) Mutational spectrum in holoprosencephaly shows that FGF is a new major signaling pathway. Hum Mutat. 37:1329–39. PMID 27363716

Dyment DA, Sawyer SL, Chardon JW, Boycott KM. (2013) Recent advances in the genetic etiology of brain malformations. Curr Neurol Neurosci Rep. 13:364. PMID 23793931

Kaliaperumal C, Ndoro S, Mandiwanza T, et al. (2016). Holoprosencephaly: Antenatal and postnatal diagnosis and outcome. Childs Nerv Syst. 32: 801–9. PMID 26767839

Kruszka P, Martinez AF, Muenke M. (2018) Molecular testing in holoprosencephaly. Am J Med Genet. 178C:187–93. PMID 29771000

Mercier S, Dubourg C, Garcelon N, et al. (2011) New findings for phenotype–genotype correlations in a large European series of holoprosencephaly cases. J Med Genet. 48:752–60. PMID 21940735

Petryk A, Graf D, Marcucio R. (2015) Holoprosencephaly: Signaling interactions between the brain and the face, the environment and the genes, and the phenotypic variability in animal models and humans. Wiley Interdisip Rev Dev Biol. 4:17–32. PMID 25339593

Roessler E, Hu P, Marino J, et al. (2018) Common genetic causes of holoprosencephaly are limited to a small set of evolutionarily conserved driver genes of midline development coordinated by TGF-β, hedgehog, and FGF signaling. Hum Mutat. 1416–1427. PMID 29992659

Solomon BD, Gropman A, Muenke M. (2013) Holoprosencephaly overview. In: Adam MP, Ardinger HH, Pagon RA et al. editors. GeneReviews [Internet]. Seattle, WA: University of Washington, Seattle; 1993–2017. PMID 20301702

# 18

# Hydrocephalus

## Clinical Consult

A male infant was born at 36 weeks' gestation by planned cesarean delivery with a head circumference of 52 cm. Other growth parameters were normal. Severe hydrocephalus had been recognized at 19 weeks' gestation. He was the first child of non-consanguineous Hispanic parents. He had ectopic calcifications in the interdigital webs between the thumbs and index fingers and abnormal bone striations with stippled metaphyseal plates (Figure 18.1). After a ventriculoperitoneal shunt was placed, he developed hepatosplenomegaly and a petechial rash that progressed to a generalized erythematous eruption, coalescing over his groin and lower limbs. He had consumptive thrombocytopenia and multiple retinal hemorrhages. C-reactive protein was elevated. CMV IgM was positive, but all CMV cultures were negative. A congenital infection was suspected, but TORCH, LCMV, and RPR studies were normal. In light of the poor prognosis, the parents elected to withdraw care, prior to which blood was obtained for exome sequencing. The diagnosis was made posthumously when gene sequencing revealed a de novo pathogenic variant in *CIAS1/NLRP3* consistent with **neonatal-onset multisystem inflammatory disorder (NOMID)** or chronic infantile neurological cutaneous articular (CINCA) syndrome.

Hydrocephalus, which is not a constant feature of NOMID, occurs when an inflammatory process obstructs CSF flow at the base of the brain. Consider NOMID/CINCA when hydrocephalus or chronic meningitis occurs with a clinical picture that mimics congenital infection.

## Definition

- Hydrocephalus, as used here, refers to a congenital or early infantile pathological accumulation of CSF within the ventricles and subarachnoid spaces of the brain that causes accelerated head growth. It is generally obstructive, progressive, and usually requires surgical intervention.
  - These disorders will not be considered here:
    - Hydrocephalus ex vacuo—primary loss of brain parenchyma with compensatory enlargement of the ventricles, without increased intracranial pressure

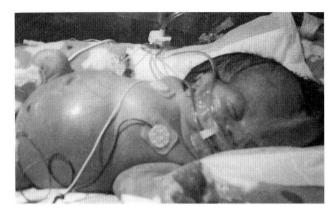

FIGURE 18.1 This infant with neonatal-onset multisystem inflammatory disorder (NOMID) had massive hydrocephaly, retinal hemorrhages, ectopic calcifications, and thrombocytopenia with negative viral studies.

- Hydranencephaly—little brain parenchyma remains after bilateral obstruction of blood flow to the brain
- Porencephaly—a fluid-filled cyst replacing brain parenchyma
- Nonobstructive hydrocephalus—ventricular enlargement due to increased CSF production (e.g., choroid plexus papilloma)
- Communicating hydrocephalus—an obstruction to CSF flow in the subarachnoid space (e.g., hemorrhage, sinovenous thrombosis, CNS tumors, intracranial teratoma)
- Incidence 3/1,000 live births
  o 2.6 M:1 F, males predominate
- Risk factors
  o Maternal obesity, hypertension, preeclampsia, diabetes mellitus, low socioeconomic status
- Etiology
  o Among those without a clear etiology, approximately one-third are nonsyndromic and two-thirds are syndromic.
    - Overall, ~20% have a known cause; in the syndromic group, 29%.
  o Genetic factors contribute to both syndromic and nonsyndromic hydrocephalus.
    - Recurrence risk for first-degree relatives: 6%
    - The risk is higher with maternal transmission, suggesting X-linked inheritance in some cases.
    - Family history positive: 3–11%
  o Chromosome anomalies
    - Microarray abnormality ~25% of fetuses prenatally diagnosed with ventriculomegaly; percentage varies with the severity of the lesion and other anomalies
      - Isolated ventriculomegaly: 9.5%
      - Ventriculomegaly with other congenital anomalies: 37.9%
      - Severe ventriculomegaly >15 mm: 66%
      - Deletions: 1p36, 2q37, 6p, 6q

- Trisomy 9
- Diploid/triploid mosaicism, triploidy

## Differential Diagnosis

### Nonsyndromic Hydrocephalus Due to Extrinsic and Acquired Causes

- Hemorrhage, including microhemorrhage, most common cause
  o Prematurity, neonatal alloimmune thrombocytopenia, maternal vitamin K deficiency (can be secondary to hyperemesis gravidarum, gastric bypass surgery), trauma
  o Mutations in *COL4A1* and *COL4A2* can cause prenatal hemorrhage.
- Teratogens*: isotretinoin, maternal diabetes*, misoprostol
- In utero infection: CMV, toxoplasmosis, enterovirus, LCMV, parvovirus B19, mumps, parainfluenza, Zika virus

### Hydrocephalus with CNS Malformations

- Commonly occurs with Dandy–Walker malformation (Figure 18.2), Chiari I malformation, holoprosencephaly,* rhomboencephalosynapsis, lissencephaly, periventricular polymicrogyria.

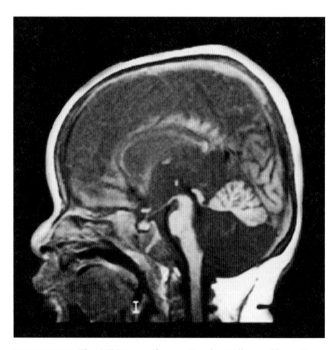

FIGURE 18.2 This MRI image shows a Dandy–Walker malformation with upward displacement of a hypoplastic cerebellum and cystic dilation of the fourth ventricle.
SOURCE: Courtesy of Drs. William Dobyns and Ghayda Mirzaa, University of Washington, Seattle, WA.

- Arachnoid cysts
  - Most are nonsyndromic.
  - They also occur in many genetic syndromes.
    - Orofacialdigital syndrome I (OFD1, MIM 300170)
    - Acrocallosal syndrome (MIM 200990)
    - Pallister–Hall syndrome (MIM 146510)
    - Greig cephalopolysyndactyly (MIM 175700)
  - May be an asymptomatic, incidental finding
- Hydrocephalus with polymicrogyria
  - **Macrocephaly–capillary malformation–polymicrogyria syndrome** (MCAP, MIM 602501)
    - Mosaic disorder, due to somatic, tissue-specific heterozygous pathogenic variant in *PIK3CA*
    - Usually detectable in affected tissue rather than blood
    - Clinical features: megalencephaly, somatic overgrowth, vascular abnormalities, syndactyly, hydrocephalus 46% (Figure 14.3)
  - **Megalencephaly–polymicrogyria–polydactyly–hydrocephalus I** (MPPH, MIM 603387)
    - Autosomal dominant disorder, caused by heterozygous pathogenic variant in *PIK3R2*
      - Other genes in the same pathway are responsible for MPPH2 (*AKT3*) and MPPH3 (*CCND2*).
    - Clinical features: megalencephaly and somatic overgrowth of prenatal onset, hydrocephaly, broad corpus callosum, thick gray matter, polymicrogyria, polydactyly, hypotonia, developmental delay, seizures
      - There is some overlap with MCAP.
- Hydrocephalus with Chiari malformation
  - Neural tube defects (NTDs)*
    - Incidence 1/1,000
    - Multifactorial trait, caused by environmental and genetic factors
    - Some familial cases have pathogenic variants in genes that affect planar cell polarity: *VANGL1, VANGL2, CCL2, FUZ.*
    - Gene testing is not indicated in sporadic isolated NTD.
    - NTDs occur more often in **infants of diabetic mothers*** with pregestational diabetes, obese mothers, and after first trimester exposure to valproic acid.
    - Clinical features: The majority of infants with open spina bifida have hydrocephalus, and most have Chiari II malformation.

## Syndromic Hydrocephalus Without Other Major Non-CNS Anomalies

- **Aqueductal stenosis, X-linked** (MIM 307000)
  - X-linked disorder impacts neural adhesion, caused by hemizygous pathogenic variant in *L1CAM*
    - Accounts for ~10% of all males with congenital hydrocephalus

    - Patients with aqueductal stenosis and a positive family history have a pathogenic variant in ~70%.
    - Test all affected males regardless of family history.
  - Clinical features: aqueductal stenosis, agenesis of the corpus callosum, hypoplasia of corticospinal tracts, hypoplasia of the anterior cerebellar vermis, fused thalami, adducted thumbs
    - **MASA syndrome** (spastic paraplegia 1, MIM 303350) is allelic to X-linked aqueductal stenosis, but it has a later onset with shuffling gait and spasticity.
- **Hydrocephalus, nonsyndromic, autosomal recessive 1** (MIM 236600)
  - Autosomal recessive trait, affects WNT signaling, caused by biallelic pathogenic variants in *CCDC88C*
- **Hydrocephalus, nonsyndromic, autosomal recessive 2** (MIM 603785)
  - Autosomal recessive trait, affects planar cell polarity, caused by biallelic pathogenic variants in *MPDZ*
- **Pettigrew syndrome** (Fried–Pettigrew syndrome, MIM 304340)
  - X-linked syndrome, caused by hemizygous pathogenic variant in *AP1S2* that affects vesicle trafficking
  - Clinical features: highly variable phenotype, hydrocephalus, aqueductal stenosis, Dandy–Walker malformation, callosal abnormalities, periventricular nodular heterotopias, microcephaly, nonspecific dysmorphic features, hypotonia, seizures, mild–profound ID
  - Deposition of iron or calcium in the basal ganglia—may not be visible in infancy

## Syndromic Hydrocephalus with Non-CNS Anomalies

- At least 100 genes have been associated with hydrocephalus. Only a few of these syndromic causes are discussed here.
  - **Achondroplasia*** (MIM 100800)
    - A large head is typical and often raises concern for hydrocephaly. (Figure 8S.2)
    - True hydrocephalus occurs in ≤5% and rarely in the newborn period.

*Pearl*: Ventriculomegaly can be a normal finding in achondroplasia. Consult specific growth charts for normal range of ventricle size in achondroplasia.

    - Foramen magnum stenosis: no consensus that this is a common cause of hydrocephalus in achondroplasia
    - Stenosis of the jugular foramen: causes increased intracranial pressure and hydrocephalus
  - Ciliopathies associated with hydrocephalus
    - **COACH syndrome** (MIM 216360)
      - Autosomal recessive disorder, associated with pathogenic variants in three ciliary genes: *TMEM67, CC2D2A, RPGRIP1L*

- Clinical features: cerebellar vermis hypo-/aplasia, congenital ataxia, coloboma, hepatic fibrosis
  - **Hydrolethalus 1** (MIM 236680)
    - Autosomal recessive disorder, caused by biallelic pathogenic variants in *HYLS1*
    - Clinical features: polydactyly and CNS anomalies, primarily hydrocephalus; similar to Meckel syndrome but lacks cystic renal and hepatic changes
  - **Joubert syndromes 2 and 9** (JBTS2, MIM 608091; JBTS9 612285)
    - Autosomal recessive conditions, caused by biallelic pathogenic variants in *TMEM216* (JBTS2) and *CC2D2A* (JBTS9)
    - Clinical features: "molar tooth" sign on brain MRI (Figure 16.3), cerebellar vermis hypo-/aplasia, polydactyly, retinal anomalies, hepatic fibrosis, renal cysts. Hydrocephalus is infrequent.
  - **Meckel syndrome** (MIM 249000)
    - A group of autosomal recessive ciliopathies caused by biallelic pathogenic variants in at least a dozen genes that cause ciliary dysfunction
    - Clinical features: occipital encephalocele and other CNS anomalies, not primarily hydrocephalus, cystic renal disease, hepatic abnormalities, portal fibrosis, polydactyly, usually postaxial (Figure 26.2)
  - **Short rib thoracic dysplasia polydactyly syndrome 14** (MIM 616546)
    - Lethal autosomal recessive disorder, due to biallelic pathogenic variants in *KIAA0586*
    - Clinical features: hydrocephalus, occipital bone defect, tongue hamartoma, cleft palate, poly-/syndactyly and other skeletal defects, narrow thorax
- **Craniosynostosis\*** syndromes associated with hydrocephalus
  - The risk for hydrocephalus is highest in multiple suture synostoses and in **Crouzon syndrome** (MIM 123500).
  - Cloverleaf skull, which has many syndromic causes, is often accompanied by hydrocephalus.
  - **Loeys–Dietz syndrome I** (MIM 609192)
    - Autosomal dominant aortic aneurysm syndrome with arterial tortuosity and systemic involvement, caused by heterozygous pathogenic variant in *TGFBR1* and other related genes
    - Hydrocephalus occurs in 15%.
  - **Shprintzen–Goldberg syndrome** (MIM 182212)
    - Autosomal dominant trait, due to heterozygous pathogenic variant in *SKI*
    - Severe progressive musculoskeletal phenotype and ID
    - Hydrocephalus uncommon
- **Fanconi anemia, complementation group B** (MIM 300514)
  - X-linked disorder, caused by hemizygous pathogenic variant of *FANCB*

- Clinical features: affects males with a similar spectrum of anomalies as VACTERL-H association, hydrocephalus. Anemia develops in later childhood.
- Increased chromosome breakage is detected with diepoxybutane.
- **Neonatal-onset multisystem inflammatory disorder** (NOMID, chronic infantile neurological cutaneous articular [CINCA], MIM 607115; see Clinical Consult)
  - Autosomal dominant syndrome, caused by a heterozygous pathogenic variant in *CIAS1/NLRP3*, which encodes cryopyrin
    - Mutations in ~50%; most are de novo.
    - Somatic mosaicism occurs in the "mutation negative" group.
  - This is a cryopyrinopathy, an autoinflammatory disorder of inflammatory cytokines and their receptors, mimicking congenital infection.
  - Clinical features: rash, fever, arthropathy, skeletal changes; aseptic chronic meningitis obstructs CNS flow causing prenatal hydrocephalus. (Figure 18.1)
  - Therapy with IL-1 blocking agents (anakinra/Kineret, rilonacept/Arcalyst, canakinumab/Ilaris) should be started as soon as possible, even before genetic studies are complete. Consult with pediatric rheumatology.
- **Noonan syndrome\*** (MIM 163950) and related disorders
  - Autosomal dominant defect, a RASopathy, caused by heterozygous pathogenic variant in *PTPN11* and other genes in the pathway
  - Clinical features: excess nuchal skin; webbed neck; cardiac anomalies, especially pulmonic stenosis, hypertrophic cardiomyopathy. Characteristic facial features: hypertelorism, down-slanting palpebral fissures. Hydrocephalus related to cervical stenosis, Arnold–Chiari malformation, syringomyelia
  - Related disorders in the RAS/MAP-kinase pathway, such as **cardiofaciocutaneous syndrome** (MIM 115150), have similar features. Hydrocephalus is reported occasionally.
- **VATER association with hydrocephalus** (MIM 276950)
  - Rare autosomal recessive disorder, caused by biallelic pathogenic variants in *PTEN*
  - Clinical features: tracheoesophageal fistula, radial ray hand anomalies, macrocephaly, hydrocephaly
- **Walker–Warburg syndrome** (hydrocephalus, agyria, retinal dystrophy with or without encephalocele [HARD+/–E], muscle–eye–brain disease, Fukuyama congenital muscular dystrophy, MIM 236670, 613155, 609308)
  - A frequently lethal group of autosomal recessive dystroglycanopathies. More than 11 genes have been identified: *POMT1, POMT2, POMGNT1, B3GNT1, FKTN, FKRP, ISPD* and *GTDC2, B3GALNT2, LARGE* and *DAG1*, and others.

- Clinical features: abnormal brain migration, cobblestone lissencephaly, cerebellar hypoplasia, congenital muscular dystrophy (elevated creatine kinase level)
  - Eye abnormalities: cataracts, shallow anterior chamber, microcornea, microphthalmia, lens defects, retinal detachment or dysplasia, hypoplasia or atrophy of the optic nerve and macula and coloboma, glaucoma
  - Poor prognosis
- Other dystroglycanopathies cause hydrocephalus: **Peters plus syndrome** (MIM 261540), **lissencephaly 5** (MIM 615191), **congenital disorder of glycosylation type Is** (MIM 300884).

*Pearl*: Order a creatine kinase in any infant with hydrocephalus of unknown etiology. When it is strikingly elevated, it suggests Walker–Warburg syndrome or a related disorder.

- ○ **X-linked heterotaxy** (MIM 306955) and **X-linked VACTERL association** (MIM 314390)
  - Both X-linked conditions are caused by hemizygous pathogenic variant in *ZIC3*.
  - Clinical features: overlapping phenotypes, complex cardiac defects, situs ambiguous, imperforate anus, branchial arch defects, vertebral anomalies, radial ray anomalies, agenesis of kidneys, sacral anomalies. Hydrocephalus is variable.
- ○ **X-linked lissencephaly with abnormal genitalia** (MIM 300215)
  - An X-linked disorder of brain migration, caused by a hemizyygous pathogenic variant in *ARX*.
  - Clinical features: hydrocephaly, lissencephaly with a posterior to anterior gradient, intractable, agenesis corpus callosum, hydranencephaly, early onset seizures, males are severely affected, undermasculinized male external genitalia. (Figure 18.3)

## Evaluation and Management

- Take pregnancy history: illness, travel, infection, trauma, alcohol, medication use. Ask about rashes, fevers, ill contacts, contact with animals or rodent-infested areas, occupational exposures (farm work, pet store), or high-risk habits such as eating raw meat and handling cat litter.
- Document family history: consanguinity, affected relatives with hydrocephalus (note sex of affected individuals to identify X-linked pedigrees), macrocephaly, intellectual disability, cerebral palsy, or infant death.
- Examine for associated anomalies.
  - ○ Consult ophthalmology for suspected congenital infection to document retinal changes or hemorrhage and to rule out cataracts or other helpful ocular findings.

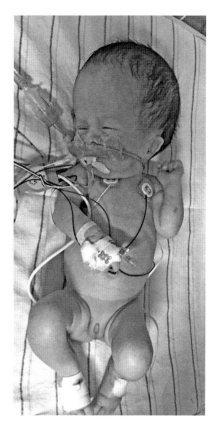

FIGURE 18.3 This male with hydranencephaly and genital hypoplasia has a pathogenic variant in *ARX*. He had a similarly affected brother, who died in infancy. His mother is an unaffected carrier.

- Imaging studies
  - ○ Head US is not adequate for detailed assessment of CNS anatomy.
  - ○ Brain MRI is preferred.
- Laboratory studies
  - ○ Creatine kinase level (Walker–Warburg syndrome and other dystroglycanopathies)
  - ○ Serology and cultures for TORCH, parvovirus, Zika, and congenital lymphocytic choriomeningitis virus
- Genetic studies
  - ○ Chromosomal microarray routinely
  - ○ Perform chromosome breakage studies (with diepoxybutane [DEB]) to rule out Fanconi anemia whenever VATER/VACTERL syndrome with hydrocephalus is suspected.
  - ○ Perform *L1CAM* gene analysis for aqueductal stenosis in a male or in either sex with a positive family history consistent with X-linked transmission.
  - ○ Consider skin biopsy for gene analysis when suspecting syndromes due to somatic mosaic mutations. Biopsy an affected area if dermatologic/pigmentary changes are present.
  - ○ Other gene testing, gene panels, or exome sequencing may be indicated for syndromes or patterns of malformation that elude clinical diagnosis.

# Further Reading

Anderson JL, Levy PT, Leonard KB, et al. (2014) Congenital lymphocytic choriomeningitis virus: When to consider the diagnosis. J Child Neurol. 29:837–42. PMID 23666045

Cacciagli P, Desvignes JP, Girard N, et al. (2014) AP1S2 is mutated in X-linked Dandy–Walker malformation with intellectual disability, basal ganglia disease and seizures (Pettigrew syndrome). Eur J Hum Genet. 22:363–8. PMID 23756445

Kalyvas AV, Kalamatianos T, Pantazi M, et al. (2016) Maternal environmental risk factors for congenital hydrocephalus: A systematic review. Neurosurg Focus. 41:E3. PMID 27798989

Kousi M, Katsanis N. (2016) The genetic basis of hydrocephalus. Annu Rev Neurosci. 39:409–35. PMID 27145913

Munch TN, Rostgaard K, Rasmussen ML, et al. (2012) Familial aggregation of congenital hydrocephalus in a nationwide cohort. Brain. 135:2409–15. PMID 22763745

Paccaud Y, Berthet G, Von Scheven-Gête A, et al. (2014) Neonatal treatment of CINCA syndrome. Pediatr Rheumatol Online J. 12:52. PMID 25584041

Tully, HM, Dobyns WB. (2014) Infantile hydrocephalus: A review of epidemiology, classification and causes. Eur J Med Genet. 57:359–68. PMID 24932902

Tully HM, Ishak GE, Rue TC, et al. (2016) Two hundred thirty-six children with developmental hydrocephalus: Causes and clinical consequences. J Child Neurol. 31:309–20. PMID 26184484

Verhagen JM, Schrander-Stumpel CT, Krapels IP, et al. (2011) Congenital hydrocephalus in clinical practice: A genetic diagnostic approach. Eur J Med Genet. 54:e542–7. PMID 21839187

# 19

# Neural Tube Defects

## Clinical Consult

A newborn girl had a lumbosacral meningomyelocele and a Chiari II malformation. Her primigravida 25-year-old mother had been treated for many years for bipolar manic episodes with Depakote (divalproex sodium) at 1,000 mg/day with reasonably good results. She had no prenatal care until 25 weeks' gestation, when Depakote was discontinued. A fetal ultrasound revealed the NTD and hydrocephalus. At 3 months, her repaired NTD was well healed. She had a long, poorly grooved philtrum and a thin upper vermillion border consistent with **valproate embryopathy syndrome** (Figure 19.1).

Depakote was approved by the U.S. Food and Drug Administration for bipolar disorder in 1995 and is still widely used for this and other indications in women of childbearing age. The risk for an NTD (almost always spina bifida) is 10–20× greater than in the general population and is not reduced by supplemental folic acid. Drugs of lower teratogenic potential, such as Lamictal, are recommended for treating bipolar disorder in women of childbearing age. Depakote should be the drug of last resort in women during their reproductive years.

## Definition

- Neural tube defects result from failure of fusion of the neural folds into a tube in the first 28 days of gestation.
  - An "open" NTD is not skin-covered; a "closed" NTD is skin-covered.
- Types of NTDs
  - Anencephaly (MIM 206500): Absence of most of the brain, skull, and scalp, a lethal disorder, results from failure of fusion of the cranial portion of the neural tube.
    - Intrauterine fetal demise (23%) and intrapartum death (35%) are common among ongoing pregnancies with anencephaly.
    - Live-born infants with anencephaly have median survival of less than 1 hour, ranging to 8 days (Obeidi et al., 2010).
  - Meningomyelocele, or spina bifida (SB): herniation of spinal cord and meninges through a vertebral defect, after

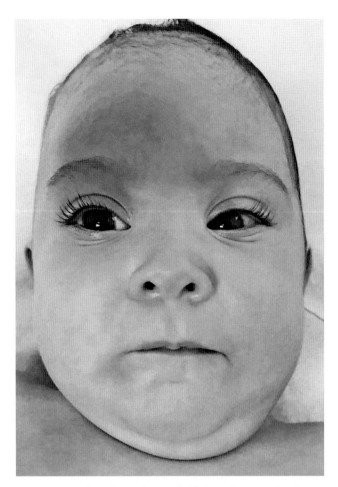

FIGURE 19.1 This infant with spina bifida has a thin upper lip, flat vermillion border, and long shallow philtrum—features consistent with the history of first trimester exposure to valproic acid.

failure of fusion of the thoracic, lumbar, or sacral portion of the neural tube

- Chiari II hindbrain malformation ~90%. The cerebellum develops in a small posterior fossa and herniates through the foramen magnum. Midbrain is distorted in 65%.
- Corpus callosal dysgenesis occurs in one-third.

o Meningocele: herniation of CSF-filled meninges, without neural elements, through a vertebral defect; typically skin-covered or "closed"

o Encephalocele: protrusion of brain and meninges through an anterior, parietal, or posterior skull defect. Prognosis varies with the size and contents of the encephalocele sac (Figure 19.2).

- A small occipital meningocele with alopecia, that does not include brain parenchyma, usually has a good prognosis (Figure 19.3)

o Sacral agenesis: lack of sacral or lumbar spine and caudal spinal cord, variable bowel and bladder innervation

o Anterior meningocele: rare spinal dysraphism; meninges protrude into retroperitoneal and presacral area through an anterior, usually sacral defect

- Infection (meningitis), constipation, urinary incontinence, or neurologic signs

o Occult spinal dysraphism: deficiency of ≥2 vertebral arches, often with overlying flat hemangioma, tuft of hair or lipoma (Figure 19.4)

- Spinal cord may be tethered.

o Complex lethal NTDs

- Craniorachischisis, a rare disorder (1/100,000 in the United States), occurs when the entire neural tube fails to fuse.
- Iniencephaly occurs with a closed cranium, an enlarged foramen magnum, a retroflexed spine, and absent neck. Spina bifida with or without encephalocele may accompany the defect.

o Spina bifida occulta: common, asymptomatic vertebral defect from which meninges do not protrude

- Common: 10–20% of the general population
- Considered a normal variant, does not confer a significant risk for serious types of NTDs

- Incidence 1/1,000 in the United States; 3,000 babies per year are born with an NTD.
- Prevalence varies with ethnicity, geography, diet, and socioeconomic level.

o Highest prevalence: Egypt, India, Northern China, Northern Ireland ≤8/1,000 live births

o Hispanics in the United States and Latin America have a higher prevalence of NTDs (anencephaly and SB) compared to non-Hispanics.

- Hispanics 1.2/1,000; non-Hispanic Caucasians 0.96/1,000; Blacks and Asians: 0.75/1,000 (California)

o Females predominate in isolated, nonsyndromic NTDs.

- Anencephaly 4 F:1 M

- Positive family history: 5%

o Isolated nonsyndromic NTD: 70–80% of all NTDs

- Typically sporadic, with multifactorial, non-Mendelian inheritance pattern, implicating both genetic and environmental risk factors
  - Recurrence risk—2–4% after one affected child
  - Recurrence risk—12% after two affected children
- Rare families have X-linked (MIM 301410) or autosomal recessive NTD (MIM 206500)

o Syndromic NTD—20%

- Causes vary and recurrence risk is determined by diagnosis: chromosomal, teratogenic, maternal disorders, single gene disorders.

- Prenatal diagnosis

o Highest prenatal detection rate: maternal serum α-fetoprotein (MSAFP) test combined with fetal US

- Elevated MSAFP detects 90% of "open" NTDs.
  - "Closed" or skin covered NTDs cannot be detected by MSAFP screening.
- Fetal US: In experienced hands, virtually all anencephalic fetuses and >90% of SB are detected.

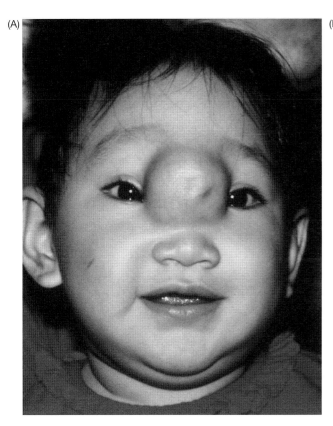

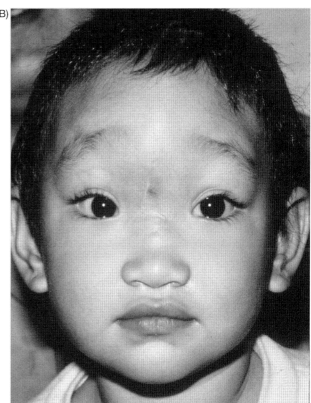

FIGURE 19.2 (A) A toddler with a nasal encephalocele. (B) The same child after surgery.

○ Prenatal US findings of SB: vertebral splaying, ventriculomegaly, banana sign—inferior displacement of the cerebellum, lemon sign   bifrontal narrowing of the skull
  ■ Fetal US may not distinguish between fetuses with isolated NTDs and those with associated anomalies.

● Prenatal US detected 73% of associated anomalies that were found at autopsy in fetuses with NTDs (Ekin et al., 2014).
○ Chromosome abnormalities: 2–10% of fetuses with isolated NTDs
  ■ Anencephalic fetuses without other anomalies have fewer chromosome anomalies—2%.
  ■ Fetuses with SB and associated anomalies have more—27%.

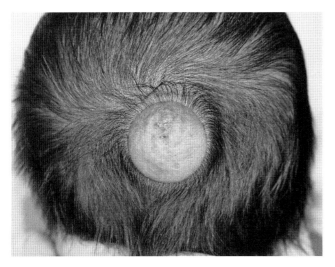

FIGURE 19.3 This small occipital defect did not include brain parenchyma. Note the well-formed "halo" of scalp hair around the encephalocele.

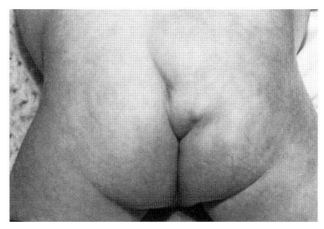

FIGURE 19.4 A lipoma overlies an occult neural tube defect.

*Pearl*: Trisomy 18 syndrome can, uncommonly, present prenatally as an apparently isolated NTD.

- ○ In a randomized prospective trial, in utero repair of meningomyelocele reduced postnatal shunts and improved motor development at 30 months but increased prematurity and uterine dehiscence at delivery (MOMS: Management of Meningomyelocele Study).
    - No significant benefit when lateral ventricle exceeded 15 mm
    - Criteria for fetal surgery: singleton pregnancy, upper limit of the spine lesion between T1 and S1, gestational age 19–26 weeks, normal fetal karyotype, Chiari II malformation by fetal MRI, no fetal anomaly unrelated to SB, maternal BMI < 35
- Associated non-CNS malformations: oral clefts, musculoskeletal, GI (imperforate anus), renal (renal agenesis, bladder exstrophy), genital and cardiac anomalies (Parker et al., 2014)
    - ○ Non-CNS anomalies occur more often with encephalocele (38%) than with anencephaly (11%) or SB (24%).
- Risk factors
    - ○ Known risk factors contribute to <50% of cases.
        - In the United States, for SB, maternal diabetes and obesity jointly account for 10% of cases.
        - In the United States, for anencephaly, Hispanic ethnicity is the major factor, contributing to 15% of cases.
    - ○ Twins increase the risk for anencephaly (OR 3–5).
        - Concordance for anencephaly is higher in MZ twins.
        - Twins conceived by ART may have a higher risk compared to spontaneously conceived twins.
    - ○ Positive family history of NTD
    - ○ Variants in the folate metabolism pathway (MIM 601634)
    - ○ Maternal smoking, active or passive smoking
    - ○ Maternal hyperthermia (hot tub, sauna use), RR 2
    - ○ Maternal dietary deficiency of micronutrients: folate, vitamin $B_{12}$, zinc, inositol, or elevated plasma homocysteine
    - ○ Maternal pregestational diabetes*
    - ○ Maternal history of gastric bypass
    - ○ Maternal pregestational obesity
        - Prepregnancy BMI >29 kg/m², RR 1.5–3.5
- Periconceptional folic acid dietary supplementation reduces the occurrence and recurrence of anencephaly and SB up to 70%.
    - ○ Food fortification is the most effective strategy to prevent NTDs, reducing mostly isolated forms by ≤50%.
    - ○ Not all NTDs are folate sensitive (MIM 182940).
        - Isolated NTDs—30% are not responsive to folic acid
        - Syndromic NTDs
        - Encephaloceles
        - Inositol prevents folate-resistant NTDs in the mouse. Human studies (PONTI study: Prevention of Neural Tube Defects Through Inositol) are in progress.

# Differential Diagnosis

- An NTD that occurs with other anomalies can be caused by chromosome anomalies, single gene disorders, maternal conditions, or teratogenic exposures.
    - ○ Chromosome anomalies
        - Aneuploidy: **trisomy 13,** * **18,** * **21,** * triploidy
        - **Deletion 22q11.2 syndrome*** (MIM 188400)
            - Meningomyelocele has been reported with **atypical distal deletions of 22q11.2** (MIM 611867) between low copy repeat areas C and D (Leoni et al., 2014).
        - Structural anomalies (inversions), microdeletions (1p36), and duplications (Lynch, 2005)
            - Anencephaly with holoprosencephaly has been reported together in association with **ring chromosome 18**.
    - ○ Environmental and teratogenic exposures
        - **Maternal pregestational diabetes***—risk increases with first trimester $HbA_{1c}$.
        - **Valproic acid exposure**: 1–2% risk for SB (see Clinical Consult)
            - Risk increases with rising dose of valproic acid (>750 mg/day) and with polytherapy.
            - Risk for anencephaly does not appear to be increased.
        - **Carbamazepine exposure** slightly increases the risk for SB—0.2%.
        - **Methotrexate** and other folate antagonists—aOR 6.5 for NTDs
        - **Warfarin embryopathy** causes encephalocele in ~10% of affected patients.
        - Maternal consumption of **mycotoxins** (fumonisins) in contaminated cornmeal in early pregnancy
            - In mice, there is a dose–response relationship between maternal fumonisin exposure and NTD rate.
    - ○ Disorders causing syndromic anencephaly
        - **Amniotic band sequence** and **Limb–body wall complex** sometimes involve attachment of the placenta to the open skull defect.
    - ○ Single gene disorders causing isolated NTDs
        - In mice, mutations in >200 genes cause NTDs (*Pax3, T (brachyury)*), but few have been identified in affected humans (Agopian et al., 2013).
        - Maternal genes associated with hyperglycemia and insulin resistance and fetal genes involved in glucose homeostasis may interact to increase the risk of NTDs.
        - Genes responsible for planar cell polarity have a role in neural tube closure and are being studied in humans with folate-resistant NTDs (*VANGL1* and *VANGL2*, MIM 182940).
    - ○ Disorders causing syndromic SB
        - **Currarino syndrome** (MIM 176450)
            - Autosomal dominant form of sacral dysgenesis, caused by heterozygous pathogenic variant in *MNX1*

- Clinical features: hemisacral vertebral defect with a "sickle" shape on radiographs, anorectal malformation, presacral mass, anterior meningocele, hydronephrosis, tethered cord, constipation
  - Often concordant in twins: MZ > DZ
- **Omphalocele–exstrophy–imperforate anus–spinal defects complex** (OEIS, MIM 258040)
  - Sporadic and rare
    - Rare recurrent CNVs: dup 22q11.21.
  - Clinical features: extensive lower abdominal wall defect, exstrophy of the cloaca and bladder, musculoskeletal defects, genital malformations, spinal defects with or without meningomyelocele, imperforate anus, omphalocele
    - NTDs in 90%; may be occult
- **Waardenburg syndrome, type 1** (MIM 193500)
  - Autosomal dominant disorder of neural crest, caused by pathogenic variant or deletion of *PAX3*
    - Responsible for 2% of apparently isolated NTDs
  - Clinical features: white forelock, hypopigmentation, heterochromia, hypertelorism, telecanthus (dystopia canthorum), deafness 20%, spina bifida
- Disorders causing syndromic encephalocele
  - **Adams–Oliver syndrome** (MIM 100300)
    - Autosomal dominant disorders with variable expression, caused by a heterozygous pathogenic variant in *ARHGAP31, RPBJ, NOTCH1,* or *DLL4*
      - Autosomal recessive forms are caused by biallelic pathogenic variants in *DOCK6* and *EOGT.*
    - Clinical features: aplasia cutis of the scalp can extend into the cranium, limb defects, syndactyly, amputations, cardiac defects 20%, pulmonary hypertension (Figure 30.3)
      - Rarely, presents as anencephaly/exencephaly and limb defects.
  - **Amniotic band sequence** (MIM 217000)
    - Encephalocele/exencephaly due to early attachment of cranium to the placenta
  - **Frontonasal dysplasia** (MIM 136760)
    - Most commonly sporadic, caused by homozygous pathogenic variants in *ALX3*
      - Up to seven subtypes of frontonasal dysplasia, some with mutations in *ALX1* (FDN3) and *ALX4* (FDN2)
    - Clinical features: anterior cranium bifidum, widow's peak, ocular hypertelorism, broad nasal bridge, midline facial cleft of the nose, upper lip and palate, notching of alae nasi, frontal (sphenoethmoidal) encephalocele, lipoma of the corpus callosum, intranasal dermoid
  - **Knobloch syndrome** (MIM 267750)
    - Autosomal recessive trait, caused by biallelic pathogenic variants in *COL18A1*

- Clinical features: ocular anomalies, congenital myopia, lens dislocation, retinitis pigmentosa, retinal detachment with or without occipital encephalocele, skull defect, cutis aplasia
  - **Meckel–Gruber syndrome** (MIM 249000)
    - Severe autosomal recessive trait, caused by biallelic pathogenic variant s in *MKS1*, interferes with function of primary cilia during embryogenesis
      - At least 12 subtypes, including *TMEM216, TMEM67, RPGRIP1L, CEP290*
    - Clinical features: postaxial or preaxial polydactyly, renal cysts, hepatic fibrosis, occipital encephalocele, Dandy–Walker malformation (Figure 26.2)
  - **Walker–Warburg syndrome** (MIM 236670)
    - Autosomal recessive congenital muscular dystrophy, caused by bialleic pathogenic variants in *POMT1* and other dystroglycanopathy genes
    - Clinical features: various brain and eye anomalies including hydrocephaly, occipital encephalocele, lissencephaly, cerebellar and retinal anomalies

# Evaluation and Management

- Obtain pregnancy history: dietary deficiencies, teratogens (especially valproic acid, carbemazepine), smoking, maternal diabetes mellitus, gastric bypass, obesity.
- Take a family history: consanguinity and affected relatives.
- When spina bifida is prenatally diagnosed, offer early in utero repair.
- Evaluate for associated anomalies: e.g. hypopigmentation in Waardenburg syndrome.
  - Eye exam, echocardiogram, renal US
- Perform neurosurgical evaluation and detailed neuroimaging.
- Anticipate and manage neurogenic bladder and bowel during intial hospitalization.
- Genetic testing
  - Chromosome analysis when trisomy is suspected; otherwise microarray.
  - Gene analysis (sequencing and deletion/duplication testing) should be guided by the differential diagnosis.
  - Consider exome sequencing when multiple congenital anomalies do not suggest a particular syndrome.
- Counsel parents regarding 3% recurrence risk. Recommend daily maternal multivitamin with additional folic acid supplementation (4 mg/day) beginning several months prior to each future pregnancy and continuing through the first trimester to reduce recurrence risk.
- Refer to multidisciplinary spina bifida clinic.
- Refer parents to patient support groups and other resources for spina bifida.

o http://spinabifidaassociation.org
o https://www.cdc.gov/ncbddd/spinabifida/index.html
- Refer syndromic NTD for genetic counseling.

## Further Reading

Agopian AJ, Tinker SC, Lupo TJ, et al.; National Birth Defects Prevention Study. (2013) Proportion of neural tube defects attributable to known risk factors. Birth Defects Res A Clin Mol Teratol. 97:42–6. PMID 23427344

Copp AJ, Adzick NS, Chitty LS, et al. (2015) Spina bifida. Nat Rev Dis Primers. 1:15007. PMID 27189655

Ekin A, Gezer C, Taner CE, et al. (2014) Chromosomal and structural anomalies in fetuses with open neural tube defects. J Obstet Gynaecol. 34:156–9. PMID 24456437

Hull S, Arno G, Ku CA, et al. (2016) Molecular and clinical findings in patients with Knobloch syndrome. JAMA Ophthalmol. 134:753–62. PMID 27259167

Leoni C, Stevenson DA, Geiersbach KB, et al. (2014) Neural tube defects and atypical deletion on 22q11.2. Am J Med Genet A. 164A:2701–6. PMID 25123577

Lynch SA. (2005) Non-multifactorial neural tube defects. Am J Med Genet C Semin Med Genet. 135C:69–76. PMID 15800854

Obeidi N, Russell N, Higgins JR, O'Donoghue K. (2010) The natural history of anencephaly. Prenat Diagn. 30:357–60. PMID 20198650

Parker SE, Yazdy MM, Mitchell AA, et al. (2014) A description of spina bifida cases and co-occurring malformations, 1976–2011. Am J Med Genet A. 164A:432–40. PMID 24357196

Peranteau WH, Adzick NS. (2016) Prenatal surgery for myelomeningocele. Curr Opin Obstet Gynecol. 28:111–18. PMID 26866841

Toru HS, Sanhal CY, Uzun OC, et al. (2016) Associated anomalies with neural tube defects in fetal autopsies. J Matern Fetal Neonatal Med. 29:798–802. PMID 25800566

# 20

# Perinatal Arterial Stroke

## Clinical Consult

A term male, born to an 18-year-old primigravida, developed seizures at 24 hours of age. His birth was complicated by prolonged ruptured membranes, a long second stage of labor, and high birth weight (LGA). Vacuum extraction was successful with one gentle pull. Birth weight was 3800 g, with a head circumference of 37.5 cm. Apgar scores were 3 and 7 at 1 and 5 minutes, respectively. The placenta was discarded. Seizures were controlled with phenobarbital. The infant remained lethargic and fed poorly. He breathed spontaneously in ambient air without other complications. Brain CT, at 36 hours of age, revealed a moderately large nonhemorrhagic ischemic infarct in the distribution of the left middle cerebral artery. At 3 months, he was seizure-free, feeding well, and smiling with mild hypertonicity, R > L. A follow-up brain CT revealed unilateral ventricular dilation and a large area of porencephaly. A genetic evaluation for thrombophilia in mother and infant was negative.

**Perinatal arterial stroke** is often the result of cumulative per inatal risk factors; in this case, possible contributors included a long second stage of labor, prolonged rupture of the membranes, and LGA with macrocephaly. An uncomplicated vacuum extraction is unlikely to affect stroke risk. This infant is at high risk for neurocognitive sequelae including hemiparesis, developmental delay and visual issues. The appropriate thrombophilia evaluation, is important, albeit controversial, because a thrombophilic factor in mother or infant or both may affect management. The chance for another stroke for the infant or parents is low (but not zero), and in the absence of thrombophilia, recurrence risks for an adverse outcome in another pregnancy are also low.

## Definition

- Perinatal arterial stroke (PAS) occurs between 28 weeks' gestation and 7 days of life. Some studies use a broader time frame of 20 weeks' gestation to 28 days of life.
- Incidence ~1/4,000 live births and is stable despite increased use of fetal monitoring and liberal utilization of Cesarean section.
  - o Mostly in term infants
- **Etiology**

○ Most commonly accepted cause for ischemic stroke is embolic with placental thrombi entering the fetal circulation via a patent foramen ovale (PFO) and reaching the circle of Willis through the left side of the heart via the carotid arteries.
- Recurrence risk for perinatal stroke ~1%
- Three main types of perinatal stroke
  ○ Arterial ischemic stroke (PAS) ~70%
  ○ Hemorrhagic stroke 20%
  ○ Cerebral sinus venous thrombosis (CSVT) 10%
- **Risk factors**
  ○ Risk factors for perinatal and pediatric strokes are distinct.
  ○ Many cases have more than one risk factor, but some have none.
    ■ The cumulative effect (number and severity) of these factors, more than any one single factor, impacts the occurrence of stroke.
    ■ Risk of stroke is higher when both infant and maternal risk factors are present.
  ○ Prothrombotic factors (e.g., factor V Leiden, factor II G20210A)
    ■ The relevance of prothrombotic gene mutations for stroke risk is an area of controversy, with evidence for and against increased risk.
      • Relatively common in the general population
      • A large meta-analysis of 22 pediatric stroke studies (1,764 patients, 2,799 controls) identified prothrombotic factors in as many as 50% of PAS and CSVT cases (Kenet et al., 2010).
      • A population-based prospective case–control study of perinatal stroke, including 212 children (135 cases, 77 controls), showed minimal differences in frequency of thrombophilic factors between cases and controls. However, mothers were not tested (Curtis et al., 2017).
    ■ Prothrombotic factors may be less significant risk factors in low-risk individuals ("just one straw") and more consequential in high-risk individuals with other risk factors, such as preeclampsia, twins, or LGA ("the straw that broke the camel's back").
  ○ Maternal risk factors
    ■ Pregnancy: primiparity, post-dates, preeclampsia, oligohydramnios, chorioamnionitis
    ■ Delivery: maternal fever, prolonged rupture of membranes, prolonged second stage of labor, vacuum extraction (borderline significance)
    ■ Health: infertility, smoking
  ○ Infant/fetal risk factors
    ■ Twins, large and small fetal size, macrocephaly
    ■ Resuscitation, 5 minute Apgar score of <7
      • Asphyxia by itself is a relatively uncommon risk factor.
    ■ Hypoglycemia, polycythemia, cardiac defect, infection
- **Brain imaging**
  ○ Most perinatal stroke is arterial in distribution.
    ■ Unilateral 80%, bilateral 20%

■ Lesions are more commonly in the distribution of the left middle cerebral artery > right middle cerebral artery.
■ Although strokes are ischemic, bleeding that occurs as a secondary phenomenon can complicate interpretation.
○ Imaging can estimate stroke timing.
  ■ A porencephalic cyst(s) forms when ischemic injury precedes birth, usually by several weeks.
- **Clinical features**
  ○ Presentation within the first 24–72 hours of life
    ■ Focal seizures are the most common presenting sign of perinatal stroke.

*Pearl:* Approximately 10% of all newborn seizures are caused by PAS. Neonatal seizures due to stroke increase the risk for later seizures.

  ■ Apnea, hypotonia, lethargy, poor feeding
  ■ When asphyxia is a contributing cause (rare), multiorgan failure may occur.
○ Delayed presentation at 3–9 months of life, after normal neonatal course
  ■ Developmental delay
  ■ Seizures
  ■ Early hand preference
  ■ Hemiparesis
  ■ Decelerating growth in head circumference
- Sequelae are common.
  ○ Risks not completely delineated
  ○ Natural history
    ■ PAS is the most important cause of hemiplegic cerebral palsy.
    ■ Initial infancy period may appear deceptively normal.
      • The severity of the lesion may not correlate with clinical severity, perhaps due to the "plasticity" of the neonatal brain.
    ■ Epilepsy, ID, learning and behavioral problems
      • These may occur long after the sentinel event, even in the later school years.
      • Neonatal seizures significantly increase risk for recurrent seizures.

# Differential Diagnosis

- **Cerebral sinus venous thrombosis** (SVT): 10% of all neonatal stroke
  ○ Occurs when venous blood flow is impaired or absent, causing increased venous pressure, increased capillary hydrostatic pressure, edema, and secondary hemorrhagic infarction
  ○ Several risk factors are similar to PAS.
    ■ Preeclampsia, chorioamnionitis, gestational diabetes, complicated delivery, thrombophilic factors
  ○ Additional risk factors

- Meningitis, sepsis, dehydration
- Congenital heart disease, extracorporeal membrane oxygenation (ECMO)
- Other congenital malformations

- **Perinatal hemorrhagic stroke**: ~20% of neonatal stroke
  - Approximately half are spontaneous and idiopathic.
  - One-third occur as secondary complicating events after ischemic stroke, sinovenous thrombosis, or HIE.
  - Incidence ~1/6,000 to 1/9,500 term births
  - Risk factors:
    - Severe thrombocytopenia (most common), neonatal alloimmune thrombocytopenia, coagulopathy, hemophilia A or B, vascular malformations, AVMs, aneurysm, significant trauma
    - Primiparity, young maternal age, low Apgar scores, low birth weight for gestational age, refusal of vitamin K prophylaxis
  - Neurologic outcome abnormal in >40%
- **Severe hypoxic ischemic encephalopathy** (HIE)
  - Localized PAS is unlikely to be due to HIE. Infarcts in HIE are usually in watershed areas.
- **Encephalitis**
  - Autoimmune mediated: neonatal lupus
  - TORCH infections and "pseudo-TORCH" syndromes
- Other causes: vasculopathy (vasculitis, Moyamoya), non-accidental trauma, severe hypoglycemia, brain tumor
- **Syndromes-rare causes of PAS**
  - **Aicardi–Goutieres syndrome** (MIM 225750)
    - Autosomal recessive and dominant forms, caused by variants in *TREX1* (most severe form), *RNASEH2A, RNASEH2B, RNASEH2C, SAMHD1*, and others
      - May simulate stroke or one of the genetically heterogeneous pseudo-TORCH syndromes
      - Consider when infection evaluation is negative and brain imaging is not typical for PAS.
      - Consider when there is more than one affected child.
    - Clinical features: progressive microcephaly, encephalopathy, spasticity, and rarely, hepatomegaly, abnormal liver function tests, and thrombocytopenia
    - Brain imaging
      - CT: basal ganglia calcifications; MRI: white matter attenuation, leukodystrophy-like
  - **Autosomal dominant porencephaly** (MIM 175780)
    - Caused by heterozygous variants in *COL4A* or *COL4A2*, leading to microangiopathy and ischemic/hemorrhagic stroke in utero, perinatally, or later in life
      - Highly variable age of onset: Stroke may occur in utero, in childhood, or in adulthood.
      - Family history is helpful.
    - Clinical features: congenital hemiplegia, hemiparesis, hydrocephalus, dystonia, seizures
      - Developmental delay, ID

- Ocular findings: congenital cataract, retinal abnormalities, iris hypoplasia, posterior embryotoxon
- Other less common findings include elevated CK, muscle cramps, renal cysts and hematuria, and hemolytic anemia.
  - Brain imaging findings
    - Porencephaly, schizencephaly, hydranencephaly
    - Cerebellar hypoplasia, cortical malformations
    - Hemorrhagic stroke
    - Diffuse white matter findings: leukoencephalopathy, periventricular leukomalacia
    - Lacunar infarcts
  - **Multisystemic smooth muscle dysfunction syndrome** (MIM 613834)
    - Autosomal dominant disorder, caused by heterozygous mutation in *ACTA2*, which encodes alpha actin, the primary actin in smooth muscle cells
      - Predisposition to vascular disease, including thoracic aortic aneurysm
      - Strokes occur less commonly in neonates; they are more common at older ages. Family history is helpful.
    - Clinical features: respiratory distress, tachypnea, pulmonary hypertension, congenital mydriasis—fixed dilated pupils
      - Aortic coarctation, PDA
      - Malrotation
    - Brain imaging
      - Periventricular white matter lesions; vascular anomalies in the CNS
        - Moyamoya disease
  - **Mitochondrial encephalopathies**—rare cause of stroke in the newborn
    - **MELAS** (*m*itochondrial myopathy, *e*ncephalopathy, *l*actic *a*cidosis, and *s*troke-like episodes, MIM 540000)
      - Rare in infancy but family history of this variable clinical phenotype may suggest diagnosis. Due to mtDNA deletions/variants
    - Other rare mitochondrial depletion syndromes include **Pearson syndrome** (MIM 557000) with sideroblastic anemia, multisystem involvement, lactic acidosis, and early death.

# Evaluation and Management

- Document family history: cerebral palsy, deep vein thrombosis, pulmonary embolism, early stroke, seizures, delayed milestones, neurologic problems, history of bleeding in males in the mother's family (e.g., hemophilia).
- Review pregnancy and birth histories: smoking, maternal trauma, SLE, preeclampsia, large or small babies, antiphospholipid antibodies, infant's platelet count.

- ○ Length of second stage of labor, placental abruption, length of rupture of membranes
- ○ Apgar scores, blood gases, liver function tests (LFT), BUN, creatinine, CK, CBC, lactate
- Retrieve and review placental pathology for evidence of vasculopathy, thrombosis in placental veins, infarction, chorioamnionitis, chronic villitis, maternal floor infarction
- Evaluate for cardiac lesions, and neonatal lupus.
- Neurology consultation for seizure management
- Brain imaging, preferably MRI, optimally within 24–36 hours of birth
  - ○ Document type of injury, pattern of vascular distribution to date the stroke as prenatal, perinatal, postnatal
  - ○ Consider MR angiography and MR venography
- Consider thrombophilia evaluation in mother (complete) and infant (limited to minimize blood volume)
  - ○ Newborn evaluation
    - ■ Factor V Leiden variant, Factor II/prothrombin G20210A variant
    - ■ Protein C and S activity levels: Must correct for age. Levels normalize by several months of age. Consider deferring for several months to limit volume of blood needed.
  - ○ Mother's evaluation
    - ■ Antiphospholipid antibodies
      - Lupus anticoagulant
      - Anticardiolipin antibodies
      - $\beta_2$ glycoprotein antibodies
    - ■ Factor V Leiden variant, Prothrombin G20210A variant
    - ■ Protein C activity: not significantly changed in pregnancy
    - ■ Protein S activity: normally depressed in pregnancy
      - If low, repeat 6 weeks postpartum. Only levels below 25% suggest true protein S deficiency.
      - Confirm with total, activity, and free S levels.
    - ■ Antithrombin III activity: suspect if positive family history for thrombosis; otherwise unlikely.
    - ■ MTHFR 677 and 1298 polymorphisms of limited utility, no longer recommended
  - ○ Father's evaluation
    - ■ Protein C and S activities, if baby is not tested
    - ■ Factor V Leiden and prothrombin G20210A, if baby is positive and mother is not
  - ○ Abnormal thrombophilia test results
    - ■ Newborn: Refer to hematologist for management and further family testing.
    - ■ Mother: Refer to perinatologist for management and recommendations for subsequent pregnancies.
    - ■ Father: Possible referral to hematology for lifestyle recommendations. Anticoagulation is not indicated unless there is a personal history of recurrent thrombosis.
    - ■ Recurrence risk for perinatal stroke is low; there is a low increased risk for other adverse pregnancy outcomes.

- Gene testing guided by family history and clinical features
  - ○ COL4A1 and COL4A2, for a positive family history for cerebral palsy, seizures, or brain hemorrhage, especially in infants with hemorrhagic stroke, porencephaly, schizencephaly, and hydranencephaly
  - ○ TORCH testing
  - ○ Aicardi–Goutieres gene testing with basal ganglia calcifications and pseudo-TORCH presentation
  - ○ Exome sequencing and/or SNP microarray in rare instances in which a genetic cause seems likely and/or there is a recurrence
- Treatment: Few studies have addressed treatment.
  - ○ Supportive treatment indicated
  - ○ Neuroprotective strategies under examination
  - ○ Anticoagulation
    - ■ Consult hematology for persistent or recurring thrombosis, to consider anticoagulation or thrombolysis. Controversial: No clinical guidelines exist.
    - ■ Consider long-term medication (e.g., low-dose [baby] aspirin, antiplatelet medications) only in cases of proven systemic hypercoagulability or cardiac factors that increase risk of recurring stroke (PFO, etc.). Chronic treatment is usually not indicated.
- Refer for early infant intervention and physical therapy. Long term neuropsychological follow up indicated.
- Follow up with pediatric ophthalmology within first few months of life and regularly: Many children with PAS have ocular dysfunction.

# Further Reading

Armstrong-Wells J, Ferriero DM. (2014) Diagnosis and acute management of perinatal arterial ischemic stroke. Neurol Clin Pract. 4:378–85. PMID 25317375

Bernson-Leung ME, Boyd TK, Meserve EE, et al. (2018) Placental Pathology in Neonatal Stroke: A Retrospective Case-Control Study. J Pediatr. 195:39–47. PMID 29397159

Cole L, Dewey D, Letourneau N, et al. (2017) Clinical characteristics, risk factors, and outcomes associated with neonatal hemorrhagic stroke: A population-based case–control study. JAMA Pediatr. 171:230–8. PMID 28114647

Curtis C, Mineyko A, Massicotte P, et al. (2017) Thrombophilia risk is not increased in children after perinatal stroke. Blood. 129:2793–2800. PMID 28258054

Fox CK, Glass HC, Sidney S, et al. (2016) Neonatal seizures triple the risk of a remote seizure after perinatal ischemic stroke. Neurology. 86:2179–86. PMID 27164703

Kenet G, Lütkhoff LK, Albisetti M, et al. (2010) Impact of thrombophilia on risk of arterial ischemic stroke or cerebral sinovenous thrombosis in neonates and children: A systematic review and meta-analysis of observational studies. Circulation. 121:1838–47. PMID 20385928

Lehman LL, Rivkin MJ. (2014) Perinatal arterial ischemic stroke: Presentation, risk factors, evaluation, and outcome. Pediatr Neurol. 51:760–8. PMID 25444092

Meuwissen ME, Halley DJ, Smit LS, et al. (2015) The expanding phenotype of COL4A1 and COL4A2 mutations: Clinical data on 13 newly identified families and a review of the literature. Genet Med. 17:843–53. PMID 25719457

Wagenaar N, Martinez-Biarge M, van der Aa NE, et al. (2018) Neurodevelopment After Perinatal Arterial Ischemic Stroke. Pediatrics. 142(3) e20174164. PMID 30072575

# Part V

## Gastrointestinal System

# 21

# Diaphragmatic Hernia

## Clinical Consult

A perinatologist requested a genetics consultation for a 36-year-old G3 mother admitted in preterm labor at 34 weeks' gestation. Fetal US revealed mild polyhydramnios and a left-sided mass in the chest containing liver and stomach consistent with congenital diaphragmatic hernia (CDH). The fetus was large for dates, although humeri were mildly short. The mother's glucose tolerance test was normal at 20 weeks' gestation. The family history was noncontributory. Chromosome analysis and FISH studies on amniocytes revealed that 50% of the cells contained a small additional isochromosome for the short arm of chromosome 12: mosaic tetrasomy 12p or **Pallister–Killian syndrome**. At birth at 39 weeks, BW was 3800 g. The female infant had striking bitemporal alopecia, a high boxy forehead, long philtrum, coarse appearance, and small ears (Figure 21.1). She survived the CDH repair but died of postoperative complications. Chromosomal microarray confirmed mosaicism for two extra copies of 12p.

Pallister Killian syndrome is a multisystem disorder, often with large BW, that is associated with CDH in up to 50%. The prognosis is for severe intellectual disability with a high frequency of visual and hearing loss, feeding problems, and seizures in approximately 50%.

## Definition

- Congenital diaphragmatic hernia (MIM 142340) occurs when abdominal contents herniate into the chest through a defect in the diaphragm.
  - Posterior lateral defect (Bochdalek) most common: 95%
    - Left-sided 85%, right-sided 10%
  - Parasternal defects (Morgagni) ~2%
  - Rare types: central hernias and anterior hernias, as in **pentalogy of Cantrell** (MIM 313850)
  - Bilateral CDH is rare, ~5%, often syndromic.
  - From 5–10% of infants with diaphragmatic defects are not symptomatic in the newborn period.
- Incidence 1/3,000 live births. Some studies have found more affected males.
- Prenatal diagnosis identifies 50–80%.

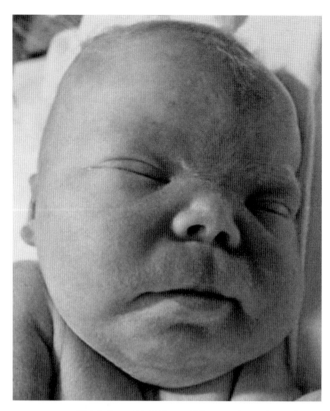

FIGURE 21.1 This infant with Pallister–Killian syndrome has a short nose and long philtrum. Bitemporal alopecia is typical.

○ Chromosome anomalies are more prevalent among the prenatally diagnosed.
• Etiology unknown ~80%
  ○ Positive family history in 1% for Bochdalek-type CDH
  ○ Multifactorial inheritance likely in nonsyndromic cases
  ○ MZ twins often discordant, implying epigenetic or developmental rather than genetic etiology
• Isolated CDH 60%; better prognosis
  ○ Recurrence risk 2%
  ○ Genetic etiology is likely and recurrence risk is higher in familial isolated CDH, including **X-linked CDH** (MIM 306950)
• CDH with associated malformations: 40%
  ○ Cardiac defects, 20%, are most frequent associated anomaly
  ○ Urogenital, musculoskeletal, CNS defects

## Differential Diagnosis

• Other intrathoracic lesions can mimic CDH.
  ○ Congenital cystic adenomatoid malformation
  ○ Bronchopulmonary sequestration, usually solid mass

  ○ Bronchopulmonary atresia
  ○ Lung teratoma
• Chromosome disorders that cause CDH
  ○ Conventional cytogenetic analysis is abnormal in 10-35%.
    ■ **Down syndrome\*** is the most frequent chromosome anomaly in Morgagni-type CDH.
      • <1% of patients with Down syndrome
    ■ **Trisomy 18\*** accounts for 2–5% of all CDH.
    ■ Other trisomies: mosaic 2, mosaic 8, 9, **13\***, 16, 22; monosomy (**Turner syndrome\***) and trisomy X
    ■ **Pallister–Killian syndrome** (mosaic tetrasomy 12p, MIM 601803)
      • Due to additional mosaic isochromosome 12p (i12p)
      • The degree of mosaicism, which is caused by loss of i12p in some cells, does not correlate with severity.
      • Causes 2–5% of CDH

*Pearl:* Pallister–Killian syndrome is most reliably diagnosed in skin fibroblasts or amniocytes because lymphocytes with the isochromosome 12p disappear from blood with age. Normal chromosome analysis in peripheral blood does not rule out Pallister–Killian syndrome.

• Clinical features: large birth weight, frontal balding, coarse face, hypertelorism, short nose, anteverted nares, streaky pigmentation, short limbs, CNS anomalies, intellectual disability, seizures (Figures 3.2, 21.1)
  • CDH occurs in ≥50%.

*Pearl:* On conventional cytogenetic banding, the isochromosome 12p can resemble an isochromosome 21q. Occasionally, infants with Pallister–Killian syndrome are misdiagnosed with a translocation variant of Down syndrome.

  ○ Microarray identifies abnormalities in an additional 3–13% with normal karyotypes.
    ■ Deletions: 1q41–42, **Wolf–Hirschhorn syndrome\*** (4p-, MIM 194190), 8p23.1 (MIM 222400), 15q26.1 (MIM 142340), 16p11.2, 17q12, Xp22-ter
    ■ Duplications: 11q23.2, 16p11.2
• Single gene disorders account for ~10% of CDH.
  ○ More than 70 syndromes have CDH as a common or rare feature.
  ○ **CHARGE syndrome\*** (MIM 214800)
    ■ A multiple congenital anomaly syndrome caused by a heterozygous pathogenic variant in *CHD7* or *SEMA3E*
    ■ Clinical features: cranial nerve deficits, facial palsy, coloboma, choanal atresia, hearing loss, inner ear and external ear anomalies and cardiac, genital, and other anomalies.

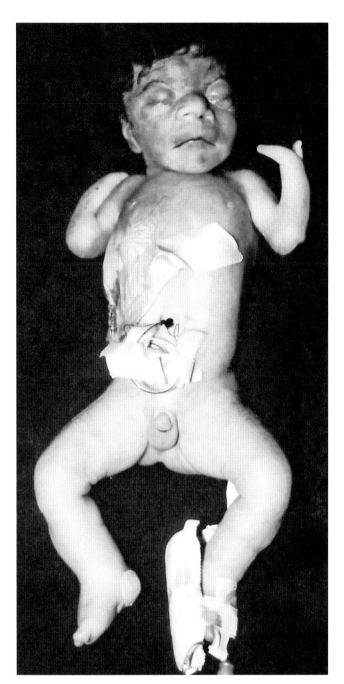

FIGURE 21.2 This deceased infant with Cornelia de Lange syndrome has characteristic arched eyebrows, prominent long philtrum, thin upper lip, oligodactyly, and diaphragmatic hernia.

o **Cornelia de Lange syndrome\*** (MIM 122470)
  ▪ An autosomal dominant disorder, caused by a heterozygous pathogenic variant in NIPBL or other genes in that function in the cohesin complex
  ▪ Clinical features: CDH ~1–5%—may be underascertained (Figure 21.2). Arched eyebrows, synophrys, long philtrum, thin and prominent upper lip, crescent shaped mouth, hypertrichosis, upper limb deficits. Poor growth.

o **Craniofrontonasal syndrome** (MIM 304110)
  ▪ X-linked disorder, caused by hemizygous pathogenic variant in *EFNB1*
  ▪ Females are more severely affected than males; both sexes can have CDH.
  ▪ Clinical features: coronal craniosynostosis, frontal bossing, hypertelorism, down-slanting palpebral fissures, bifid nasal tip, syndactyly of fingers and toes. CDH is rare.
o **Donnai–Barrow syndrome** (MIM 222448)
  ▪ Autosomal recessive disorder, caused by biallelic pathogenic variants in *LRP2*
  ▪ Clinical features: enlarged anterior fontanel, agenesis of corpus callosum, hypertelorism, eye anomalies (myopia, retinal detachment, optic atrophy), hearing loss. omphalocele. CDH >70% (Figure 21.3)
o **Fryns syndrome** (MIM 229850)
  ▪ Autosomal recessive syndrome, caused in some by biallelic pathogenic variants in *PIGN*
  ▪ Clinical features: cloudy corneas, broad nasal bridge, cleft palate, absence of lung lobation, nail hypoplasia, hypoplasia of the distal fingers, duodenal atresia; GI, CNS, renal, and genital anomalies (Figure 21.4). CDH >80%.
o **Goltz syndrome** (focal dermal hypoplasia, MIM 305600)
  ▪ X-linked condition, caused by pathogenic variant in *PORCN*
  ▪ Affects primarily females, presumed lethal in males

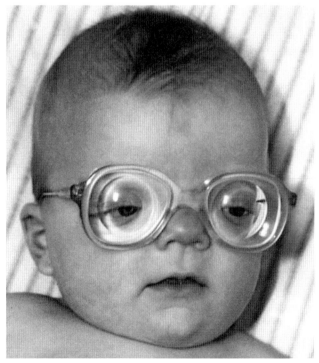

FIGURE 21.3 This infant with Donnai–Barrow syndrome has hypertelorism, eye anomalies, and a short nose.
SOURCE: Courtesy of Dr. Dian Donnai, Manchester, UK.

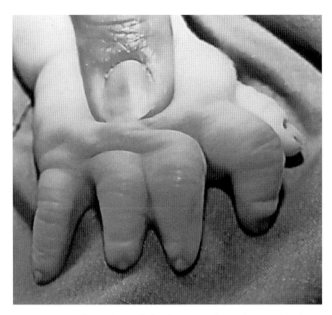

FIGURE 21.4 This infant with diaphragmatic hernia has syndactyly and hypoplastia of the distal fingers and fingernails, which are characteristic of Fryns syndrome.

- Clinical features: linear and swirling skin pigmentation, focal fatty herniation, ocular, digital defects. CDH is rare.
  ○ **Kabuki syndrome** (MIM 147920)
    ■ Autosomal dominant disorder, caused by heterozygous pathogenic variant in *KMT2D*; typically de novo, sporadic
      • X-linked form caused by pathogenic variant in *KDM6A* (Figures 7.4, 12.3)
    ■ Clinical features: long palpebral fissures, everted lower lids, sparse lateral eyebrows, large prominent ears, cleft palate, prominent fingerpads, cardiac defects, poor growth, developmental delay. CDH 15%
  ○ **Matthew–Wood syndrome** (MIM 601186)
    ■ Autosomal recessive trait, caused by biallelic pathogenic variants in *STRA6* or *RARB*
    ■ Clinical features: IUGR, anophthalmia or microphthalmia; cardiac, renal anomalies. CDH >50%
  ○ Overgrowth syndromes*
    ■ **Beckwith–Wiedemann syndrome*** (MIM 130650)
      • Overgrowth disorder caused by pathogenic variant or deletion of imprinted genes on chromosome 11q15.5.
      • Clinical features: CDH uncommon. Somatic overgrowth, visceromegaly, umbilical hernia, omphalocele, macroglossia, ear creases. Predisposed to Wilms and other embryonal tumors.
    ■ **Perlman syndrome** (MIM 267000)
      • Autosomal recessive disorder, caused by pathogenic variants in *DIS3L2*

- Clinical features: LGA, inverted V-shaped upper lip, flat nasal bridge, hypotonic, organomegaly, nephroblastomatosis, hyperinsulinism, early Wilms tumor, can be bilateral. CDH is rare.
  ■ **Simpson–Golabi–Behmel syndrome** (MIM 312870)
    • X-linked recessive disorder, caused by pathogenic variant in *GPC3*
    • Clinical features: CDH occasional. Large birth weight, polydactyly, syndactyly, pectus excavatum, vertebral anomalies, cardiac arrhythmias, predisposed to Wilms and other embryonal tumors

## Evaluation and Management

- Document family history: consanguinity, other affected relatives, note sex of affected relatives to identify X-linked inheritance.
- Prenatal management
  ○ Families may consider in utero surgical intervention for isolated CDH with normal echocardiogram and microarray.
    ■ Fetal treatment is tracheal occlusion followed by an EXIT procedure.
    ■ Investigational, available at specialized fetal therapy centers
  ○ No definite benefit for cesarean delivery
  ○ When liver is in the chest or lung volume is unfavorable, deliver in a tertiary center where ECMO is available.
- Evaluate for dysmorphic features, digital anomalies, and other structural malformations.
  ○ Echocardiogram, abdominal US
  ○ Obtain Head MRI *before* surgical repair or ECMO because CNS anomalies may influence decision-making
- Genetic testing
  ○ Chromosome microarray
  ○ When CDH is isolated and family history is negative, no further generic testing is need if microarray is normal.
  ○ Syndromic CDH: After a normal microarray, offer gene studies or exome sequencing depending on the pattern of anomalies.
- Multidisciplinary follow-up is optimal to manage common complications: gastroesophageal reflux disease (GERD), developmental delay, hearing loss.

## Further Reading

Ackerman KG, Vargas SO, Wilson JA, et al. (2012) Congenital diaphragmatic defects: Proposal for a new classification based on observations in 234 patients. Pediatr Dev Pathol. 15:265–74. PMID 22257294

Badillo A, Gingalewski C. (2014) Congenital diaphragmatic hernia: Treatment and outcomes. Semin Perinatol. 38:92–6. PMID 24580764

McInerney-Leo AM, Harris JE, Gattas M, et al. (2016) Fryns syndrome associated with recessive mutations in PIGN in two separate families. Hum Mutat. 37:695–702. PMID 27038415

Rocha G, Baptista MJ, Correia-Pinto J, Guimarães H. (2013) Congenital diaphragmatic hernia: Experience of 14 years. Minerva Pediatr. 65:271–8. PMID 23685378

Slavotinek AM. (2014) The genetics of common disorders—Congenital diaphragmatic hernia. Eur J Med Genet. 57:418–23. PMID

Stoll C, Alembik Y, Dott B, Roth MP. (2008) Associated malformations in cases with congenital diaphragmatic hernia. Genet Couns. 19:331–9. PMID 18990989

Tovar JA. (2012) Congenital diaphragmatic hernia. Orphanet J Rare Dis. 7:1–15. PMID 22214468

Turek JW, Nellis JR, Sherwood BG, et al. (2017) Shifting risks and conflicting outcomes: ECMO for neonates with congenital diaphragmatic hernia in the modern era. J Pediatr. 190:163–8. PMID 29144241

Vrecenak JD, Flake AW. (2013) Fetal surgical intervention: Progress and perspectives. Pediatr Surg Int. 29:407–17. PMID 23552956

Wynn J, Yu L, Chung WK. (2014) Genetic causes of congenital diaphragmatic hernia. Semin Fetal Neonatal Med. 19:324–30. PMID 25447988

# 22

# Gastroschisis

## Clinical Consult

A 20-year-old G3P2 pregnant woman had an 18-week fetal US that revealed a typical pattern of gastroschisis, with abdominal contents floating freely in the amniotic cavity. There was no spontaneous movement of either arm at the shoulders or elbows. The wrists were flexed facing backwards with no movement of the fingers. Genetic consultation suggested the diagnosis of gastroschisis with amyoplasia, the most common form of arthrogryposis and a finding in approximately 3-10% of infants with gastroschisis. The family was counseled about the need for multiple surgeries, intensive physical therapy, and assistive devices. The family elected to continue the pregnancy. The diagnosis was confirmed at birth (Figure 22.1). Early physical therapy improved range of motion within weeks. The gastroschisis repair was uneventful. The baby was discharged on full feedings at 6 weeks. At 8 months, her cognitive development was normal, and she had gained some use of her fingers on one hand. The prognosis for normal development with both conditions is good. Early and intensive physical therapy and referral to a major center for limb anomalies improves the outcome.

## Definition

- **Gastroschisis** (MIM 230750) is an abdominal wall defect that usually occurs as an isolated anomaly.
- Gastroschisis is anatomically distinct from omphalocele.
  - The defect in gastroschisis is on the right side of the umbilicus.
  - Abdominal contents are exposed, without a covering membrane.
    - Usually only intestines, but rarely stomach, liver, and other organs, are extruded.
  - Umbilical cord inserts normally, to the left of the defect and normal skin typically bridges the area between the defect and the umbilicus.
  - Rarely, a ruptured omphalocele may present in a similar way, but diagnostic confusion is unusual.
- Inheritance is multifactorial.
  - Usually occurs sporadically

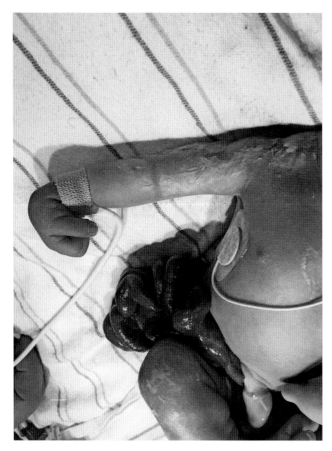

FIGURE 22.1 Gastroschisis with amyoplasia. Note intervening bridge of normal skin between cord and defect and the extended straight arm with a "policeman's tip" hand positioning.

- Surgical complications, intestinal atresias with loss of bowel and short bowel syndrome
  - Risk factors associated with mortality: male gender, low birth weight, IUGR, prematurity, low 5-minute APGAR score, vasopressor use, high oxygen requirements
  - The recurrence risk is ~4%, suggesting that genetic factors play some role in this malformation.

*Pearl*: The association of IUGR with gastroschisis does not imply a more generalized syndrome or another etiology. It is a frequent finding seen in at least half of these infants.

- Isolated malformation 80%
- Comorbidities
  - GI strictures and atresias, defects in muscles of the lateral abdominal wall ~6%. Likely due to vascular disruption
  - IUGR—at least 50% of infants with gastroschisis are <10% for weight at birth.
- Associated congenital anomalies (~10%)
  - Amyoplasia, the most common type of arthrogryposis, suggests a common vascular disruptive etiology (~3–10% incidence).
  - Other limb anomalies, such as transverse reduction defects/hypoplasia, are reported (~2%).
  - CNS anomalies (~3%) occur that also have a vascular etiology e.g. porencephaly, schizencephaly
  - Amniotic band disruption sequence—rare association
  - A deceased monozygotic co-twin—rare association

- Positive family history 2.5%
  - Recurrence risk ~4%
- Incidence 1/10,000 live births; 7/10,000 in mothers younger than age 20 years
  - 1.5 M:1 F
  - Increasing prevalence documented after 1980 in birth defects registries in several countries. In the United States, the greatest increase has been among young Black mothers (263% increase from 1995 to 2012; Jones et al., 2016).
- Most patients are prenatally diagnosed either by an elevated α-fetoprotein (AFP) on a maternal serum screening test (MSAFP) or by a routine fetal US.
- Etiology is unknown, but a vascular cause is suspected.
- Risk factors
  - Maternal age <25 years, change in paternity, interpregnancy interval <12 months, including miscarriages and elective termination
  - Nutrition: possible maternal micronutrient depletion
  - Environmental agents: tobacco, ibuprofen, aspirin, alcohol
  - Medications with first trimester exposure: inhaled asthma medication ($\beta_2$ agonists), oral contraceptives, paroxetine
- Outcome is generally favorable.
  - Mortality <5%

## Differential Diagnosis

- Chromosome anomalies are uncommon, but they are somewhat more common when other anomalies are present.
  - **Trisomy 13*** and **trisomy 18***, **Turner syndrome*** and **Down syndrome*** reported but rare
    - Chromosomal aneuploidy occurs much less often in gastroschisis than in omphalocele
- Defects in body wall formation and lateral folding may have overlapping features with gastroschisis.
  - **Omphalocele–exstrophy–imperforate anus–spinal defects (cloacal exstrophy)** (OEIS, MIM 258040)
    - Rare sporadic lower abdominal wall defect
    - Clinical features: omphalocele, failure of fusion of the pubic rami, exstrophy of the bladder, imperforate anus, spinal defects, including spina bifida, abnormal genitalia
  - **Limb–body wall complex**
    - Clinical features: severe scoliosis is characteristic; limb involvement with abnormal angulation of a limb, missing limb frequent but not invariable (Figure 22.2)

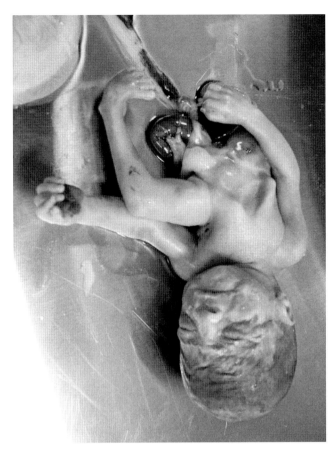

FIGURE 22.2 Limb–body wall defect with severe scoliosis, extrusion of multiple organs, and absent leg.

- Body wall defect with extrusion of stomach, intestines, liver, and, rarely, thoracic organs; Exencephaly and oral clefting seen.
  - A lethal disorder: Distinguishing it prenatally from isolated gastroschisis is important.

## Evaluation and Management

- Document family history: other affected relatives.
- Review pregnancy history: environmental and teratogenic exposures.
- Prenatal management
  - Monitor for IUGR, oligohydramnios, and polyhydramnios.
  - US findings of thickened bowel wall, gastric dilation, and bowel dilation are unfavorable prognostic indicators.
  - Consult pediatric surgery prenatally.
  - Prematurity is common. Arrange delivery at a hospital with pediatric surgery capabilities.
  - No firm evidence that cesarean delivery improves survival, lessens morbidity, or decreases length of hospitalization.
- Examine infant for other associated anomalies: amniotic band constriction rings, limb contractures.
  - Head US to rule out disruptive defects especially if there are any neurologic findings
- Genetic testing is not indicated for isolated gastroschisis.
  - Consider microarray when there are other primary malformations.

## Further Reading

Benjamin B, Wilson GN. (2015) Registry analysis supports different mechanisms for gastroschisis and omphalocele within shared developmental fields. Am J Med Genet A. 167A:2568–81. PMID 26138114

Clark RH, Walker MW, Gauderer MW. (2011) Factors associated with mortality in neonates with gastroschisis. Eur J Pediatr Surg. 21:21–4. PMID 21328190

D'Antonio F, Virgone C, Rizzo G, et al. (2015) Prenatal risk factors and outcomes in gastroschisis: A meta-analysis. Pediatrics. 136:e159–69. PMID 26122809

Feldkamp ML, Carey JC, Pimentel R, et al. (2011) Is gastroschisis truly a sporadic defect? Familial cases of gastroschisis in Utah, 1997 to 2008. Birth Defects Res A Clin Mol Teratol. 91:873–8. PMID 21987464

Given JE, Loane M, Garne E, et al. (2017) Gastroschisis in Europe— A case-malformed–control study of medication and maternal illness during pregnancy as risk factors. Paediatr Perinat Epidemiol. 31:549–59. PMID 28841756

Jones AM, Isenburg J, Salemi JL, et al. (2016) Increasing prevalence of gastroschisis—14 States, 1995–2012. MMWR Morb Mortal Wkly Rep. 65:23–6. PMID 26796490

Ruano R, Picone O, Bernardes L, et al. (2011) The association of gastroschisis with other congenital anomalies: How important is it? Prenat Diagn. 31(4):347–50. PMID 21413033

Skarsgard ED. (2016) Management of gastroschisis. Curr Opin Pediatr. 28:363–9. PMID 26974976

Werler MM, Guéry E, Waller DK, Parker SE. (2018) Gastroschisis and Cumulative Stressor Exposures. Epidemiology. 29(5):721–8. PMID 29863532

# 23

# Omphalocele

## Clinical Consult

A preterm dysmorphic male with respiratory distress had an omphalocele and short extremities. His chest was narrow and bell-shaped. He required mechanical ventilation for severe pulmonary hypoplasia and pulmonary hypertension. A genetic consultation was requested for suspected skeletal dysplasia. A radiograph showed "coat-hanger" ribs (Figure 23.1) characteristic of **paternal uniparental disomy for chromosome 14** (UPD14pat). DNA methylation studies confirmed the diagnosis. He failed several trials of extubation. After counseling about his poor prognosis, his parents chose comfort care. He expired after extubation.

A bell-shaped thorax with "coat-hanger" ribs is characteristic of UPD14pat. Several genes on distal chromosome 14q are differentially expressed depending on the parent of origin. Maternally expressed genes on chromosome 14q are inactive in UPD14pat. The diagnosis can be made by SNP microarray when the chromosomes 14 are identical (isodisomy). Methylation analysis is the preferred test.

## Definition

- Omphalocele (exomphalos) is a common congenital abdominal wall defect due to failure of herniated gut to return from the umbilical cord to the abdomen after 10 weeks' gestation.
- Incidence 1/4,000 live births
- 1.2 M:1 F
- Most are sporadic and multifactorial, but familial cases have been reported with autosomal recessive, dominant and X-linked patterns of transmission.
- Omphalocele is centered at umbilicus, covered by amnion, lined with peritoneum; cord inserts into defect; covering membrane may rupture (Figure 23.2)
  - In contrast, the defect in gastroschisis* is to the right of the umbilicus.

- Usual contents are intestines and liver; other organs are less common.
  - "Giant" omphalocele: diameter of the defect is ≥5 cm or >75% of the liver herniated into the sac

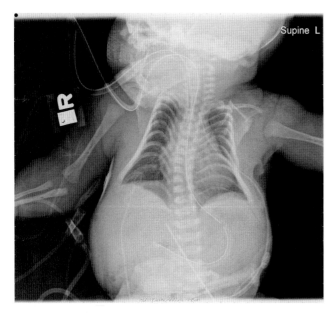

FIGURE 23.1 These "coat hanger" ribs are a cardinal sign of UPD14pat.

- Caused by major disruption of abdominal wall formation
- Most are prenatally diagnosed by elevated maternal serum AFP screening test and/or fetal US as early as 11 or 12 weeks.
- Periconceptional folic acid supplementation reduces the birth prevalence of omphalocele by 20%
- Risk factors
  - ART
  - Maternal age: young <25 years, OR 1.77; and older >35 years, OR 1.34
  - Multiple gestation has twice the singleton rate.

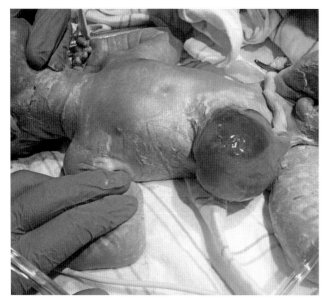

FIGURE 23.2 The umbilical cord inserts directly into the defect in an omphalocele.

  - Teratogens*
- Outcome
  - High mortality: 28.7% die in infancy
  - Best prognosis
    - Isolated malformation: 1-year survival ~90%
    - Normal chromosome microarray
  - Poor prognosis
    - Chromosome anomaly
    - Low birth weight
    - Giant omphalocele, 50% fatality rate
  - Routine cesarean delivery does not improve prognosis.
  - Primary closure, when possible, improves outcome.
- Isolated omphalocele 25%
  - Gastroschisis, in contrast, is typically isolated ~84%
  - Distinguish from umbilical hernia
    - Umbilical hernia is a common isolated anomaly, especially in African populations
    - Present in many genetic syndromes, including mucopolysaccharidoses

*Pearl*: The pattern of anomalies, not the size of the defect, determines whether a genetic evaluation is needed. Suspect a syndrome when associated anomalies are present, even when the abdominal defect is small.

- Syndromic omphalocele 70%
  - Omphalocele with associated malformations: 44% have a recognizable syndrome.
  - Cardiac anomalies 32%
    - TOF, ASD, PDA, VSD, coarctation
    - Two-thirds are syndromic.
  - CNS anomalies 8%
    - Spina bifida, anencephaly
  - Gastrointestinal
    - Hirschsprung disease, biliary atresia, pyloric stenosis
  - Common: GU and musculoskeletal anomalies

## Differential Diagnosis

- Chromosomal disorders: 17% in newborns, 50% in fetuses
  - **Trisomy 18\***: 50% of chromosomally abnormal group
  - **Trisomy 13\***: 29%
  - **Down syndrome\***: 8%
  - **Turner syndrome\*** and other sex chromosome aneuploidies: 47,XXX, 47,XXY, 47,XYY
  - Duplication 1p31.3 (Autosomal omphalocele, MIM 164750), 3q
  - **Tetrasomy 12p** mosaicism (Pallister–Killian syndrome, MIM 601803)

*Pearl*: Chromosome anomalies are more common when the liver is not included in the sac.

- o **Paternal uniparental disomy for chromosome 14** (UPD14pat, Kagami–Ogata syndrome, MIM 608149)
  - ▪ Sporadic disorder caused by loss of maternally derived copy of chromosome 14
    - • Paternal isodisomy or heterodisomy produces a paternal DNA methylation pattern (methylation-sensitive MLPA).
      - • UPD14pat may be segmental.
    - • Other 14q32 errors produce the same phenotype.
      - • Malsegregation of Robertsonian translocation 13;14
      - • Terminal deletion of maternally derived chr 14q
  - ▪ Clinical features: IUGR, dysmorphic facial features, omphalocele, narrow bell-shaped thorax, short limbs, joint contractures, hypospadias
  - ▪ Radiographs: classic "coat hanger" ribs
- • Teratogens*
  - o ART
  - o **Maternal diabetes mellitus***
  - o Maternal obesity
  - o **Misoprostol**
  - o Selective serotonin reuptake inhibitors
  - o **Valproic acid** (Figures 6.2, 19.1)
- • Single gene disorders associated with omphalocele
  - o **Beckwith–Wiedemann syndrome*** (MIM 130650)
    - ▪ Usually sporadic overgrowth disorder, caused by pathogenic variants or methylation errors in the imprinted region on 11q15.5.
      - • Autosomal dominant in 15%
    - ▪ Risk factors
      - • ART
    - ▪ Prenatal findings 50%: large fetal size, long umbilical cord, placental mesenchymal dysplasia, polyhydramnios, prematurity
    - ▪ Clinical features: large birth weight, ear creases, macroglossia, posterior ear pits, diastasis recti, hemihypertrophy, renal anomalies. Omphalocele may be large (Figure 23.3), small, or only an umbilical hernia.
    - ▪ Comorbidities
      - • Hypoglycemia
      - • Poor feeding, obstructive sleep apnea, other breathing issues resolve as macroglossia improves
      - • Increased risk for embryonal tumors (Wilms tumor, hepatoblastoma)
  - o **CHARGE syndrome*** (MIM 214800)
    - ▪ Autosomal dominant trait, caused by heterozygous pathogenic variants in *CHD7* or *SEMA3E*
    - ▪ Clinical features: coloboma, choanal atresia, hearing deficit, cleft palate, facial palsy, characteristic abnormal ear morphology, cardiac and genital defects
  - o **Donnai–Barrow syndrome** (MIM 222448)
    - ▪ Autosomal recessive trait, caused by biallelic pathogenic variants in *LRP2*
    - ▪ Clinical features: hypertelorism, prominent eyes, large fontanelle, omphalocele, absence of corpus callosum,

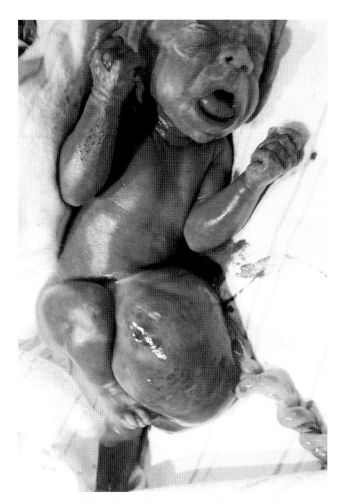

FIGURE 23.3 This infant with Beckwith–Wiedemann syndrome has a large omphalocele. Note the macroglossia.

diaphragmatic hernia, myopia, sensorineural deafness, low-molecular-weight proteinuria (Figure 21.3)
  - • Rare: iris hypoplasia, iris coloboma, cataract, retinal detachment; may have only an ocular phenotype
- o **Focal dermal hypoplasia** (Goltz syndrome, MIM 305600)
  - ▪ X-linked trait, caused by hemizygous pathogenic variant in *PORCN*
  - ▪ Predominantly females; lethal in utero in males
  - ▪ Clinical features: asymmetric limb, eye, streaky, and focal skin defects (Figure 33.4)
    - • ID common
- o **Fryns syndrome** (MIM 229850)
  - ▪ Autosomal recessive trait, usually lethal, due to biallelic pathogenic variants in *PIGN* in some families
  - ▪ Clinical features: omphalocele, genitourinary abnormalities, diaphragmatic hernia, CNS abnormalities, coarse face, hypoplastic distal fingers and nails
- o **Gershoni–Baruch syndrome** (MIM 609545)
  - ▪ Autosomal recessive trait, usually lethal; no responsible gene

- Clinical features: large omphalocele, diaphragmatic hernia, radial ray defects
  - **Hydrolethalus syndrome** (MIM 236680)
    - Autosomal recessive lethal ciliopathy, due to biallelic pathogenic variants in *HYLS1* or *KIF7*
      - Overlaps with "pseudotrisomy 13"
    - Clinical features: hydrocephalus, holoprosencephaly, keyhole-shaped foramen magnum, cleft lip/palate, small mandible, small eyes, postaxial polydactyly (hands), preaxial polydactyly (feet)
      - Stillbirth and polyhydramnios
  - **Manitoba oculotrichoanal syndrome** (MOTA, MIM 248450)
    - Autosomal recessive trait, due to biallelic pathogenic variants in *FREM1*
      - Phenotype overlaps **Fraser syndrome** (MIM 219000)
    - Clinical features: cryptophthalmos, eyelid colobomas, GI anomalies
  - **Meckel syndrome** (Meckel–Gruber syndrome, MIM 249000)
    - Autosomal recessive lethal disorder. Multiple ciliopathy genes have been implicated.
  - **Otopalatodigital syndrome, type II** (MIM 304120)
    - X-linked trait, often lethal in males, due to hemizygous pathogenic variant in *FLNA*
    - Clinical features: cleft palate, hearing loss, omphalocele, bowed long bones, hypertelorism, prominent down-slanting eyes, micrognathia, characteristic digital and skeletal findings
- Severe abdominal wall defects
  - Rare, usually sporadic, often lethal disorders
    - Recurrence risk is typically low.
  - **Cloacal exstrophy/OEIS complex** (*o*mphalocele, *e*xstrophy of the bladder, *i*mperforate anus, *s*pinal defects/*s*pina bifida, MIM 250040)
    - Usually sporadic
    - Increased in MZ and conjoined twins
    - Prenatal diagnosis 50%: nonvisualization of bladder, sacral mass; elevated maternal serum AFP
    - Clinical features: variable omphalocele, spinal, anal, genital, and bladder defects. Prolapsed ileum resembles an "elephant trunk." (Figure 26.4)
    - Requires experienced specialty management
      - Gender assignment in XY individuals requires multidisciplinary approach.
  - **Limb–body wall complex**
    - Sporadic, lethal defect of embryonic disc ectoderm
    - Usually detected by early fetal US
    - Clinical features: major body wall defect of thorax and/or abdomen (Figure 22.2); extrusion of multiple organs; scoliosis; limb defects: amelia, distortion, syndactyly
      - Oral clefts, exencephaly, encephalocele

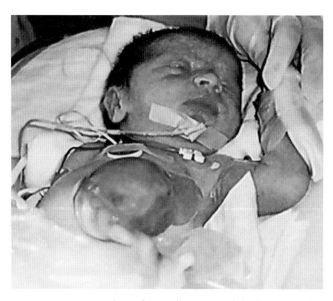

FIGURE 23.4 In pentalogy of Cantrell, a supraumbilical omphalocele occurs with defects in the sternum (with or without ectopia cordis), anterior diaphragm, diaphragmatic pericardium, and heart.

- Placental attachment to body parts or connected by skin tubes, short umbilical cord
- Cardiac defects, absent gallbladder, vertebral or genitourinary defects
  - **Pentalogy of Cantrell** (MIM 313850)
    - Usually sporadic and isolated
      - Rare in trisomy 18* and Goltz (focal dermal hypoplasia) syndromes
    - Clinical features: supraumbilical omphalocele, lower sternal defect, ectopia cordis, deficiency of anterior diaphragm, defect of diaphragmatic pericardium (Figure 23.4)

# Evaluation and Management

- Document family history: consanguinity, abdominal defects, high birth weight, overgrowth.
- Obtain pregnancy history: ART, multiple gestation, teratogens, maternal diabetes.
- Review fetal findings: increased nuchal thickness, cystic enlargement of placenta (placental histology if available), polyhydramnios, large for gestational age.
- Identify associated anomalies: ear pits, creases, macroglossia, rib shape, long umbilical cord.
  - Echocardiogram
  - Abdominal US
  - Skeletal survey
  - Ophthalmologic exam
  - Audiology assessment
  - Intracranial imaging

- Genetic testing
  - Chromosomal SNP microarray: preferred first test
  - Chromosome analysis when aneuploidy is suspected (e.g. positive cell-free DNA)
  - Methylation analysis (methylation-sensitive multiplex ligation probe amplification, MS-MLPA) for suspected Beckwith–Wiedemann syndrome (11q15.5) or UPD14pat (distal 14q)
  - Genetic testing should be considered when an infant with an omphalocele has an unusual pattern of multiple congenital anomalies.

# Further Reading

Christison-Lagay ER, Kelleher CM, Langer JC. (2011) Neonatal abdominal wall defects. Semin Fetal Neonatal Med. 16:164–72. PMID 21474399

Donnai D, Barrow M. (1993) Diaphragmatic hernia, exomphalos, absent corpus callosum, hypertelorism, myopia, and sensorineural deafness: A newly recognized autosomal recessive disorder? Am J Med Genet. 47:679–82. PMID 8266995

Gamba P, Midrio P. (2014) Abdominal wall defects: Prenatal diagnosis, newborn management, and long-term outcomes. Semin Pediatr Surg. 23:283–90. PMID 25459013

Hunter AGW, Seaver LH, Stevenson RE. (2011) Limb–body wall defect: Is there a defensible hypothesis and can it explain all the associated anomalies? Am J Med Genet A. 155:245–59. PMID 21815262

Marshall J, Salemi JL, Tanner JP, et al; National Birth Defects Prevention Network. (2015) Prevalence, correlates, and outcomes of omphalocele in the United States, 1995–2005. Obstet Gynecol. 126:284–93. PMID 26241416

Ogata T, Kagami M. (2016) Kagami–Ogata syndrome: A clinically recognizable upd(14)pat and related disorder affecting the chromosome 14q32.2 imprinted region. J Hum Genet. 61:87–94. PMID 26377239

Shuman C, Beckwith JB, Weksberg R. (2016) Beckwith–Wiedemann syndrome. In: Pagon RA, Adam MP, Ardinger HH, et al., editors. GeneReviews [Internet]. Seattle, WA: University of Washington, Seattle; 1993–2017. PMID 20301568

Stoll C, Alembik Y, Dott B, Roth MP. (2008) Omphalocele and gastroschisis and associated malformations. Am J Med Genet A. 146A:1280–5. PMID 18386803

Wilkins-Haug L, Porter A, Hawley P, Benson CB. (2009) Isolated fetal omphalocele, Beckwith–Wiedemann syndrome, and assisted reproductive technologies. Birth Defects Res A Clin Mol Teratol. 85:58–62. PMID 19107956

# 24

# Anorectal Malformations

## Clinical Consult

After an uneventful pregnancy and delivery, a term male infant was delivered at a community hospital with normal BW and APGAR scores. He roomed in with his mother until 12 hours of life, when he became dusky. A pulse oximeter showed poor $O_2$ saturation. When re-examined, anal atresia was noted. He developed hypoxemic respiratory distress that did not respond to blow-by $O_2$ or continuous positive airway pressure (CPAP). An echocardiogram showed pulmonary hypertension without a cardiac defect. After transfer to a tertiary care facility, he continued to deteriorate after sildenafil treatment, ventilation with nitric oxide, and high-frequency oscillator ventilation. Within 24 hours of delivery, he was cannulated for ECMO. The common causes of pulmonary hypertension—perinatal asphyxia, cardiac defect, pneumonia, and Down syndrome—were ruled out. At 2 days of age, a genetics consultant documented a negative family history and lack of dysmorphic features and suggested the diagnosis of **alveolar capillary dysplasia with misalignment of pulmonary veins** (ACD/MPV). After a failed attempt at decannulation, he tolerated a lung biopsy while he was on ECMO, despite anticoagulation. Lung histology showed pulmonary veins coursing with pulmonary arteries in the same adventitial sheath, confirming the diagnosis of ACD/MPV. The infant expired after ECMO was discontinued. A postmortem skin biopsy was obtained for *FOXF1* analysis. Unexplained respiratory distress with GI atresias should suggest this disorder.

*Pearl*: When congenital anomalies are present, take a blood sample for possible gene analysis *prior* to starting ECMO.

## Definition

- Anorectal malformations (ARM) include
  - Anterior (ectopic) placement of the anus
  - Persistent anal membrane
  - Anal stenosis
  - Anal and rectal atresias with or without a fistula
  - Persistent cloaca
- Incidence 1:2,500 live births

- 1.06 M:1 F; slight male preponderance for isolated ARM (EUROCAT study)
  - Females predominate when there is ectopic anus with perineal fistula.
  - Males predominate when there is anal atresia without fistula.
- High lesions 26%; atresia occurs above levator muscles
  - More common in syndromic ARM; less common, 10%, in isolated ARM.
  - More common in males
  - Tethered cord 25%
- Low lesions 57%
  - More common in girls
  - Tethered cord in 50%, higher in males
  - Ribbon-like stools indicate an internal membrane or stenotic canal.
- Associated anomalies >50%
  - When ARM occurs with associated anomalies, high lesions are up to 13× more common than low lesions.
  - Most common associated malformations: GU (renal agenesis, hypospadias), vertebral, extremities, cardiac (VSD)
    - An upper limb anomaly more than doubles the likelihood of a genetic disorder: 23% versus 9%
    - Sacral vertebral anomalies are associated with incontinence and abnormal innervation to the levator ani muscle
- Risk factors: assisted reproductive technology, consanguinity, infertility, obesity, pregestational maternal diabetes mellitus, twins. Maternal smoking and maternal respiratory disease have been implicated in some studies.
- Genetic etiology
  - Increased consanguinity
  - Familial aggregation
    - Among patients with ARM, 2–8% have an affected first- or second-degree relative.
  - Recurrence risk: 2–5% in first-degree relatives, who are also at increased risk for non-anorectal anomalies
- Preconceptional folic acid supplementation taken by the mother reduces the incidence of imperforate anus.

## Differential Diagnosis

- Chromosome abnormalities 4.5–11%. Microarray studies have identified various submicroscopic deletions and duplications.
  - **Down syndrome***
    - ARM occurs in ~1% of infants with Down syndrome
    - Makes up 40% of the chromosome abnormalities in ARM
    - 2–5% of all ARM
  - **Cri du chat syndrome*** (5p minus syndrome, MIM 123450)

*Pearl:* Rare copy number variants are often seen in isolated ARM.
  - Microduplication of 8p11.2–12.1, locus of *DKK4*

  - **Microdeletions 15q24.1–q24.2 and 16q24.1** *FOXF1*
  - **Trisomy 18***
  - **Deletion of chromosome 22q11.2*** (velocardiofacial syndrome, MIM 192430; DiGeorge syndrome, MIM 188400)
    - Clinical features: ARM ~3%, asymmetric crying face, hypocalcemia, absent thymus, cardiac or ear anomalies
  - **Cat eye syndrome** or tetrasomy 22p (MIM 115470)
- Syndromes
  - **Alveolar capillary dysplasia with misalignment of the pulmonary veins** (MIM 265380; see Clinical Consult)
    - Lethal disorder, caused by heterozygous pathogenic variant or deletion of *FOXF1*, on chromosome 16q24
      - Pathogenic variant detected ~50%
      - Maternal uniparental disomy for chromosome 16 (matUPD16) or a chromosome 16p anomaly can affect *FOXF1* transcription.
    - Clinical features: unexplained respiratory distress, pulmonary hypertension, unresponsive to aggressive treatment, cardiac anomalies, gastrointestinal atresias, VATER/VACTERL-like anomalies
    - Lung histology is diagnostic: Alveolar capillaries do not make contact with the respiratory epithelium tract.
  - **Currarino syndrome** (MIM 176450)
    - Autosomal dominant trait, caused by heterozygous pathogenic variant or deletion in *MNX1* (*HLXB9*)
    - Clinical features: triad of anorectal stenosis (primarily), atresia or fistula, presacral mass, usually an anterior meningocele, and bony defects of the sacrum; dermoid cysts and tethered cord
  - **Fanconi anemia** (FA, MIM 227650)
    - Autosomal recessive disorders of increased chromosome breakage. Many genes have been identified.
    - Clinical features: IUGR, café au lait spots, microphthalmia, and microcephaly. Limb anomalies, especially radial ray/thumb defects, are common, but may be subtle.
      - Children with FA are often misdiagnosed with **VATER/VACTERL* association**.
  - **Fraser syndrome** (MIM 219000)
    - Rare, distinctive, and variable autosomal recessive syndrome, caused by biallelic pathogenic variants in *FRAS1*, *FREM2*, or *GRIP1*
    - Clinical features: anorectal malformations 42%, cryptophthalmos 75%, other eye anomalies, cutaneous syndactyly 58%, renal/urinary, laryngeal 25% and respiratory tract anomalies, ambiguous genitalia, ear anomalies 20% and oral clefts 8% (Figure 24.1)
  - **Johanson–Blizzard syndrome** (MIM 243800)
    - Autosomal recessive trait, caused by pathogenic variants in *UBR1*

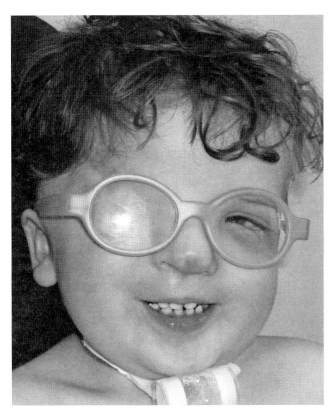

FIGURE 24.1 This boy with Fraser syndrome has unilateral cryptophthalmos and a bulbous nasal tip.

- Clinical features: hypoplastic nares, scalp defects, exocrine pancreas insufficiency
  - Anorectal malformations ~50%, most commonly imperforate anus
  - Congenital hearing loss, hypothyroidism, malabsorption, postnatal growth retardation, intellectual disability, absent permanent teeth
- **Omphalocele–exstrophy–imperforate anus–spinal defects association** (OEIS, MIM 258040)
  - Usually sporadic; consists of the major features listed in its name. (Figure 26.4)
- **Pallister–Hall syndrome** (MIM 146510)
  - Autosomal dominant disorder, due to biallelic pathogenic variants in *GLI3*
  - Clinical features: hypothalamic hamartomoblastoma, imperforate anus, postaxial or mesoaxial polydactyly
- **Persistent cloaca**
  - Usually genetic; occurs in females.
  - Accounts for ≤10% of anal atresia
  - Clinical features: The rectum, urethra, and vagina drain into a common channel onto the perineum. GI, GU, and sacral anomalies, including tethered cord, are common.
    - Features may overlap with **VATER/VACTERL association**.
    - High rate of renal failure in childhood

- Townes–Brocks syndrome (MIM 107480)
  - Variable autosomal dominant disorder, caused by heterozygous pathogenic variant or deletion in *SALL1*
  - Clinical features: classic triad of ear anomalies, anal atresia (>80%), and thumb anomalies. All elements need not be present in every affected person. Also malformations in kidney, heart, hands, feet, eyes (Figure 24.2)
- **Urorectal septum malformation sequence (URSMS)**
  - Rare disorder, no known genetic cause
  - Clinical features: anal atresia, absent perineal openings, aphallia (absent penis) or ambiguous genitalia. Colonic and lumbosacral anomalies are frequent. Cardiac anomalies have been reported.
    - Renal malformations (present in all): agenesis, cystic dysplasia, hydronephrosis
    - Partial URSMS: single perineal or anal opening draining a common cloaca
    - Smooth perineum often with a knob-like protuberance instead of genital structures (Figure 24.3). Occasional phallic-like structure occurs in a 46,XX infant
  - Generally lethal due to pulmonary hypoplasia. Increasingly recognized prenatally

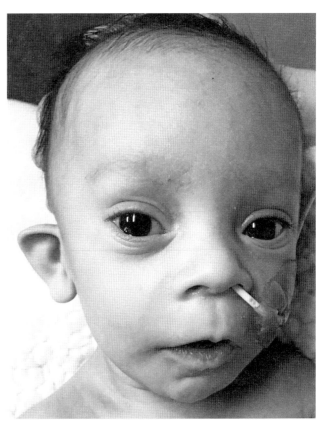

FIGURE 24.2 This infant with ear anomalies and anal atresia has Townes–Brocks syndrome caused by a deletion of 16q12.1 that includes *SALL1*. The diagnosis was established by a chromosome microarray test.

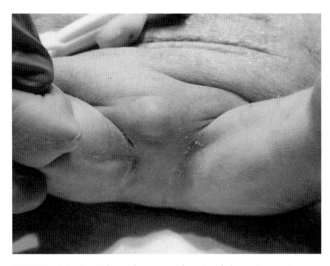

FIGURE 24.3 Genitalia and anus are absent and the perineum is smooth in urorectal septum malformation sequence.

- ○ **VATER/VACTERL association*** (MIM 192350)
  - ▪ Relatively common, sporadic disorder
  - ▪ Clinical features: normal facial features and birth weight. These anomalies occur together more often than expected: vertebra, anus, cardiac, trachea–esophagus, renal, limb (Figure 18S.1)
  - ▪ Consider **Fanconi anemia** (MIM 226650) in these patients.
- ○ Other syndromes with ARM: **FG syndrome** (MIM 305450), **Kabuki syndrome** (MIM 147920), **Mullerian–renal-cervicothoracic somite association** (MURCS, MIM 601076), sirenomelia, and **STAR syndrome** (MIM 300707)

## Evaluation and Management

- Obtain pregnancy history: smoking, obesity, diabetes mellitus, respiratory disease, infertility, ART.
- Document family history: consanguinity, affected relatives with malformations, constipation.
- Evaluate for other anomalies.
  - ○ Echocardiogram, head and abdominal US
  - ○ Check for IUGR, microcephaly, café au lait spots, and subtle limb anomalies (for VATER/VACTERL and Fanconi anemia).
  - ○ Assess urine stream and voiding pattern for evidence of bladder innervation and function.
  - ○ Include a perineal skin prick to elicit a response from the anal sphincter ("anal wink").
- Use imaging studies to delineate the rectal anatomy.
  - ○ Voiding cystourethrogram, fistulogram, US, X-rays, CT and MRI imaging studies
- Laboratory tests

- ○ Chromosome breakage studies with DEB to rule out Fanconi anemia, when considering VATER/VACTERL
- Genetic tests
  - ○ Chromosome microarray analysis
  - ○ Consider UPD16 testing (for suspected ACD/MPV) and chromosome analysis when the microarray is normal and the baby has associated anomalies.
  - ○ Base gene tests on differential diagnosis, or consider exome sequencing.
- Utilize educational resources on microarray abnormalities from https://www.rarechromo.org.
- Counsel family that preconceptional folic acid supplementation reduces the risk for imperforate anus in a future pregnancy.

## Further Reading

Barisic I, Odak L, Loane M, et al. (2013) Fraser syndrome: Epidemiological study in a European population. Am J Med Genet A. 161A:1012–8. PMID 23532946

Caro-Domínguez P, Bass J, Hurteau-Miller J. (2017) Currarino syndrome in a fetus, infant, child, and adolescent: Spectrum of clinical presentations and imaging findings. Can Assoc Radiol J. 68:90–95. PMID 27887934

Faivre L, Portnoï MF, Pals G, et al. (2005) Should chromosome breakage studies be performed in patients with VACTERL association? Am J Med Genet A. 137:55–8. PMID 16015582

Huang KY, Kuo KT, Li YP, et al. (2016) Urorectal septum malformation sequence—Fetal series with the description of a new "intermediate" variant: Time to refine the terminology? Am J Med Genet A. 170:2479–82. PMID 27273846

Marcelis C, de Blaauw I, Brunner H. (2011) Chromosomal anomalies in the etiology of anorectal malformations: A review. Am J Med Genet A. 155:2692–2704. PMID 21990113

Reutter H, Hilger AC, Hildebrandt F, Ludwig M. (2016) Underlying genetic factors of the VATER/VACTERL association with special emphasis on the "renal" phenotype. Pediatr Nephrol. 31:2025–33. PMID 26857713

Sukalo M, Fiedler A, Guzmán C, et al. (2014) Mutations in the human *UBR1* gene and the associated phenotypic spectrum. Hum Mutat. 35:521–31. PMID 24599544

Szafranski P, Gambin T, Dharmadhikari AV, et al. (2016) Pathogenetics of alveolar capillary dysplasia with misalignment of pulmonary veins. Hum Genet. 135:569–86. PMID 27071622

van den Hondel D, Wijers CH, van Bever Y, et al. (2016) Patients with anorectal malformation and upper limb anomalies: Genetic evaluation is warranted. Eur J Pediatr. 175:489–97. PMID 26498647

Wijers CH, van Rooij IA, Marcelis CL, et al. (2014) Genetic and nongenetic etiology of nonsyndromic anorectal malformations: A systematic review. Birth Defects Res C Embryo Today. 102:382–400. PMID 25546370

Zwink N, Rissmann A, Pötzsch S, et al.; CURE-Net Consortium. (2016) Parental risk factors of anorectal malformations: Analysis with a regional population-based control group. Birth Defects Res A Clin Mol Teratol. 106:133–41. PMID 26690556

# 25

# Hirschsprung Disease

## Clinical Consult

A 1-day-old Pakistani female born to young unrelated parents was referred for failure to pass meconium, IUGR, mild dysmorphic features, and a large cisterna magna on prenatal US. She had microcephaly and down-slanting palpebral fissures (Figure 25.1). Her brain MRI was remarkable for decreased gyral pattern, abnormal corpus callosum, and mildly hypoplastic cerebellar vermis. Rectal biopsy demonstrated long-segment Hirschprung disease (L-HSCR). She underwent surgery with subsequent pull-through at 7 months.

The parents' first child died at 3 months of diarrhea and dehydration in Pakistan. His early history was significant for intermittent severe constipation and small size at birth.

An autosomal recessive condition with intellectual disability, **Goldberg–Shprintzen syndrome** was suspected, and the diagnosis was confirmed by homozygous pathogenic variants in *KIAA1279*. The family has had prenatal diagnosis in three subsequent pregnancies, all with normal outcomes. The patient has made slow, steady progress but remains significantly delayed at age 5 years.

## Definition

- Hirschsprung disease is characterized by incomplete innervation along a variable length of the gastrointestinal tract. Typically, parasympathetic enteric ganglion cells in the submucosal and myenteric plexuses of the distal intestine are absent. Vagal and sacral neural crest cell proliferation and migration into the hindgut at 4–7 weeks' gestation are disrupted.
  - Short segment (S-HSCR) 80%: from anal sphincter up to upper sigmoid
  - Long segment (L-HSCR) 12%: extends to sigmoid
  - Total colonic aganglionosis 7%: involves entire colon
  - Total intestinal aganglionosis involves both small intestine and colon
  - Segmental or zonal aganglionosis
  - In variant HSCR, ganglion cells are present but abnormal in number or function.

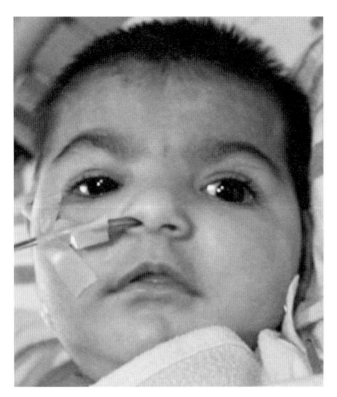

FIGURE 25.1 This female infant with Goldberg–Shprintzen syndrome has microcephaly, hypertelorism, down-slanting palpebral fissures, and Hirschsprung disease.

- Incidence 2/10,000 live births
  - Hispanics: 1/10,000
  - Asians: 2.8/10,000
- 3.5 M:1 F; males predominate
  - L-HSCR: no male preponderance, 1 M:1 F
- Prenatal diagnosis is uncommon: hyperechoic bowel, polyhydramnios, other anomalies.
- Clinical presentation: delayed passage of meconium beyond 24–48 hours, abdominal distention, vomiting, enterocolitis. When total colonic aganglionosis presents in the newborn, the features can be severe with dilated small bowel, microcolon, intestinal obstruction, and peritonitis following intestinal perforation.
  - Accounts for ~10% of intestinal obstruction in the newborn

*Pearl*: 85–90% of affected patients are diagnosed in infancy, but others may take years. Consider HSCR in severe constipation and overflow diarrhea.

- Positive family history ~7%
  - Severe L-HSCR: 15% have autosomal dominant trait with incomplete penetrance.
- Isolated HSCR 70%
  - Usually sporadic and multifactorial. Epigenetic factors also contribute.
  - Pathogenic variants, often multiple, are identified in ~50%.

- Heterozygous loss-of-function pathogenic variants in *RET* cause 3–10% of isolated S-HSCR, 50% of familial cases, and 70–80% of L-HSCR.
- Pathogenic variants in *RET* pathway genes that promote neural crest proliferation cause HSCR: *GDNF, GFR alpha-1, NRTN.*
- Pathogenic variants in *EDNRB* or *EDN3* cause 10% of HSCR.

*Pearl*: Co-occurrence of HSCR and multiple endocrine neoplasia 2A in the same family (or the same individual) is caused by a "Janus" (two-faced) pathogenic variant in *RET* exon 10 with both gain-of-function and loss-of-function qualities.

- Hirschsprung disease is associated with other malformation in 15–20%
  - More often in affected males; 6 M: 1 F
  - Most common associated malformations: CNS, GU, skeletal, GI, cardiovascular
- Chromosome abnormalities 12%
  - **Down syndrome**\* accounts for 2–10% of HSCR.
  - **45,X/47,XXX**—Turner/triple XXX mosaicism
  - Microdeletions: **2q22** (*ZEB2*, previously called *ZFHX1B*, associated with **Mowat–Wilson syndrome**), **10q11.2** (*RET*), **13q22** (*EDNRB*), **22q11.2**

## Differential Diagnosis

- Other GI dysmotility disorders
  - **Chronic intestinal pseudo-obstruction** (MIM 300048)
    - X-linked recessive disorder, caused by hemizygous pathogenic variant or duplication of *FLNA* at Xq28
      - An autosomal recessive form also exists (MIM 243180)
    - Clinical features: malrotation, bilious vomiting, functional bowel obstruction, congenital short gut syndrome
- Syndromic HSCR
  - **Cartilage hair hypoplasia** (MIM 250250)
    - Autosomal recessive skeletal dysplasia, caused by biallelic pathogenic variants in *RMRP*
    - Clinical features: metaphyseal skeletal dysplasia, early onset anemia, serious immunodeficiency, HSCR 10%
      - May require bone marrow transplant, making early diagnosis important
  - **Goldberg–Shprintzen syndrome** (MIM 609460)
    - Autosomal recessive trait, caused by biallelic pathogenic variants in *KIAA1279*
    - Clinical features: IUGR, short stature, microcephaly, cleft palate, distinctive facial appearance, S-HSCR > L-HSCR, mild to moderate ID
      - CNS: small cerebellar vermis, gyral malformations, abnormal corpus callosum

o **Haddad syndrome** (congenital central hypoventilation syndrome with Hirschsprung disease, Ondine's curse, MIM 209880)
  ■ Rare autosomal dominant condition, due to heterozygous pathogenic variant in *ASCL1*
    ● Several other genes have been implicated in congenital central hypoventilation syndrome without Hirschsprung disease: *PHOX2B, GDNF, RET, BDNF.*
  ■ Clinical features: dysfunctional autonomic nervous system, hypoventilation due to blunted response to hypercarbia, poor thermoregulation, abnormal cardiac rhythm and abnormal gastrointestinal motility, L-HSCR 16–20%
    ● Neural crest tumors
    ● Normal intelligence but neurodevelopmental problems occur
  ■ Neonatal death is common.
    ● Tracheotomy, home ventilation, and diaphragm pacing may prolong survival.
o **Mowat–Wilson syndrome** (MIM 235730)

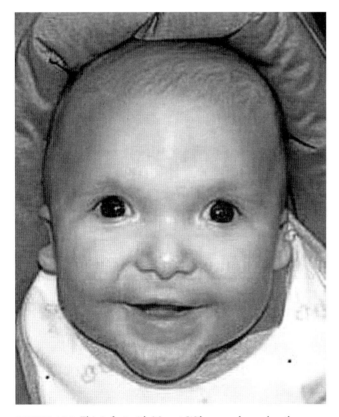

FIGURE 25.2 This infant with Mowat-Wilson syndrome has the characteristic facial features of hypertelorism, deep set eyes, wide nasal bridge, long prominent chin and uplifted ear lobules.
SOURCE: Courtesy of Margaret Adam, MD, University of Washington, Seattle, WA.

■ Autosomal dominant disorder, caused by heterozygous pathogenic variant or deletion of *ZEB2* (*ZFHX1B*)
■ Clinical features: deep-set eyes, prominent triangular pointed chin, uplifted characteristic earlobes (Figure 25.2), excess nuchal skin, cardiac defects, corpus callosum agenesis, hypospadias, severe ID, seizures, HSCR >50%. In those without HSCR, severe constipation is common.
o **Shah–Waardenburg syndrome** (Waardenburg syndrome type 4, WS4, MIM 609136)
  ■ Autosomal recessive trait, caused by biallelic pathogenic variants in *EDNRB*, less commonly in *EDN3*
    ● Autosomal dominant heterozygous pathogenic variant in *EDN3* or *SOX10* also cause WS4.
  ■ Clinical features: white forelock, no displacement of inner canthi, hypopigmented skin, lack of neural crest-derived melanocytes, hearing loss 20%, HSCR frequent
o HSCR also occurs in **Bardet–Beidl syndrome** (MIM 209900), **familial dysautonomia** (MIM 223900), **Fryns syndrome** (MIM 229850), **neurofibromatosis type 1** (MIM 613113), **Smith–Lemli–Opitz syndrome\*** (MIM 270400), **tibial hypoplasia with polydactyly syndrome** (Werner mesomelic dysplasia, MIM 188740, see Figure 32.1), and **X-linked aqueductal stenosis** (MIM 307000).

## Evaluation and Management

● Document family history: consanguinity, chronic constipation, deafness, intestinal obstruction, hypopigmentation, iris heterochromia, tumors including thyroid cancer.
● Evaluate extent of lesion.
  o Contrast enema, X-rays (showing dilated proximal colon and distal narrowing of the aganglionic segment), rectal biopsy
● Evaluate for associated anomalies: echocardiogram, brain imaging, abdominal US.
● Genetic testing
  o Chromosome microarray: recommended first test in most cases
  o Chromosomes analysis: when aneuploidy is suspected
  o Gene testing should be guided by differential diagnosis. Gene panels are available.
● Genetic counseling
● Long-term management of L-HSCR is complex, and sequelae are common.
● Stem cell therapies are under investigation.

# Further Reading

Amiel J, Sproat-Emison E, Garcia-Barcelo M, et al. (2008) Hirschsprung disease, associated syndromes and genetics: A review. J Med Genet. 45:1–14. PMID 17965226

Fattahi F, Steinbeck JA, Kriks S, et al. (2016) Deriving human ENS lineages for cell therapy and drug discovery in Hirschsprung disease. Nature. 531:105–9. PMID 26863197

Garavelli L, Zollino M, Mainardi PC, et al. (2009) Mowat–Wilson syndrome: Facial phenotype changing with age: Study of 19 Italian patients and review of the literature. Am J Med Genet A. 149A:417–26. PMID 19215041

Green HL, Rizzolo D, Austin M. (2016) Surgical management for Hirschsprung disease: A review for primary care providers. JAAPA. 29:24–9. PMID 26945276

Ivanovski I, Djuric O, Caraffi SG, et al. (2018) Phenotype and genotype of 87 patients with Mowat-Wilson syndrome and recommendations for care. Genet Med. 20:965–975. PMID 29300384s

Moore SW. (2017) Genetic impact on the treatment & management of Hirschsprung disease. J Pediatr Surg. 52:218–22. PMID 28003043

Tam PK. (2016) Hirschsprung's disease: A bridge for science and surgery. J Pediatr Surg. 51:18–22. PMID 26611330

# Part VI

## Genitourinary System

# 26

# Renal and Urinary Tract Anomalies

## Clinical Consult

A 35-year-old G2P0TAb1 woman delivered a 33-week gestation male in the breech presentation. Amniotic fluid was severely diminished, and ruptured membranes were suspected because amniotic fluid levels had previously been normal on fetal US at 16 and 19 weeks' gestation. He had severe respiratory distress and ventilated poorly despite high pressures. The geneticist noted large fontanels, widely separated sutures, and facial features that suggested Potter sequence: flat nasal tip and large ears. She suspected pulmonary hypoplasia. The infant died at 9 hours of age after support was discontinued. At autopsy, pulmonary hypoplasia was diagnosed. Although the local pathologist and a consulting renal pathologist at an academic center read the renal histology as normal, a fetal pathologist made the diagnosis of **renal tubular dysgenesis** (MIM 267430) on the basis of the paucity of proximal convoluted renal tubules.

The mother had terminated her first pregnancy at 22 weeks' gestation for anhydramnios, agenesis of the corpus callosum, and a VSD. Fetal chromosome analysis had been normal. The autopsy had not revealed a diagnosis, and kidneys were reported to be normal. The renal histology was re-examined in light of this baby's diagnosis, and renal tubular dysgenesis was confirmed in the previous fetus.

Renal tubular dysgenesis is usually lethal in the perinatal period because of pulmonary hypoplasia secondary to renal hypoperfusion, fetal anuria, and oligohydramnios. Early prenatal diagnosis may be difficult because the amniotic fluid volume can be normal until 22 weeks' gestation. This amniotic fluid pattern may raise suspicion for this diagnosis.

## Definition

- **Congenital *a*nomalies of the *k*idney and *u*rinary *t*ract** (CAKUT, MIM 610805), a heterogeneous group of structural renal disorders
  o Incidence 3–6/1,000 births
    ▪ Leading cause of end-stage renal disease in children
    ▪ Males: Renal anomalies occur with greater frequency and severity.

- CAKUT includes many different renal malformations.
    - Ureteropelvic junction obstruction is the most common renal anomaly: ~20%.
    - Others are renal agenesis/hypoplasia, multicystic dysplastic kidneys, renal cysts, obstructive uropathy and hydronephrosis, vesicoureteral reflux, megaureter, ectopic ureter, horseshoe kidney, and duplicated collecting system.
- Extrarenal anomalies occur in one-third of cases.
    - One in six infants with CAKUT has a recognizable syndrome.
    - Most common associated malformations are in the VATER/VACTERL spectrum: vertebral defects, anal atresia, cardiac anomalies, tracheoesophageal atresia, limb anomalies
- Etiology
    - **Maternal diabetes mellitus**\*
        - Present in 4.1% of the CAKUT group versus 2.3% of controls
        - Pregestational diabetes mellitus (DM) confers greater risk for CAKUT than does gestational DM.
    - Chromosome abnormalities
        - Aneuploidy or microscopically visible structural chromosome anomaly: 7%
            - **Trisomy 18**\*: 2% of all infants with renal defects
        - Microarray anomalies: most commonly **22q deletion**\* and **deletion of 17q12** (*HNF1B*)
            - Occur in 10–16% of isolated renal malformations
            - More common, 22%, when renal anomalies occur with extrarenal anomalies
    - Monogenic disorders: see Nicolaou et al. (2015)
        - Heterozygous pathogenic variants in two genes cause ~15% of CAKUT:
            - *PAX2* (MIM 120330): renal dysplasia or hypoplasia
            - *HNF1B* (MIM 137920): bilateral hyperechoic or cystic kidneys with or without a family history
        - Most sporadic CAKUT is not monogenic.
- Prenatal diagnosis
    - Renal anomalies that would not be symptomatic until later in childhood, if at all, are often recognized prenatally: hyperechoic kidneys, renal cysts, renal aplasia/hypoplasia, multicystic dysplastic kidney, hydronephrosis.
    - Incidence for major renal anomalies: 1/500 fetal US examinations
        - Pelviectasis occurs in ~2% of routine second trimester scans; ~96% resolve spontaneously.
    - Appropriate management for asymptomatic conditions is unclear.
        - Watchful waiting, regular monitoring, and surveillance are reasonable for isolated renal malformations without functional renal impairment.
- Positive family history of renal anomalies: 10%
    - Phenotypes may vary within families.

*Pearl*: Recommend renal US examination in both parents, and their other offspring, when a renal anomaly is found in their infant.

# Differential Diagnosis

## Structural and Functional Renal Anomalies

- Hydronephrosis
    - Incidence 1/1,000–1/1,500
        - Common on fetal US, often regresses during pregnancy
            - 1–4.5% of all pregnancies
            - 2% of patients with **Down syndrome** have an obstructive anomaly of the renal pelvis or hydronephrosis.
    - Commonly caused by
        - **Ureteropelvic junction obstruction** (MIM 143400)
        - Vesicoureteral reflux (VUR)
    - Syndromic hydronephrosis: >100 syndromes. One example:
        - **Genitopatellar syndrome** (MIM 606170)
            - Autosomal dominant disorder, due to a heterozygous pathogenic variant in *KAT6B*
            - Clinical findings: microcephaly, coarse facial features, joint contractures of lower extremities, absent patellae (difficult to appreciate in the newborn), absent scrotum
                - May present on fetal US as apparently isolated multicystic kidney(s) or hydronephrosis
                - Other urogenital anomalies
- Horseshoe kidney
    - Kidneys are fused across the midline, usually at the lower poles.
    - Prevalence 1/400
    - 2 M:1 F
    - Isolated renal anomaly in 30%
    - Classical finding in **Turner syndrome**\* and **trisomy 18**\*
        - Other renal anomalies are also common in these disorders.
- Isolated renal agenesis; renal aplasia/hypoplasia/dysplasia
    - **Autosomal dominant renal adysplasia** (MIM 191830), caused by a heterozygous pathogenic variant in *ITGA8, RET, PAX2*
        - First-degree relatives have renal malformations 9%
            - Many asymptomatic
        - Clinical features: continuum of severity, may be bilateral (lethal) or unilateral
            - Lethal (Potter sequence)
                - Oligohydramnios, pulmonary hypoplasia
                - Bilateral renal agenesis or unilateral renal agenesis and contralateral renal dysplasia
                - Potter facies (flattened facial features, micrognathia, semicircular depression on chin; Figure 26.1A),

(A)

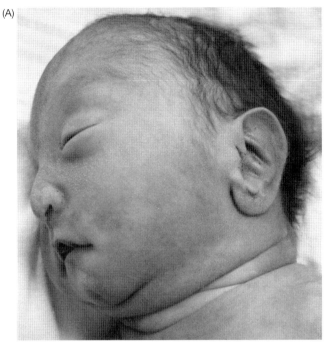

(B)

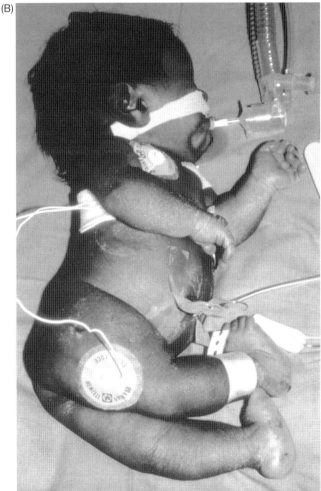

FIGURE 26.1  (A) This baby with Potter sequence had oligohydramnios and intrauterine compression causing a flat nose, micrognathia, and large ear. (B) This infant with Potter sequence had renal agenesis, oligohydramnios, pulmonary hypoplasia, genu recurvatum, and rocker bottom feet.

SOURCE: Reprinted with permission from W. B. Saunders, publishers.

large fontanels, loose skin, abnormal position of limbs (Figure 26.1B)
- Asymptomatic: unilateral renal agenesis

- Syndromic renal agenesis
  - **Fraser syndrome** (MIM 219000)
    - Autosomal recessive disorder, due to biallelic mutations in *FRAS1, GRIP1, FREM2*
      - Consanguinity common
    - Incidence 1/500,000
    - Clinical findings: renal agenesis bilateral 50%, unilateral 17%; cryptophthalmos, anophthalmia or other eye anomalies 83%, syndactyly 58%, anorectal anomalies 42%, ambiguous genitalia 13%, oral clefts, cardiac anomalies, laryngeal, and tracheal anomalies
  - ***M**ullerian duct aplasia, **u**nilateral **r**enal agenesis, **c**ervicothoracic **s**omite association* (MURCS, MIM 601076)
    - Sporadic disorder, almost exclusively in females
    - Clinical findings: absent or ectopic kidney, multicystic kidney, absent vagina, bicornuate uterus, absent ovary, fusion and segmentation defects of the C-spine (Klippel–Feil anomaly)
- **Renal tubular dysgenesis** (MIM 267430). See clinical consult
  - Autosomal recessive lethal syndrome, caused by biallelic pathogenic variants in one of four genes in the renin–angiotensin pathway: *ACE* 64%, *REN* 20%, *AGT, AGTR1* 8%
  - Nongenetic causes of this phenotype include:
    - **Twin–twin transfusion syndrome** causes hypoperfusion of the kidneys in the donor fetus.
    - Maternal use of **ACE inhibitors** during second and third trimesters
  - Prenatal findings: late second trimester onset of oligohydramnios with apparently normal kidneys on US
    - Amniotic fluid volume can be normal before 22 weeks.
  - Clinical findings: paucity or absence of differentiated proximal tubules, Potter facies, skull defects, cutis aplasia. Generally lethal because of pulmonary hypoplasia
    - Cardiac defects, absent gallbladder, absent thymus, branchial clefts, imperforate anus, choanal atresia, absent nipples and breasts, broad digits, small nails
- Congenital nephrotic syndromes
  - Prenatal presentation: prenatal onset of proteinuria causes markedly increased maternal serum AFP or amniotic fluid AFP (often >10 multiples of the median for the gesational age)
  - **Cerebral ventriculomegaly with congenital nephrosis** (MIM 219730)
    - Autosomal recessive trait, caused by biallelic pathogenic variants in *CRB2*
    - Clinical findings: echogenic kidneys, cysts at the corticomedullary junction
      - CNS: hydrocephalus, periventricular nodular heterotopias

- Cardiac: ASD, pericardial effusion
  - **Congenital nephrotic syndrome, type 1—Finnish type** (MIM 256300)
    - Autosomal recessive disorder, caused by biallelic pathogenic variants in *NPHS1*, which encodes nephrin
    - Common in Groffdale Mennonites: 1/500 live births
    - Prenatal onset of massive proteinuria
      - Progresses rapidly to renal failure
      - Steroid resistant
    - Lethal without renal transplant
      - At autopsy: Electron microscopy of renal tissue is diagnostic with diffuse podocyte foot process effacement.
  - **Galloway–Mowat syndrome** (MIM 25130)
    - Autosomal recessive trait caused by pathogenicvariants in *WDR73*
    - Clinical findings: congenital nephrosis, renal cysts at the corticomedullary junction, proteinuria, steroid resistant
      - CNS: microcephaly, gyral anomalies, paraventricular heterotopias, hydrocephalus, hypoplasia of the cerebellum
      - GI: hiatal hernia

## Renal Syndromes with Distinctive Extrarenal Anomalies

- **VATER/VACTERL association*** (MIM 192350)
  - Sporadic multiple anomaly disorder affecting *v*ertebrae, *a*nal atresia, *c*ardiac, *t*racheo*e*sophageal fistula, *r*adial ray, *r*enal and *l*imb
  - Renal anomalies 69%
    - Vesicoureteral reflux with a structural kidney anomaly 27%
    - Multicystic/dysplastic kidney 18%
      - Vesico-urethrogram (VCUG) is recommended when a structural renal anomaly is identified.
    - Unilateral renal agenesis 24%
  - Other monogenic conditions mimic VATER/VACTERL association.
    - **Fanconi anemia** (MIM 227650)
- Craniofacial disorders associated with renal anomalies
  - Some syndromes with both ear and renal anomalies
    - **Branchio-oto-renal syndrome** (MIM 113650)
    - **CHARGE syndrome*** (MIM 214800)
    - **Diabetic embryopathy***
    - **Goldenhar/facio-auricular-vertebral syndrome** (MIM 164210)
    - **Mandibulofacial dysostosis with microcephaly** (*EFTUD2* mutations or haploinsufficiency) (MIM 610536)
    - **Nager syndrome** (MIM 154400)
    - **Townes–Brocks syndrome** (MIM 107480)
  - Among patients with isolated ear anomalies, including preauricular pits or tags, up to 11% had renal anomalies in one study.

- Ear anomalies may be an indication for renal imaging, but consensus is lacking.
- Renal disorders associated with genital, hepatic, and pancreatic anomalies
  - **ARC syndrome** (Nezelof syndrome, MIM 208085)
    - Autosomal recessive disorder, caused by biallelic pathogenic variants in *VPS33B* or *VIPAR*
    - Clinical findings: renal insufficiency with proximal tubulopathy, generalized aminoaciduria, proteinuria, arthrogryposis, failure to thrive, cholestasis, jaundice, ichthyosis
      - Organ biopsy can cause life-threatening hemorrhage. Gene testing is the preferred diagnostic method.
  - **Pancreatic hypoplasia or insufficiency** (MIM 208540)
    - Autosomal recessive disorder, caused by biallelic pathogenic variants in *NPHP3*
    - Clinical findings: renal cystic dysplasia, cysts and fibrosis of liver and pancreas
  - **Renal cysts and diabetes syndrome** (MODY5, MIM 137920)
    - Autosomal dominant disorder, caused by heterozygous pathogenic variant or deletion in *HNF1B*
    - Clinical findings: variable CAKUT anomalies—cysts, small kidney, horseshoe kidney, renal failure
      - Vaginal and uterine anomalies in females. Maturity-onset diabetes mellitus can develop in childhood.
- Renal disorders associated with eye anomalies
  - **Acro-renal-ocular syndrome** (Duane–radial ray syndrome, MIM 607323)
    - Autosomal dominant disorder, due to a heterozygous pathogenic variant in *SALL4*
    - Clinical findings: horseshoe kidney, radial ray abnormalities, ocular coloboma. Deafness and imperforate anus are less common features.
  - **Lowe syndrome** (oculocerebrorenal syndrome; MIM 309000)
    - X-linked recessive disorder, caused by hemizygous pathogenic variant in *OCRL1*
      - De novo 32%
      - High rate of germ line mosaicism
    - Family history
      - Almost all carrier mothers have "snowflake" lenticular opacities on slit-lamp exam.
    - Clinical findings in affected males: renal proximal tubular dysfunction by 6–12 months, polyuria, renal tubular acidosis, aminoaciduria, proteinuria, phosphaturia, rickets
      - Usually presents with the extrarenal anomalies in the newborn
      - Congenital dense cataracts, glaucoma 50%
      - Hypotonia, areflexia, feeding problems may require nasogastric (NG) or G-tube
      - Developmental delay is universal.

- Generalized aminoaciduria and elevated phosphatidylinositol 4,5-bisphosphate
  - **Renal coloboma syndrome** (papillorenal syndrome, MIM 120330)
    - Autosomal dominant disorder, caused by heterozygous pathogenic variant in *PAX2*
    - Clinical findings: renal hypoplasia/dysplasia, vesicoureteral reflux or another structural renal anomaly; renal failure without a structural kidney anomaly
      - Eye findings vary, and some patients have no ocular findings.
        - Small cornea, microphthalmia, optic nerve coloboma, dysplastic optic disc ("morning glory anomaly")
      - Hearing loss has been reported.

## Renal Cysts Without Extrarenal Anomalies

- Renal cysts can be isolated renal anomalies (bilateral, unilateral, familial, sporadic) or part of various multiple congenital anomaly syndromes, many of which are "ciliopathies."
- **Multicystic dysplastic kidneys**
  - Prevalence 4/10,000 (Europe)
  - 3 M:2 F
  - Etiology—two theories
    - Disruption of ureteric bud branching leads to cysts and obstructive uropathy.
      - May be monogenic: *HNF1B*
      - Activating mutation in *NFAT* causes multicystic dysplastic kidney in mouse.

*or*

    - Primary urinary tract obstruction damages the renal parenchyma and causes a secondary cystic response.
  - Clinical findings: Renal cysts are of different sizes, disrupting renal architecture.
    - More often unilateral; L > R
      - When unilateral, the contralateral functioning kidney has structural or functional defects in one-third of cases.
    - Vesicoureteral reflux: 20% of unilateral group
    - Ureteropelvic junction stenosis
  - Extrarenal features uncommon
    - Unilateral multicystic kidney: 84% isolated
    - Bilateral multicystic kidney: 51% isolated
- **Polycystic kidney disease, autosomal dominant—adult type** (ADPKD, MIM 173900)
  - Autosomal dominant, typically adult-onset, disorder, due to a heterozygous pathogenic variant in *PKD1* or *PKD2*; inherited (familial) 95%
    - Infantile presentation can be caused by
      - Biallelic pathogenic variants in *PKD1,* when one or both mutations are mild (hypomorphic)

      - Digenic pathogenic variants in *PKD1* and *HNF1B*
      - Chromosome 16p deletion that removes both *PKD1* and *TSC2*
  - Prevalence 1–2.5/1,000
    - The most common single gene disorder of kidneys
  - Clinical findings in fetus or newborn: large echogenic kidneys without distinct cysts
    - Later findings: adult-onset bilateral renal cysts and enlarged kidneys, renal dysfunction, urinary tract infection, flank pain, hematuria, liver cysts, intracranial aneurysms 4–12%, cardiovascular anomalies, hypertension, left ventricular hypertrophy, mitral valve prolapse, aortic insufficiency, enlarged aortic root
  - Neonatal diagnosis of ADPKD can bring the disorder to the attention of affected family members before they are aware of their condition.
    - Parents need renal imaging.
      - Variable expression
        - ~80% of affected adults will have three or more renal cysts in at least one kidney by age 30, and 95% will by age 40.
        - End-stage renal disease occurs in approximately half of affected adults by age 60.
      - Incomplete penetrance
        - Some heterozygotes do not express the disorder.
        - An apparently unaffected individual may die prior to diagnosis of his or her renal disease.
- **Polycystic kidney disease, autosomal recessive—infantile type** (ARPKD, MIM 263200)
  - Autosomal recessive disorder, due to biallelic pathogenic variants in *PKHD1* in ~80%
    - When only one variant is identified, perform deletion/duplication testing in addition to sequence analysis.
  - Incidence 1/10,000–1/40,000
  - Prenatal diagnosis
    - Enlarged bilateral hyperechoic kidneys are commonly detected by fetal US, but some affected infants have normal renal images on fetal US.
    - Fetal urinary output is usually normal.
      - When severe, may present with oligohydramnios causing the Potter phenotype
    - ~20–30% die in the first year of life from pulmonary causes.
      - Clinical findings: nephromegaly and bilateral palpable flank masses. Renal cysts are not always evident in newborns. Hypertension, impaired renal function, liver involvement ~45%, often with hepatosplenomegaly
      - Later findings: may present in older infants and toddlers with chronic liver disease and portal hypertension rather than renal disease
  - Diagnosis is confirmed by typical renal imaging in the baby *and* at least one of the following:
    - Biliary ductal ectasia or hepatic fibrosis

■ An affected sibling
■ No renal enlargement or cysts in the parents

## Syndromes with Renal Cysts

- **Bardet–Biedl syndrome** (MIM 209900)
  - ○ Autosomal recessive group of disorders, due to biallelic pathogenic variants in ~18 responsible genes
  - ○ Clinical features: renal cysts, postaxial polydactyly
    - ■ A challenging diagnosis to make in infancy without a positive family history
    - ■ Later findings: obesity, hypogonadism, retinitis pigmentosa, learning disability
- **Short rib thoracic dysplasia with or without polydactyly** (MIM 208500)
  - ○ Autosomal recessive group of disorders, caused by biallelic pathogenic variants in *IFT80* and a dozen other genes
    - ■ **Jeune syndrome** (MIM 208500): Lethal asphyxiating thoracic dystrophy is no longer the preferred name because it is not uniformly lethal.
    - ■ **Ellis van Creveld syndrome** (MIM 225500)
  - ○ Clinical findings: renal cysts, nephritis, progressive renal failure
  - ○ Extrarenal features
    - ■ Skeletal: primarily short ribs, short long bones, polydactyly, trident appearance of acetabular roof
      - • Constricted chest can cause respiratory failure.
    - ■ Oral clefts, brain, eye, cardiac, liver (cirrhosis, portal fibrosis), intestines (malabsorption), pancreas (cysts)
- **Joubert syndrome** (MIM 213300)
  - ○ Heterogeneous group of autosomal recessive disorders, due to biallelic pathogenic variants in one of 19 genes including *NPHP1, AHI1*
    - ■ Two variants can be identified in ~50%.
    - ■ See *GeneReviews* summary (Parisi and Glass, 2017, Figure 2) for gene testing algorithm.
  - ○ Prevalence 1/100,000
    - ■ Clinical findings: renal cysts, coloboma, hypotonia, episodic tachypnea, apnea, hypoplasia or agenesis of the cerebellar vermis, characteristic "molar tooth" sign on brain MRI, retinal dysplasia, oculomotor apraxia, postaxial polydactyly, progressive renal failure
- **Meckel–Gruber syndrome** (MIM 249000)
  - ○ Lethal group of autosomal recessive disorders that cause cystic renal disease and posterior fossa abnormalities, often with polydactyly
    - ■ Death is due to pulmonary hypoplasia.
  - ○ Many genes have been identified: *TMEM67, CEP290, RPGRIP1L,* and others.
  - ○ Diagnostic triad
    - ■ Bilateral enlarged cystic kidneys, also other renal anomalies

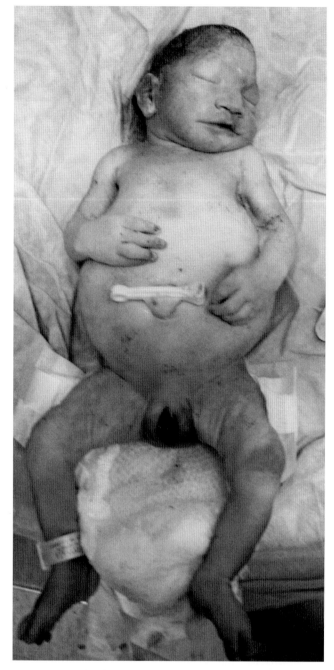

FIGURE 26.2  This deceased infant with Meckel–Gruber syndrome has bulging flanks caused by large cystic kidneys and a posterior occipital encephalocele.

- ■ CNS anomalies, especially occipital encephalocele (Figure 26.2)
- ■ Hepatic fibrosis and bile duct proliferation on liver biopsy or at autopsy
- **Zellweger syndrome** (cerebrohepatorenal syndrome, MIM 214100)
  - ○ Prototypic lethal autosomal recessive disorder of peroxisome biosynthesis, caused by biallelic pathogenic variants in *PEX1* and other peroxisome genes

- Phenotypic overlap with a large group of other peroxisomal disorders caused by related genes
- Clinical findings: polycystic kidneys, jaundice, liver dysfunction, chondrodysplasia punctata, weak suck, poor feeding, seizures
- Physical findings: absent Moro response, large fontanel, high forehead, hypotonia
  - Very long-chain fatty acids accumulate in plasma: hexacosanoic acid (C26:0) and hexacosenoic acid (C26:1).

## Disorders with an Enlarged Bladder

- **Prune belly sequence** (PBS; MIM 100100)
  - Incidence 1/30,000 live births
  - 95 M:5 F
  - Etiology is heterogeneous.
    - Defects in smooth muscle without bladder outlet obstruction
    - Mechanical obstruction of the urethra
      - Posterior urethral valves (males only)
      - Urethral atresia (both sexes affected)
    - More common in
      - **Beckwith–Weidemann syndrome\*** (MIM 130650)
      - **Down syndrome**, as are other renal and urinary tract anomalies
  - Most are sporadic, but recurrences have been reported.
  - Microarray anomalies
    - De novo chromosome 17q12 deletion including *HNF1B*, a CAKUT gene, has been reported.
  - Familial reports uncommon, often associated with consanguinity
    - Homozygous pathogenic variants in *CHRM3* in consanguineous Turkish family with several affected brothers
      - Unable to constrict pupils in response to light
  - Clinical findings: enlarged bladder, various dilated urinary tract abnormalities, urinary ascites, patent urachus, thin wrinkled abdominal skin (Figure 26.3), deficient abdominal musculature, undescended testes, lower limb hypoplasia/absence
    - Additional anomalies in two-thirds
      - Cardiac anomalies 10%: PDA, VSD, ASD, TOF
  - Neonatal mortality 20%: respiratory insufficiency; pulmonary hypoplasia secondary to oligohydramnios
    - Prognosis may be worse when prenatally diagnosed
    - Limited utility of prenatal surgical intervention
- **Megacystis–microcolon–intestinal hypoperistalsis syndrome** (MMIHS, visceral myopathy; MIM 155310, 249210)
  - Autosomal dominant disorder of smooth muscle dysfunction, caused by a missense pathogenic variant in *ACTG2*
    - Encodes a major detrusor muscle protein: α-smooth muscle actin

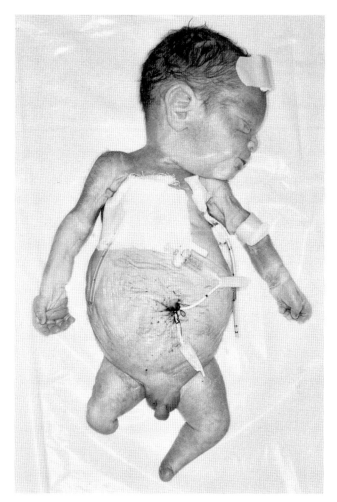

FIGURE 26.3 This deceased infant has prune belly sequence. The weight of his obstructed bladder caused vascular compromise in utero that obstructed perfusion of the lower limbs. Bilateral pneumothoraces, treated with thoracotomy tubes, are evidence of pulmonary hypoplasia.
SOURCE: Reprinted with permission from W. B. Saunders, publishers.

- Affected siblings have been born to phenotypically normal parents; parental mosaicism may be the cause of recurrence, or an autosomal recessive form may exist.
- Clinical findings: marked dilatation of the bladder, small colon, lack of effective peristalsis, abnormal pulmonary and aortic vessels
- **Urofacial syndrome** (Ochoa syndrome, MIM 236730)
  - Rare, autosomal recessive disorder, caused in some cases by biallelic pathogenic variants in *LRIG2* and *HPSE2*
  - Prenatal diagnosis: fetal megacystis on US
  - Clinical findings: bladder dysfunction with incomplete emptying without an anatomic obstruction, VUR, urosepsis
    - Characteristic grimace when smiling, laughing, or crying
- **Urorectal septum malformation sequence**
  - Rare, usually lethal, disorder; no known genetic cause; features variable but constant renal malformations, anal atresia, and absent perineal openings

## Disorders with Exstrophy of the Bladder/Cloaca

- **Bladder exstrophy epispadias complex** (BEEC, MIM 600057)
  - Prevalence 1/30,000
  - 2.3 M:1 F
  - Risk factors
    - Advanced maternal age
    - ART
    - Maternal exposures to tobacco, antacids
  - Usually sporadic, but there is evidence for a genetic contribution
    - Copy number variants in isolated cases
      - Deletion 1qter, duplication 19p13.12
    - Pathogenic variants reported in *TP63* and its target, *PERP*
      - Genes involved in the embryogenesis of the human bladder
    - Concordance is high in MZ twins: 45% MZ, 6% DZ.
  - Clinical features: Exstrophy of bladder is an isolated anomaly in 70%.
    - Extraurinary tract features infraumbilical abdominal wall defects, diastasis of symphi8sis pubis, midline genital defects, epispadias, bifid clitoris.
- *Omphalocele–exstrophy of the cloaca–imperforate anus–spinal defects* (OEIS complex, MIM 258040)
  - Prevalence 1/185,000 births
    - ~10% in like-sex twins
  - Usually sporadic; no identified genetic cause
  - Clinical findings: variable exstrophy of the cloaca through a defect in the lower abdominal wall; kidneys may be malpositioned, rotated
    - ~25% have all components: omphalocele 55%, divided pubic symphysis, imperforate anus, spinal segmentation anomalies including dysraphism, prolapsed ileum ("elephant's trunk"), biphallia, failure of fusion of the genital tubercles (Figure 26.4).

# Evaluation and Management

- Pregnancy history: ART, anhydramnios, oligohydramnios, maternal age, maternal diabetes, medication use (ACE inhibitors), teratogenic exposures.
- Family history: consanguinity, fetal losses, stillbirth, previous children with congenital anomalies, renal transplant or renal dialysis. Ask about causes of death among deceased.
- Examine parents and family members.
  - Abdominal US on parents and first-degree relatives when a renal anomaly is diagnosed in the newborn
- Imaging studies
  - Echocardiogram, head US, ophthalmology exam, hearing test to identify extrarenal anomalies

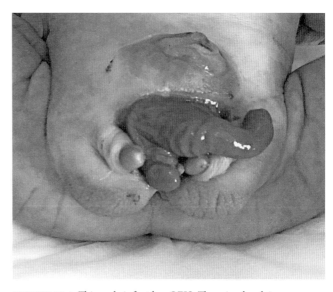

FIGURE 26.4 This male infant has OEIS. There is a low lying omphalocele, exstrophy of the bladder and an inperforate anus. Note the prolapsed ileum resembling an "elephant's trunk" and the duplicated phalluses. A testis was palpable in each scrotal sac.

- Renal and bladder US and other imaging studies
  - After prenatal diagnosis of any renal anomaly including hydronephrosis
  - When primary major congenital anomaly is identified in heart, brain, eye, and ear
  - VCUG when structural renal anomaly is diagnosed in context of other VATER/VACTERL association anomalies
- Genetic studies
  - Chromosome breakage studies with DEB when VATER/VACTERL association or Fanconi syndrome suspected
  - SNP chromosome microarray, especially when there are extrarenal anomalies and a syndromic diagnosis is not apparent
  - Gene or gene panel testing should be guided by the phenotype.
    - Gene panels for CAKUT are available
    - Consider exome sequencing in complex malformation syndromes.
- Nephrology and urology consultations for structural anomalies of the kidneys and urinary tract
  - Prophylaxis with antibiotics to prevent recurrent urinary tract infection
  - Monitor renal function, and arrange serial imaging after discharge.

# Further Reading

Barisic I, Odak L, Loane M, et al. (2013) Fraser syndrome: Epidemiological study in a European population. Am J Med Genet A. 161A:1012–8. PMID 23532956

Bekheirnia MR, Bekheirnia N, Bainbridge MN, et al. (2017) Whole-exome sequencing in the molecular diagnosis of individuals with congenital anomalies of the kidney and urinary tract and identification of a new causative gene. Genet Med. 19:412–20. PMID 27657687

Cunningham BK, Khromykh A, Martinez AF, et al. (2014) Analysis of renal anomalies in VACTERL association. Birth Defects Res A Clin Mol Teratol. 100:801–5. PMID 25196458

Dart AB, Ruth CA, Sellers EA, et al. (2015) Maternal diabetes mellitus and congenital anomalies of the kidney and urinary tract (CAKUT) in the child. Am J Kidney Dis. 65:684–91. PMID 25595566

Faguer S, Chassaing N, Bandin F, et al. (2014) The HNF1B score is a simple tool to select patients for HNF1B gene analysis. Kidney Int. 86:1007–15. PMID 24897035

Gubler MC. (2014) Renal tubular dysgenesis. Pediatr Nephrol. 29:51–9. PMID 23636579

Nicolaou N, Renkema KY, Bongers EM, et al. (2015) Genetic, environmental, and epigenetic factors involved in CAKUT. Nat Rev Nephrol. 11:720–31. PMID 26281895

Parisi M, Glass I. (2017) Joubert Syndrome. In: Adam MP, Ardinger HH, Pagon RA, et al, editors. GeneReviews® [Internet]. Seattle, WA: University of Washington, Seattle; 1993–2018. PMID 20301500

Rodriguez MM. (2014) Congenital anomalies of the kidney and the urinary tract (CAKUT). Fetal Pediatr Pathol. 33:293–320. PMID 25313840

Stoll C, Dott B, Alembik Y, Roth MP. (2014) Associated nonurinary congenital anomalies among infants with congenital anomalies of kidney and urinary tract (CAKUT). Eur J Med Genet. 57:322–8. PMID 24821302

Woolf AS, Stuart HM, Newman WG. (2014) Genetics of human congenital urinary bladder disease. Pediatr Nephrol. 29:353–60. PMID 23584850

# 27

# Hypospadias

## Clinical Consult

A very small for gestational age (SGA), nondysmorphic term male had penoscrotal hypospadias with chordee. His testes were descended, and his scrotum was fused. His mother was a 43-year-old primigravida, who conceived after in vitro fertilization and intracytoplasmic sperm injection using her egg and her 50-year-old husband's sperm. Poor fetal growth was noted from the earliest fetal US exams. Chromosome analysis was 46,XY with normal FISH for *SRY*. Testosterone and dihydrotestosterone levels were normal. The placental weight was below the third percentile for a term infant.

Hypospadias is >10 times more frequent in very low-birth-weight compared to normal-birth-weight babies. Severe hypospadias is significantly more frequent in SGA babies (~60% of all hypospadias) than among normal-birth-weight cohorts (11% of all hypospadias). **Early placental insufficiency** is the presumed cause of fetal growth restriction and hypospadias. Early testosterone levels are dependent on human chorionic gonadotropin secretion, a placental hormone.

## Definition

- Hypospadias is caused by lack of development of the ventral aspect of the penis with ectopic, usually proximal, displacement of the urethral meatus.
- *Disorders of sex development* (DSD; 46,XY DSD, 46,XX DSD) describe a spectrum of disorders that affect gonadal and genital development. Hypospadias is the most mildest DSD and the most common disorder of male external genitalia. Other common disorders of primarily male genital development are reviewed in this chapter. A comprehensive review of disorders of sexual development is beyond the scope of this chapter.
- The language describing these disorders has been revised in light of their psychological impact and the recognition that delaying sex assignment and surgery may be beneficial in some patients.
  - The term *ambiguous genitalia* is currently being replaced with *atypical genitalia* when the anatomical sex and chromosomal sex are discordant or atypical.

○ The term *hermaphrodite*, formerly used to describe patients in whom both male and female components occur in the same individual, has been replaced by 46,XX DSD or 46,XY DSD.

○ There is a growing consensus that patients with severe hypospadias and other DSD should be cared for in specialty centers by interdisciplinary teams with surgical, endocrine, gynecologic, psychosocial, and genetic expertise.

*Pearl*: Absence of the ventral aspect of the prepuce ("congenital circumcision") should prompt a careful examination for hypospadias.

- Incidence of hypospadias: 1/225 live-born males
- Caused by failure of the urethral folds to fuse at 7–14 weeks of gestation
- Mild cases may be missed in the newborn period when there is a physiologic phimosis.
- Risk factors
  ○ ART (especially *intra*cytoplasmic *s*perm *i*njection [ICSI]) and ovarian stimulation (clomiphene or progesterone)
  ○ Drugs, medications, and environmental exposures
    ■ Anticonvulsants and a variety of prescription drugs (including iron supplements)
    ■ Male offspring of diethylstilbesterol (DES)-exposed daughters (referring to mother's own intrauterine exposure to DES) have a high risk for hypospadias (OR 21.3); rare.
    ■ Endocrine-disrupting environmental chemicals
  ○ Maternal factors: advanced age, hypertension, preeclampsia, oligohydramnios
  ○ Parental smoking
  ○ Paternal subfertility
  ○ Small placental size and low birth weight
    ■ Risk for hypospadias increases, as does its severity, as birth weight decreases across all gestational ages: OR is 1.9 for the smallest compared to the largest weight for gestational age quintiles.
      • Risk increases as the gestational age decreases: For a 32-week gestation male in the lowest birth weight group, the OR is 10.4 for hypospadias.
    ■ In MZ twins discordant for hypospadias, the unaffected twin weighs 500 g (average) more than his affected co-twin.
    ■ Underlying syndromes and hormonal abnormalities are uncommon.
  ○ Twins and higher multiples
- Family history supports multifactorial inheritance for isolated hypospadias.
  ○ Positive family history 10–22%, in both maternal (31%), and paternal (59%) relatives.
  ○ Milder variants of hypospadias are more often familial.

○ Risk for hypospadias is increased significantly for sons of fathers with hypospadias: OR 9.7. Risk for brothers of an affected male 17%
- Severity
  ○ Mild hypospadias 60%; involves only the glans or corona (coronal hypospadias)
    ■ Often isolated anomaly
    ■ May not require surgery
  ○ Penile (second-degree) hypospadias 25%
  ○ Scrotal/perineal (third-degree) hypospadias 15% (Figure 27.1)
    ■ Non-genital anomalies more common in the severe groups
- Common associated genital anomalies 7%
  ○ Cryptorchidism occurs in 2% of all term males and in 5–30% of males with hypospadias; it is more prevalent in those with severe hypospadias.
  ○ Chordee, micropenis, bifid scrotum, inguinal hernia, testicular dysgenesis/agenesis: when other genital anomalies are present, it is more likely that a genetic cause is responsible for the DSD.

*Pearl*: Anogenital distance, a biomarker for fetal androgen exposure, is reduced in hypospadias and cryptorchidism. It is associated with reduced fertility, semen quality, and testosterone levels.

# Differential Diagnosis

- Chromosome abnormalities are more common in more severe hypospadias and when there are associated non-genital anomalies. May be detectable only with microarray.
  ○ Isolated hypospadias ≤5%
    ■ Severe hypospadias 5–18%
      • The higher percentage pertains to hypospadias with undescended testes.
    ■ Genitalia that are not fully masculinized ~25%
  ○ Autosomal chromosome anomalies include multiple congenital anomalies in addition to hypospadias
    ■ **Down syndrome***
    ■ Deletions: 1p36.33, 2q22, **Wolf–Hirschhorn syndrome (4p-)***, **Cri du Chat syndrome** (5p-),* 9p23p24.3, 10q26, 12p13.2, 13q32.2, 16p11.2, 19q12q13.11, 22q11.2
    ■ Duplications: 5p15, 22q11.2
  ○ Sex chromosome anomalies
    ■ **Mosaic 45,X/46,XY**: When prenatally diagnosed, most are phenotypically normal males.
      • ~3% have genital anomalies ranging from mild hypospadias with or without cryptorchidism to female external genitalia and **Turner syndrome*** phenotype.
      • Screen for cardiac anomalies that commonly involve the left outflow tract, aorta, and prolonged QTc.

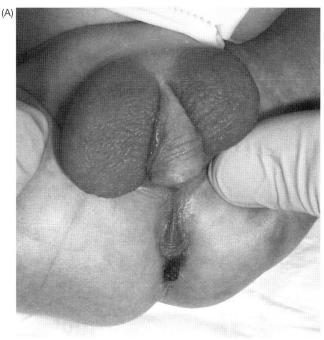

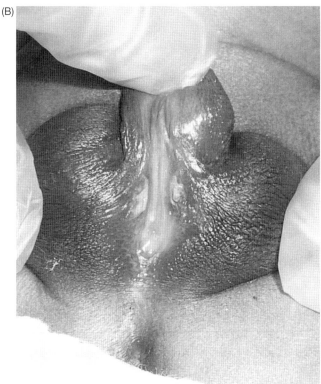

FIGURE 27.1 This infant with 5α-reductase deficiency has a bifid scrotum and severe hypospadias.

- Deletion or duplication of Xq28, Yp11.31
- Dicentric Y chromosome (idic Y): often lost during cell division can predispose to mosaic 45,X/46,XY chromosome complement
- Isolated hypospadias ~80%

o Usually not caused by single gene disorders
  o Common variants in sex hormone biosynthesis and metabolism genes cause hypospadias (Carmichael et al., 2014).
  o **X-linked isolated hypospadias 1** (MIM 300633)
    ■ X-linked disorder, caused by pathogenic variant in androgen receptor gene, *AR*
    ■ In mild hypospadias, with or without other genital defects, 2% have a pathogenic variant in *AR*.
  o **X-linked hypospadias 2** (MIM 300758)
    ■ X-linked disorder, caused by a hemizygous pathogenic variant or deletion in *MAMLD1* at Xq28
      • A contiguous gene microdeletion on Xq28, which involves both *MTM1* and *MAMLD1*, causes **X-linked myotubular myopathy with abnormal genital development** (MIM 300219)
      • Clinical features: hypospadias, microphallus
- DSD cause atypical (ambiguous) genitalia for which the anatomical, gonadal, and chromosomal sex are discordant.
  o Incidence 1/2,000–1/4,500 live births
    ■ 46,XY DSD occurs twice as often as 46,XX DSD.
  o There is no identified etiology in >50% of children with severe 46,XY DSD. For a comprehensive review, see Barbaro et al. (2011). Common causes of DSD are reviewed here.
  o **46,XX sex reversal 2** (MIM 278850)
    ■ Caused by a duplication of a *SOX9* regulatory region on chr 17q24
    ■ Clinical features: 46,XX chromosome complement with variable genital masculinization
  o **46,XY sex reversal 3** (MIM 612965)
    ■ Autosomal dominant trait, caused by heterozygous pathogenic variant or microdeletion of *NR5A1*, encoding steroidogenic factor 1 (SF1), which regulates the regression of Mullerian structures
    ■ Clinical features: 46,XY chromosome complement, genital anomalies range from severe hypospadias to complete sex reversal with uterus and streak gonads, variable adrenal hypoplasia/failure
      • Female (46,XX) carriers have premature ovarian failure.
  o **5-α-Reductase deficiency** (MIM 264600)
    ■ Autosomal recessive male-limited androgen biosynthesis disorder, caused by biallelic pathogenic variant in *SRD5A2*, disrupting the enzyme 5α-reductase type 2, which converts testosterone to dihydrotestosterone
    ■ Clinical features: 46,XY chromosome complement, atypical female genitalia without a uterus, small phallus/clitoromegaly, penoscrotal hypospadias, blind perineal pouch, bifid scrotum. Masculinization occurs at puberty.
      • In males undergoing surgery for isolated hypospadias, 7/81 (8%) had at least one pathogenic variant in *SRDA2*, and 6/7 had penile or scrotal hypospadias (Silver and Russell, 1999).

- The testosterone:dihydrotestosterone ratio is elevated after human chorionic gonadotropin (HCG) stimulation test.
  - Other androgen biogenesis disorders include the congenital adrenal hyperplasia, **3β-hydroxysteroid dehydrogenase deficiency** (MIM 201810).
- ○ **Androgen insensitivity syndrome** (testicular feminization syndrome, MIM 300068)
  - X-linked disorder of androgen sensitivity, caused by pathogenic variant in *AR*, which encodes the androgen receptor
  - Clinical features:
    - **Partial androgen insensitivity syndrome** (PAIS, MIM 312300) causes variable undermasculinization of male genitalia: micropenis, hypospadias.
      - Isolated hypospadias without micropenis or cryptorchidism: 3% have missense pathogenic variants in *AR* (Kalfa et al., 2013).
    - **Complete androgen insensitivity syndrome** (CAIS, MIM 313700) causes 46,XY sex reversal: female genitalia without a uterus or adnexal structures. Testes are undescended or inguinal. It may not be detected in newborn period.
- ○ **Campomelic dysplasia** (MIM 114290)
  - Autosomal dominant skeletal dysplasia, caused by heterozygous pathogenic variant in *SOX9*
  - Clinical features: 11 rib pairs, variably bowed long bones, clubfeet, bell-shaped thorax, cleft palate (Figure 35.2)
    - Up to 75% of affected males (46,XY) are undervirilized or have complete sex reversal.
- ○ **Congenital adrenal hyperplasia with 21-hydroxylase deficiency** (MIM 201910)
  - Autosomal recessive disorder of cortisol biosynthesis, caused by biallelic pathogenic variants in *CYP21A2*
    - Most parents are carriers: Some hirsute mothers are affected with the late-onset virilizing (nonclassical) form.
    - De novo 1%
  - Incidence 1/18,170 (New York state newborn screening data)
    - Most common etiology for 46,XX DSD; due to excess production of adrenal androgens
  - Clinical features: virilized external genitalia; females have clitoromegaly without palpable gonads (Figure 27.2); the ovaries and uterus are normal. Males: penile enlargement; hyperpigmentation of scrotum and linea alba
    - Salt-wasting form >75%; can cause life-threatening crises. Treat with glucocorticoid and mineralocorticoid replacement.
    - Other phenotypes are HLA-associated, including simple virilizing (non-salt-wasting), late postnatal onset of virilization (nonclassical), and cryptic (enzymatic defect only).

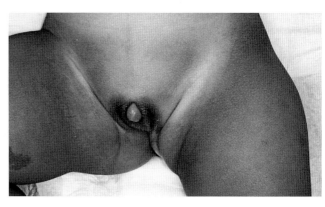

FIGURE 27.2  Congenital adrenal hyperplasia in a female with clitoromegaly and labial fusion. The gonads were not palpable. Ovaries and uterus are normal in affected females.

- Serum 17-hydroxyprogesterone (17-OHP) markedly elevated
- Plasma renin elevated in salt-wasting form
- ○ **Frasier syndrome** (MIM 136680)
  - Autosomal dominant form of 46,XY gonadal dysgenesis, caused by heterozygous pathogenic variant in *WT1*
    - Distinct from the allelic **Denys–Drash syndrome** (MIM 194080) in which Wilms tumor is common
  - Clinical features: 46,XY chromosome complement, female genitalia with streak gonads, gonadoblastoma common
    - Proteinuria at 2–6 years with progressive glomerulopathy
  - Detected in the newborn when prenatal testing identifies a 46,XY chromosome complement
- ○ **XY gonadal dysgenesis** (MIM 400044 and others)
  - Caused by deletion or pathogenic variant of *SRY*, on chromosome Yp
  - Clinical features: female external genitalia with a uterus but no ovaries
    - May be detected when amniocentesis revealed a 46,XY chromosome complement and the infant appeared to be female on US and at delivery.
    - Typically, affected female adolescents present with primary amenorrhea.
- Hypospadias associated with non-genital anomalies
  - ○ 60% have only one other anomaly; 40% have multiple anomalies.
  - ○ The most common non-genital anomalies are cardiac 14%, limb 12%, gastrointestinal 9%, and renal 6%.
- Syndromic hypospadias
  - ○ Most syndromes are recognized by the pattern of non-genital anomalies.
  - ○ Hypospadias occurs in hundreds of syndromes, only a few of which are summarized here.
  - ○ **α-Thalassemia/mental retardation syndrome** (MIM 301040)

- X-linked disorder, caused by hemizygous pathogenic variant in *ATRX*
  - Carrier females have skewed X-inactivation ratios.
- Clinical features: microcephaly, hypertelorism, anteverted nares, tented upper lip, open mouth with downturned corners, mild hemoglobin H disease (occasional), dysphagia, gastroesophageal reflux
- Small penis, cryptorchidism, female genitalia with 46,XY chromosome complement
- **Fraser syndrome** (cryptophthalmos-syndactyly syndrome, MIM 219000)
  - Autosomal recessive disorder, caused by biallelic pathogenic variants in *FRAS1, GRIP1,* or *FREM2*
  - Clinical features: variable cryptophthamos, absent lacrimal ducts, laryngeal stenosis, cleft lip, ear malformations, deafness, syndactyly, micropenis, hypospadias, undescended testes, hypertelorism, bicornuate uterus, renal agenesis, imperforate anus (Figures 10.4, 24.1)
- **Hand–foot–genital syndrome** (MIM 140000)
  - Autosomal dominant disorder, caused by heterozygous pathogenic variant in *HOXA13*
  - Clinical features: small feet, short great toes, short first metacarpal and metatarsal, short little fingers, thumb anomalies. Radiographic changes in the hands and feet are characteristic.
    - Males: variable hypospadias, with or without chordee
    - Females: duplication of the uterus, longitudinal vaginal septum
    - Both sexes: vesicoureteral reflux, multicystic dysplastic kidneys

*Pearl*: Suspect hand–foot–genital syndrome when a male with hypospadias has a mother with uterus didelphys.

- **IMAGe syndrome** (*I*UGR, *m*etaphyseal dysplasia, *a*drenal insufficiency, *ge*nital anomalies, MIM 614732)
  - Autosomal dominant trait, caused by gain-of-function heterozygous pathogenic variant in *CDKN1C,* on 11p15
    - This syndrome is expressed only when transmitted by the mother because this region is differentially methylated based on the parent of origin.
  - Clinical features: severe IUGR (birth weight −2 to −4 SD), frontal bossing, depressed nasal bridge, micrognathia, triangular face, metaphyseal and epiphyseal dysplasia; calcifications of liver, spleen. Variable failure to thrive, vomiting, hypotonia, developmental delay, hypercalcuria, hypocalcemia, cleft palate, craniosynostosis (Figure 2.4)
    - Males: cryptorchidism, hypospadias, small phallus, hypogonadotropic hypogondism. Females have normal genitalia.

- Congenital adrenal insufficiency can cause adrenal crisis within the first week: hyponatremia, hyperkalemia, elevated ACTH.
- **McKusick–Kaufman syndrome** (MIM 236700)
  - Autosomal recessive disorder, caused by biallelic pathogenic variants in *MKKS* (formerly *BBS6*)
  - Clinical features: postaxial polydactyly 60%, cardiac 15%, GI and renal anomalies, hypospadias, cryptorchidism, chordee in males. Hydrometrocolpos causes a large cystic pelvic mass in 70% of female infants.
    - Must exclude **Bardet–Biedl syndrome** (MIM 209900)
- **Mowat–Wilson syndrome** (MIM 235730)
  - Autosomal dominant syndrome, caused by a heterozygous pathogenic variant or deletion of *ZEB2* on 2q22
  - Clinical features: hypertelorism, deep-set eyes, uplifted ear lobules, round nasal tip, pointed chin, cardiac defects, agenesis of corpus callosum, hypospadias, other genitourinary anomalies, Hirschsprung disease, seizures, intellectual disability (Figure 25.2)
- **Opitz GBBB syndrome** (hypertelorism hypospadias syndrome, MIM 300000)
  - X-linked disorder, caused by hemizygous pathogenic variant in *MID1*. Females may be affected.
    - Autosomal dominant form (Opitz GBBB2, MIM 145410) is caused by heterozygous pathogenic variant of *SPECC1L.*
  - Clinical features: hypertelorism, telecanthus, hypospadias, cryptorchidism, renal anomalies; poor feeding, stridor, aspiration, and difficulty swallowing caused by laryngeal clefts and hypoplastic epiglottis; cleft lip/palate; cardiac defects. CNS anomalies: ventriculomegaly, abnormalities of the corpus callosum, cerebellar vermis hypoplasia. Intellectual disability is common in males.
- **Smith–Lemli–Opitz syndrome*** (MIM 270400)
  - Autosomal recessive disorder, caused by biallelic pathogenic variants in *DHCR7*
  - Clinical features: characteristic face, ptosis, cleft palate, polydactyly, thumb hypoplasia, undervirilized male genitalia: hypospadias, bifid scrotum, cryptorchidism, micropenis, complete sex reversal with female genitalia (Figure 27.3)
    - Elevated 7-dehydrocholesterol
- **Wilms tumor, aniridia, genitourinary anomalies, and mental retardation syndrome** (WAGR, MIM 194072)
  - Contiguous gene deletion on chromosome 11p13, including *PAX6* and *WT1*
  - Clinical features: poor growth, microcephaly, aniridia, iris dysplasia, cataracts, glaucoma, nystagmus, optic nerve hypoplasia, cardiac defects, Wilms tumor (bilateral), gonadoblastoma
    - Males: hypospadias, cryptorchidism, atypical genitalia, sex reversal.
    - Females: aniridia, Wilms tumor, gonadoblastoma

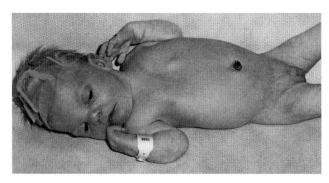

FIGURE 27.3 This undervirilized male infant with Smith–Lemli–Opitz syndrome has the typical facial features of SLOS: ptosis, short nose, long philtrum, and down-turned mouth. Note the flat thenar eminence of the left thumb.

- ○ **X-linked lissencephaly with abnormal genitalia** (XLAG, MIM 300215)
  - ■ X-linked disorder, caused by hemizygous loss-of-function pathogenic variant in *ARX*
    - • 35% of carrier females have developmental and learning problems: partial or complete agenesis of the corpus callosum, motor delay, ADHD
  - ■ Clinical features: microcephaly, lissencephaly with a posterior (agyria) to anterior (pachygyria) gradient, enlarged lateral ventricles, hydranencephaly, agenesis of corpus callosum, early onset seizures (Figure 18.3)
    - • Micropenis, hypospadias, undescended testes, abnormal genitalia, 46,XY chromosome complement
  - ■ Lissencephaly and 46,XY gonadal dysgenesis occur as an autosomal recessive trait in **muscular dystrophy-dystroglycanopathy, type A7** (MDDGA7, Walker–Warburg syndrome, MIM 614631) and **type A10** (MDDGA10, MIM 615041), caused by biallelic pathogenic variants in *ISPD* and *TMEM5*, respectively.

## Evaluation and Management

- Document pregnancy history: early IUGR, infertility, ART, ICSI, teratogens (anticonvulsants), exposures to anti-androgens, pesticides.
- Take a family history: consanguinity, hypospadias (document even minor forms in paternal and maternal relatives), infertility, miscarriages, neonatal deaths, congenital anomalies.
- With low birth weight, note placental size and histology.
- Evaluate for other genitourinary anomalies: inguinal US for undescended testes, pelvic US for persistent Mullerian structures, abdominal US for renal anomalies.
- Examine carefully for non-genital anomalies: echocardiogram, ophthalmology evaluation.

- Laboratory studies depend on clinical features: 7-dehydrocholesterol, comprehensive steroid analysis for adrenal and sex hormones.
- Genetic testing
  - ○ Chromosome analysis with FISH for X, Y, and *SRY*
    - ■ Microarray may not detect low-level mosaicism (e.g., 45,X/46,XY), which is identified more readily by FISH/chromosome analysis.
  - ○ Chromosome microarray
  - ○ Genetic testing is guided by the phenotype and differential diagnosis.
    - ■ When hypospadias is associated with other genitourinary anomalies, testing should include *AR, MAMLD1, NR5A1, SRD5A2, SRY* (FISH and sequencing).
- When genitalia are atypical or ambiguous, consult specialists before assigning sex of rearing.
  - ○ Consult Pediatric Urology and Pediatric Endocrinology to coordinate and prioritize testing strategy, especially when hypospadias occurs without palpable testes.
- Multidisciplinary team approach provides best approach when genital anomalies are complex or atypical.

## Further Reading

Audí L, Ahmed SF, Krone N, et al. (2018) GENETICS IN ENDOCRINOLOGY: Approaches to molecular genetic diagnosis in the management of differences/disorders of sex development (DSD): position paper of EU COST Action BM 1303 "DSDnet." Eur J Endocrinol. pii: EJE-18-0256. [Epub ahead of print]. PMID 29973379

Barbaro M, Wedell A, Nordenstrom A. (2011) Disorders of sex development. Semin Fetal Neonatal Med. 16:119–27. PMID 21303737

Bouty A, Ayers KL, Pask A, et al. (2015) The genetic and environmental factors underlying hypospadias. Sex Dev. 9:239–59. PMID 26613581

Hashimoto Y, Kawai M, Nagai S, et al. (2016) Fetal growth restriction but not preterm birth is a risk factor for severe hypospadias. Pediatr Int. 58:573–7. PMID 26634292

Jensen MS, Wilcox AJ, Olsen J, et al. (2012) Cryptorchidism and hypospadias in a cohort of 934,538 Danish boys: The role of birth weight, gestational age, body dimensions and fetal growth. Am J Epidemiol. 175:917–25. PMID 22454385

Kalfa N, Philibert P, Werner R, et al. (2013) Minor hypospadias: The "tip of the iceberg" of the partial androgen insensitivity syndrome. PLoS One. 8(4):e61824. PMID 3640041

Ollivier M, Paris F, Philibert P, et al. (2018) Family history is underestimated in children with isolated hypospadias: a French multicenter report of 88 families. J Urol. 200:890–894. PMID 29723568

Silver RI, Russell DW. (1999) Five alpha reductase type 2 mutations are present in some boys with isolated hypospadias. J Urol. 162:1142–5. PMID 10458450

Tannour-Louet M, Han S, Corbett ST, et al. (2010) Identification of de novo copy number variants associated with human disorders of sexual development. PLoS One. 5(10):e15392. PMID 21048976

# Part VII

## Skeletal System

# 28

# Arthrogryposis

## Clinical Consult

A 23-year-old pregnant G3 woman reported that her first male baby died at 30 weeks after a pregnancy marked by polyhydramnios, decreased to absent fetal activity, and no respiratory effort at birth. Photographs demonstrated bilateral equinovarus feet, contracted knees, flexed hands with overlapping fingers, and mild generalized edema (Figure 28.1). Clinically, the baby had the **fetal akinesia deformation sequence** (FADS). No autopsy or other studies had been performed.

At 20 weeks' gestation, her current female fetus appeared to be similarly affected with generalized contractures and lack of fetal movement. At delivery, the infant failed to breathe and died at a few minutes of age. Clinical findings were similar to those seen in the first infant. DNA was collected from cord blood and sent for exome sequencing on a research basis.

Several months later, compound heterozygous variants in *CHRNG* were reported, confirming a lethal autosomal recessive form of arthrogryposis most consistent with **lethal multiple pterygia syndrome**. Pathogenic variants in this gene also cause Escobar syndrome, which may be compatible with long-term survival with significant pulmonary and skeletal disability.

Increasingly, exome sequencing can achieve a molecular diagnosis in patients with these usually lethal arthrogryposis syndromes that have been previously "lumped" together in a clinically heterogeneous group called "fetal akinesia sequence."

## Definition

- Arthrogryposis describes a heterogeneous group of disorders causing congenital contractures, affecting multiple joints in more than one body area.
  - This "catch-all" term does not imply a particular etiology or diagnosis. "Arthrogryposis multiplex congenita" is a nondiagnostic umbrella term that should not be used if a more specific diagnosis can be made.
- Incidence 1/3,000–1/12,000
- More than 400 discrete conditions and more than 150 genes with pathogenic variants have been described to date.

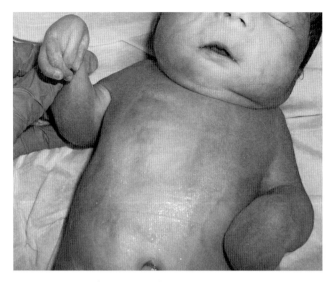

FIGURE 28.1 Fetal Akinesia Deformation Sequence in the deceased second affected sibling. The diagnosis was reinterpreted as lethal multiple pterygia syndrome after exomes revealed homozygous variants in *CHRNG*.

- Defects in the CNS, spinal cord, anterior horn cells, axons, muscle, connective tissue, or abnormalities at the neuromuscular junction cause arthrogryposis.
  - Fetal factors: multiple gestation, oligohydramnios, fetoplacental vascular compromise
  - Maternal factors: myasthenia gravis, other illnesses or drugs
- Arthrogryposis may involve limbs only (40%), limbs and other body organs (36%), or limbs with CNS dysfunction (24%).
- Prenatal diagnosis is frequent, but only when fetal limb movement is routinely and critically assessed.
- Accurate clinical descriptions and diagnostic assessment are essential for appropriate diagnosis and management.
- Intensive physical therapy may vastly improve outcome in many different types of arthrogryposis, except when the CNS is severely involved.

## Differential Diagnosis

- A general classification should be possible in ~50%. Commonly encountered disorders are reviewed here. Collagen VI disorders and myotonic dystrophy are reviewed in Chapter 1. These rare conditions require the expertise of a clinical geneticist and neurologist and usually genetic testing is required.

- **AMYOPLASIA** (amyoplasia congenita)
  - Sporadic condition, caused by early vascular compromise at critical early stage in the development of anterior horn cells
    - Many individuals with amyoplasia have had children; no recurrences have been reported.
    - Increased frequency in MZ twins or history of "vanishing twin"

- Most common form of arthrogryposis, accounting for approximately one-third of cases.
- This is a *clinical* diagnosis that should be made early because physical therapy is essential, and normal intelligence is anticipated.
- Clinical features: alert interactive infant
  - Nevus flammeus on forehead and IUGR (BW <10%) are almost always present, but head circumference is preserved.
  - All limbs involved in 56%, upper only 17%, lower only 15%, asymmetric 5%
    - Severe in 7%: hyperextended neck, head and spine, scoliosis, respiratory problems
  - Internally rotated shoulders, straight elbows, and flexed fingers (Figure 28.2)
  - "Policeman's tip" hand position very common but not pathognomonic (see Figure 28.2), finger flexion creases absent or very faint
  - Severe equinovarus feet
  - Muscles essentially absent with replacement by fibrous, fatty tissue
  - Affected limbs usually shortened by ~10%
  - Deep dimples over the joints

*Pearl*: The nevus flammeus over the glabellar region of the forehead, nose, and philtrum is a common feature in almost all syndromes with abnormal limb development including absence of long bones, skeletal dysplasias and syndromes with lack of limb movement.

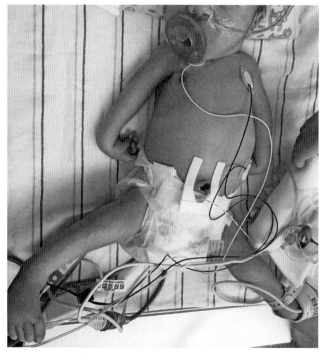

FIGURE 28.2 Infant with amyoplasia, the most common form of arthrogryposis. Note straight arms and legs, clubfeet, and characteristic hand positioning.

- ○ Associated findings suggest vascular disruption.
  - ■ Abdominal wall defects (gastroschisis) or bowel atresia in 10%
  - ■ Distal limb abnormalities from wrapping of limbs by the umbilical cord are seen in ~10% (Figure 28.3).

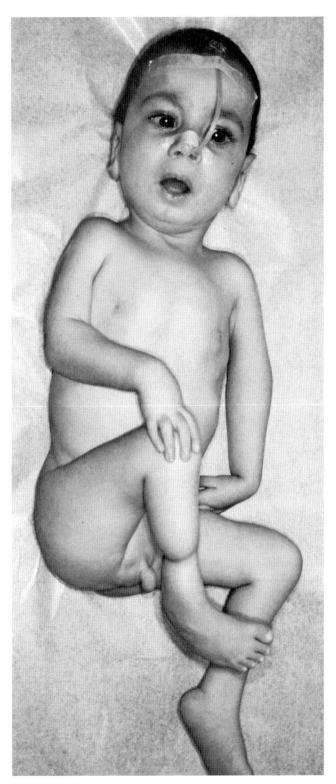

FIGURE 28.3 Amyoplasia with typical hand positioning and cord wrapping evident on lower leg.

- ■ Amniotic bands cause distal digital amputations in ~10%.
- ○ Natural history
  - ■ 30–40% have early feeding problems; most resolve.
  - ■ 1% die in first year (prematurity, respiratory, anesthesia).
  - ■ Fractures at birth are common and can be iatrogenic at delivery.
    - • Osteoporosis common later due to disuse
  - ■ Relatively independent in activities of daily living
    - • 85% are ambulatory by age 5 years.

- • **DISTAL ARTHROGRYPOSIS** (DA, MIM 108120)
  - ○ A large group of disorders that cause congenital hand and foot contractures
  - ○ Comprise ~20% of patients with arthrogryposis
  - ○ Genetically and clinically heterogeneous with dominant, recessive, and sporadic causes. Generally classified as DA 1–10
    - ■ It is likely that several of the numbered DA syndromes form a spectrum and are not discrete entities.
    - ■ Mutations in the same gene can cause more than one DA phenotype. Common DA disorders are below.
  - ○ **Variants in *PIEZO2* cause several DA phenotypes**
    - ■ **Congenital contractures with impaired proprioception and touch** (MIM 613629)
      - • Autosomal recessive trait due to biallelic pathogenic variants in *PIEZO2*; documents an important role for *PIEZO2* in mechanosensation
      - • Clinical features: hand contractures, clubfeet, dislocated hips. Contractures and scoliosis are progressive.
      - • Normal intelligence
    - ■ **Distal arthrogryposis type 5** (DA5, MIM 108145) overlapping features with Gordon syndrome and Marden Walker. No cleft palate.
      - • heterozygous variants in *PIEZO2*
    - ■ **Gordon syndrome** (DA3, MIM 114300)
      - • Autosomal dominant disorder; gain-of-function variants in *PIEZO2*
      - • Clinical features: Hand and foot contractures occur with cleft palate or bifid uvula, short stature, and ptosis. Restrictive lung disease late in course
    - ■ **Marden–Walker syndrome** (MIM 248700)
      - • Heterozygous de novo variants in *PIEZO2* described in two patients with this rare phenotype.
      - • Clinical features: immobile facies, blepharophimosis, scoliosis, significant motor delay but at least one child is cognitively normal at age 3 (Figure 28.4)
      - • CNS abnormalities occur: vermian hypoplasia, defects in the Dandy–Walker spectrum.
  - ○ **Variants in *MYH3* and related genes cause other types of DA**
    - ■ **Freeman–Sheldon syndrome** (whistling face syndrome, DA2A, MIM 193700)

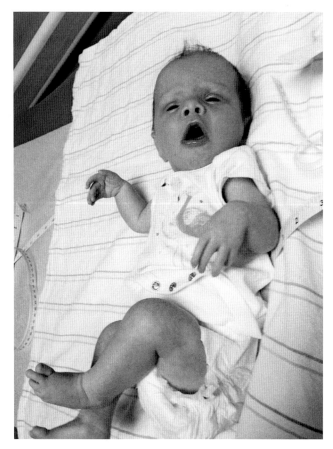

FIGURE 28.4 Marden–Walker syndrome. Findings included multiple contractures, dimples on extremities, ptosis, and a Dandy–Walker malformation. A de novo variant in *PIEZO2* is causative in this child.

- Autosomal dominant syndrome, caused by heterozygous variants in *MYH3*
- Clinical features: blepharophimosis, long philtrum with H-shaped cutaneous dimpling of the chin, high palate, small tongue
  - ID, microcephaly in 30–50%
- **Sheldon–Hall syndrome** (DA2B, MIM 601680)
  - Autosomal dominant syndrome, caused by heterozygous variants in one of several genes encoding fast-twitch skeletal muscle isoforms of troponin I (*TNNI2*) and troponin T (*TNNT3*), embryonic myosin (*MYH3*), *TPM2* and others
  - Clinical features: small mouth and micrognathia with high palate (similar to Freeman–Sheldon syndrome), short neck with webbing, severe contractures at birth and progressive scoliosis (see Figure 29.3)
    - Intelligence is normal.

- **FETAL AKINESIA SEQUENCE** (FADS MIM 208150)
  - A genetically and clinically heterogeneous, usually lethal group of disorders, sometimes called the **Pena–Shokeir phenotype**. Absence of fetal movement from any cause can produce a similar phenotype. This phenotype includes IUGR, lack of fetal movement, pulmonary

hypoplasia, variable facial findings, contractures and short umbilical cord.
- Multiple etiologies include single gene disorders, metabolic diseases and environmental agents that cause myopathies, defects at the neuromuscular junction, spinal muscular atrophy, and CNS defects.
- Pathogenic variants in one responsible gene, *CHRNG*, may cause a variable phenotype ranging from lethal (see Clinical Consult) to a presentation compatible with a longer life with significant handicaps and pulmonary disease (e.g., Escobar syndrome).
  - Many are autosomal recessive disorders; recurrence risk approaches 25%.
  - Prenatal findings: fetal akinesia, IUGR, polyhydramnios, hydrops/cystic hygroma, short umbilical cord
Clinical features:
- Micrognathia, microcephaly, small mouth, cleft palate, depressed tip of nose, high nasal bridge
- Congenital contractures, pterygia (webs) across joints may occur
- Pulmonary hypoplasia causes lethality
  - Selected disorders that cause fetal akinesia deformation sequence
    - **Cerebro-oculo-facio-skeletal syndrome I** (COFS, MIM 214150)
      - Variants in *ERCC6* and other excision repair genes
      - Allelic to Cockayne syndrome
      - Progressive neurodegenerative disorder with photosensitivity, cataracts, microphthalmia, and other features of FADS
    - **Congenital myopathies**
      - Variants in several genes: *RYR1, DMPK, LMNA, ACTN3, TNN12*
    - **Congenital myasthenic syndromes** (MIM 254210)
      - Clinically and genetically heterogeneous; most involve pathogenic variants in genes involved in the acetylcholine endplate.
      - May have neonatal presentation
      - Clinical features: hypotonia, ventilatory failure, ptosis, ocular palsies, contractures
        - Targeted treatments based on the molecular defect have shown promise in some of the myasthenic syndromes (Engel A, 2018)

*Pearl*: Some asymptomatic mothers with myasthenia syndromes produce antibody to fetal muscle or neural proteins such as fetal AChR. They may have recurrent arthrogryposis in their offspring. This can only be diagnosed by testing the mother for antibody to fetal AChR.

- **Lethal multiple pterygia syndromes** (MIM 253290)
  - Autosomal recessive lethal syndromes associated with pathogenic variants in the fetally expressed CHRN genes: *CHRNG, CHRNA1, CHRND*

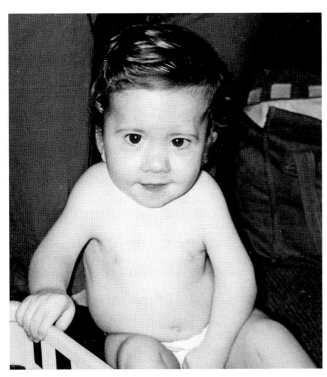

FIGURE 28.5 Escobar syndrome in this child with multiple pterygia, limited joint excursion, normal intelligence, and pulmonary problems.

- Those without pterygia may be due to variants in *RAPSN, DOK7,* and others.
- Clinical features: pterygia, hydrops, cystic hygroma
- **Nonlethal multiple pterygia syndromes** (Escobar syndrome, MIM 265000)
  - Autosomal recessive disorders, due to mutations in *CHRNG* and likely other genes
  - Clinical features: pterygia, craniofacial dysmorphic features, short stature, progressive scoliosis, respiratory issues (Figure 28.5)
- **Proliferative vasculopathy and hydranencephaly–hydrocephaly syndrome** (Fowler syndrome, MIM 229790)
  - Lethal autosomal recessive disorder caused by homozygous or compound heterozygous variants in *FLVCR2*
  - Clinical features: early onset fetal akinesia with contractures, pterygia, cystic hygroma, destruction of the cerebral hemispheres with microcalcifications
- **Congenital disorders of glycosylation** (MIM 212065) various sub-types increasingly reported with FADS
- **Perinatal lethal Gaucher disease** (MIM 608013)
  - Autosomal recessive disorder, due to biallelic pathogenic variants in *GBA;* causes absence of glucocerebrosidase
  - Clinical features: fetal akinesia, ichthyosis, hepatosplenomegaly, hydrops

- CNS abnormalities such as hydranencephaly and rarely in utero infections may present with features of FADS.
- **OTHER SYNDROMES WITH CONTRACTURES**
  - **ARC syndrome** (*a*rthrogryposis, *r*enal dysfunction, *c*holestasis syndrome; Nezelof syndrome; MIM 208085)
    - Neonatal lethal autosomal recessive disorder, caused by biallelic variants in *VPS33B* or *VIPAR*
    - Clinical findings: congenital contractures, osteopenia, renal Fanconi syndrome with generalized aminoaciduria and proteinuria, failure to thrive
      - Cholestasis with paucity of bile ducts and conjugated hyperbilirubinemia, jaundice
      - Ichthyosis, paucity of white matter in CNS
    - Gene testing is the preferred diagnostic test over liver or renal biopsy. Biopsy can cause life-threatening hemorrhage.
  - **Schaff–Yang syndrome** (MIM 615547)
    - Variable disorder caused by a heterozygous truncating variant in *MAGEL2,* a paternally expressed gene located within the imprinted Prader–Willi syndrome critical region on chromosome 15q11.2. May be paternally transmitted
    - Clinical features: Prader–Willi-like phenotype, severe microretrognathia, short palpebral fissures, hypertelorism, camptodactyly, contractures of the elbows and knees, clubfoot
      - Prenatal features: polyhydramnios, decreased fetal movement
    - Death may occur in utero in the third trimester.
  - **X-linked spinal muscular atrophy 2** (SMAX2, MIM 301830)
    - X-linked recessive form of arthrogryposis, caused by hemizygous variant in *UBA1*
    - Clinical features: severe hypotonia, generalized weakness and muscle atrophy, areflexia; multiple joint contractures associated with loss of anterior horn cells; mildly elevated CK levels; periventricular white matter changes
    - Progressive and frequently lethal course from respiratory insufficiency
    - Promising therapeutic tools under investigation

# Evaluation and Management

- Document family history: consanguinity, fetal losses, infant deaths (note the sex), cleft palate, clubfeet, maternal myotonia.
- Take detailed pregnancy history: medication use, oligohydramnios, fetal movements.
- Examine parents for trismus (limited jaw excursion), unusual hand or foot position, hand and finger creases; findings may be subtle.

- Diagnosis is *clinical* for infants with classic phenotype of amyoplasia.
- Genetic testing for other forms of arthrogryposis
  - Chromosome microarray
  - Single gene testing: spinal muscular atrophy
  - Gene sequencing panels are appropriate for distal arthrogryposis syndromes and fetal akinesia sequence depending on panel composition and number of genes covered
  - Exome sequencing (WES) trio testing (includes parental blood samples): infants with complex arthrogryposis syndromes with negative NGS panel testing or other atypical features
    - If exome trio test is not possible, save DNA from blood or tissue.
    - Delineation of the genetic basis of arthrogryposis will evolve rapidly with gene discovery and improved knowledge of their pathways.
- Genetic counseling
  - Lethal forms of arthrogryposis are most often autosomal recessive. Knowledge of the specific molecular diagnosis will allow targeted prenatal diagnosis.
- Therapy
  - Early physical therapy is key to optimal joint mobilization and maximizing function.
    - Maximizing muscle strength may be more important than increasing range of motion in achieving functional goals.
    - Avoid immobilizing joints.
    - Consider night splints to maintain functional position of joints and reduce recurrent contractures.
    - Use appropriate pain control with procedures to achieve the best results.
  - Later, orthopedic procedures may improve functionality.
  - New customizable assistive devices are increasingly available due to 3D printers.
    - See "Magic Arms" video at www.youtube.com/watch?v=Pqsd2tm0HdQ.
    - Enroll appropriate patients in clinical therapeutic trials. www.clinical trials.gov
- Refer to a specialty center utilizing a multidisciplinary team-based approach.

## Further Reading

Beck AE, McMillin MJ, Gildersleeve HI, et al. (2013) Spectrum of mutations that cause distal arthrogryposis types 1 and 2B. Am J Med Genet A. 161A:550–5. PMID 23401156

Bissinger RL, Koch FR. (2014) Nonlethal multiple pterygium syndrome: Escobar syndrome. Adv Neonatal Care. 14:24–9. PMID 24472885

Chesler AT, Szczot M, Bharucha-Goebel D, et al. (2016) The role of PIEZO2 in human mechanosensation. N Engl J Med. 375:1355–64. PMID 27653382

Engel AG. (2018) Genetic basis and phenotypic features of congenital myasthenic syndromes. Handb Clin Neurol. 148:565–589. PMID:29478601

Hall JG. (2014) Arthrogryposis (multiple congenital contractures): Diagnostic approach to etiology, classification, genetics, and general principles. Eur J Med Genet. 57:464–72. PMID 24704792

Hall JG, Aldinger KA, Tanaka KI. (2014) Amyoplasia revisited. Am J Med Genet A. 164A:700–30. PMID 24459070

Kowalczyk B, Feluś J. (2016) Arthrogryposis: An update on clinical aspects, etiology, and treatment strategies. Arch Med Sci. 12:10–24. PMID 26925114

Meyer E, Ricketts C., Morgan NV, et al. (2010). Mutations in FLVCR2 are associated with proliferative vasculopathy and hydranencephaly–hydrocephaly syndrome (Fowler syndrome). Am J Hum Genet. 86: 471–8. PMID 20206334

Todd EJ, Yau KS, Ong R, et al. (2015) Next generation sequencing in a large cohort of patients presenting with neuromuscular disease before or at birth. Orphanet J Rare Dis. 10:148. PMID 26578207

# 29

## Clubfoot

## Clinical Consult

A male infant with prenatally diagnosed bilateral clubfoot (Figure 29.1) had a family history of a connective tissue disorder. His sister had a marfanoid habitus, mildly dilated aortic root, and pectus excavatum. The parents appeared to be unaffected. Her *FBN1* gene analysis was negative. The family had declined further testing.

His clubfeet responded well to therapy with the Ponseti method. At 6 weeks, a bifid uvula was appreciated. His sister was re-examined, and she had the same finding. This combination of features was consistent with **Loeys–Dietz syndrome**. *TGFBR1* gene analysis confirmed the diagnosis. Parental testing was negative, suggesting that one parent had a germ line mutation. Further imaging in both children revealed widespread arterial tortuosity. Parents declined treatment with a beta blocker or losartan.

Loeys–Dietz syndrome is an autosomal dominant connective tissue disorder. It can occur in siblings when an unaffected parent has germ line mosaicism. Aggressive treatment of the arterial tortuosity can modify the vascular consequences of this condition.

## Definition

Clubfoot is used interchangeably with talipes equinovarus here.

- A clubfoot is rigid, typically fixed in equinus and cannot be manually corrected to a neutral position.
  - An affected foot is stiffer and usually smaller than an unaffected one.
  - The calf and peroneal muscles are small and remain so after corrective therapy.
- Incidence 1/1,000 live births in Caucasians
  - More common among Pacific Islanders, 6–7/1,000
  - Less common among East Asians, 0.5/1,000
  - 2 M:1 F; male predominance
  - More common in first pregnancies
- Isolated clubfoot in 80%
  - Bilateral 50%
    - Associated with early amniocentesis or chorionic villous sampling

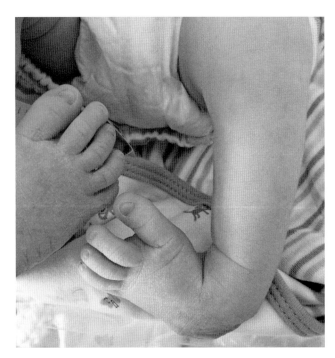

FIGURE 29.1 Bilateral clubfoot in a newborn with Loeys–Dietz syndrome.

○ Genetic and environmental factors contribute to multifactorial etiology in most cases.
  ■ Concordance in MZ twins 33% versus DZ twins 3–4%
  ■ Consanguinity increases risk.
    • Offspring of first cousin parents have four times the population risk.
  ■ Chromosome microdeletions and microduplications
    • Common in familial isolated clubfoot: 60%: 17q23 copy number variants (including *TBX4*) cause >5% of familial isolated clubfoot
    • Less common in apparently isolated clubfoot diagnosed prenatally: 5%
  ■ Maternal gestational diabetes, obesity (BMI >30; OR 1.46), maternal or household smoking (first trimester), OR 2.67
○ Positive family history 25%
  ■ Affected first-degree relatives 7–21%
○ Affected females are more likely to have a positive family history.
○ Recurrence risk for isolated clubfoot: 4%
  ■ Higher for affected females and when there is a positive family history of clubfoot

*Pearl*: The "Carter effect," discovered by geneticist Cedric Carter, describes that there are more affected relatives when the proband is of the less commonly affected sex.

○ Serial casting using the Ponseti method can correct 70–80% of isolated and syndromic clubfeet.

• Other structural and positional anomalies of the foot that are not rigid can be mistaken for clubfoot.
  ○ Risk factors for positional foot deformities
    ■ Bicornuate uterus
    ■ Breech or other malpresentation
    ■ Nulliparity
    ■ Oligohydramnios
    ■ Twins and higher multiples

*Pearl*: Positional variants occur five times as often as true clubfoot.

  ○ Metatarsus adductus: deformation due to in utero molding and constraint occurs later in gestation
  ○ **Congenital vertical talus** (CVT, rocker-bottom foot deformity, MIM 192950)
    ■ Incidence 1/10,000 live births
    ■ Unlike clubfoot, most patients with CVT have other anomalies.
    ■ In isolated CVT, 20% have an autosomal dominant trait (MIM 192950), caused by a heterozygous pathogenic variant in *HOXD10*.
    ■ CVT can be present in one foot while clubfoot is present in the other.

# Differential Diagnosis

## Syndromic Clubfoot

• Associated anomalies are present in 5–20% of all patients with clubfoot.
  ○ Chromosome anomalies
    • Aneuploidy: **Down syndrome,**\* **Trisomy 18,**\* Klinefelter syndrome, and its variants: 47,XXY, 48,XXYY, 49,XXXXY
    • **Deletion 22q11.2 syndrome\*, deletion of 12q13.13** (5' HOXC gene cluster region), **deletion of 18q** (MIM 601808), and other copy number variants
  ○ Teratogens\*
    • **Alcohol**
    • **Maternal or household smoking**
    • **Methotrexate** (treatment for misdiagnosed ectopic pregnancy), phenytoin, **valproate** and other anticonvulsant medications, serotonin reuptake inhibitors
    • **TORCH infections** that affect CNS function

## Neuromuscular Disorders

• CNS anomalies are found in 50% of syndromic clubfoot.
  ○ **Spina bifida** and associated brain anomalies Chiari II and hydrocephalus
    ■ Clubfoot in spina bifida may be rigid and severe.

- More common in those with thoracic or lumbar lesions
- Dandy–Walker malformation and variants, absence of the corpus callosum, lissencephaly
- **Congenital myotonic dystrophy** (type I, MIM 160900)
  - Autosomal dominant trait, caused by expanded number of CTG repeats in *DMPK*
  - Severity is correlated with number of CTG repeats. Expanded number of repeats usually occurs with transmission from an affected mother; rarely, expansion may occur via an affected father.
  - Clinical features: myopathic face, tented mouth, respiratory insufficiency, contractures, hypotonia, "frog leg" position (Figure 29.2)
  - Affected mothers may be asymptomatic or mildly affected.
    - Delayed grip release can cause difficulty releasing an object such as a steering wheel or frying pan, or hands can "get stuck" after picking up a heavy object.
    - Examine for cataracts, weakness, temporal hair loss, mildly decreased facial expression, and unconcerned attitude, described as "la belle indifférence."
- **Arthrogryposis**\*
  - Heterogeneous group of disorders with congenital contractures affecting multiple joints
  - Many have clubfeet.
    - Lethal syndromes: **fetal akinesia sequence** (MIM 208150), **lethal multiple pterygium syndrome** (MIM 253290)
    - **Distal arthrogryposes** (MIM 108120), **Sheldon–Hall** (MIM 601680) (Figure 29.3), **Escobar syndrome** (MIM 265000), amyoplasia congenita.

- **Spinal muscular atrophy** (SMA)
  - Heterogeneous group of disorders characterized by muscle weakness and degeneration of anterior horn cells
  - **Werdnig–Hoffman syndrome** (SMA1, MIM 253300)
  - **Spinal muscular atrophy with respiratory distress** (SMARD, MIM 604320)
  - **SMA affecting the lower extremities** (SMALED-2, MIM 615290)

- **TARP syndrome** (*t*alipes, *a*trial septal defect, *R*obin sequence, *p*ersistence of left superior vena cava, MIM 311900)
  - X-linked recessive trait, caused by hemizygous pathogenic variant in *RBM10*
  - Usually lethal in affected males during infancy
  - Clinical features: brain anomalies, cerebellar vermis hypoplasia, partial absence of corpus callosum, hearing loss, cleft palate, pulmonary hypertension
    - Severe ID
    - All features in acronym may not be present.

## Connective Tissue Disorders

- **Ehlers–Danlos type IV syndrome** (MIM 130050)
  - Autosomal dominant due to pathogenic variant in *COL3A1*
  - Infants usually do not have a striking phenotype, but fragile skin, easy bruising, and prominent veins may be seen.
  - Clubfoot in 8%

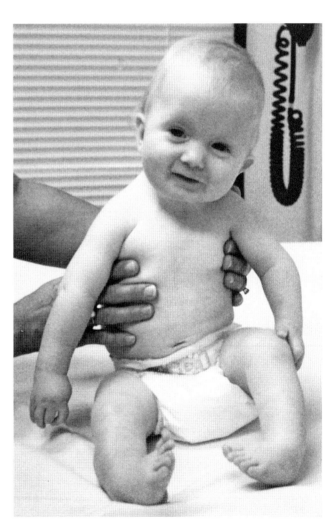

FIGURE 29.3 Clubfeet in an infant with arthrogryposis due to a de novo variant in *TPM2* (Sheldon–Hall syndrome, also called distal arthrogryposis type 2B).

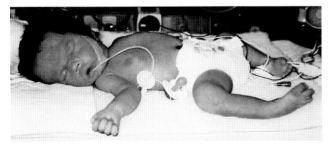

FIGURE 29.2 Clubfoot in a newborn with hypotonia due to congenital myotonic dystrophy.

- **Loeys–Dietz syndrome** (MIM 609192)
  - ○ Autosomal dominant connective tissue disorder, caused by heterozygous pathogenic variant in *TGFBR1*, *TGFBR2*, and related genes
  - ○ Clinical features: hypertelorism, blue sclerae, cleft palate, bifid uvula, submucous cleft palate, craniosynostosis, joint laxity, Marfanoid habitus, arachnodactyly, aortic enlargement, vascular tortuosity and aneurysms, hernias, scoliosis, pectus deformities, mild ID (Figure 29.1)
- **Marfan syndrome** (MIM 154700)
  - ○ Autosomal dominant connective tissue disorder due to heterozygous pathogenic variant in *FBN1*
  - ○ Classical features of arachnodactyly, aortic dilation, ectopia lentis, scoliosis, and many musculoskeletal findings uncommon in neonates
  - ○ Severely affected infants can be long at birth and have striking arachnodactly, dolichocephaly, long narrow face, deep-set eyes, joint laxity, and contractures with clubfeet.

## Skeletal Dysplasias

- **Campomelic dysplasia** (MIM 114290)
  - ○ Autosomal dominant trait caused by heterozygous pathogenic variant in *SOX9* (Figure 35.2)
  - ○ Clinical features: short bowed long bones, talipes, hypoplastic scapulae and iliac wings, 11 pairs of ribs. Some affected males have sex reversal with female external genitalia, vagina, uterus, and fallopian tubes. Tracheobronchial hypoplasia can cause respiratory compromise.
- **Diastrophic dysplasia** (MIM 222600)
  - ○ Autosomal recessive short-limbed dwarfism, caused by biallelic pathogenic variants in *SLC26A2*
  - ○ Clinical features: "hitchhiker thumbs," clubfeet (Figure 29.4), cystic swellings in ear cartilage, spine anomalies, cervical kyphosis, scoliosis, stenosis, lumbar lordosis

*Pearl*: Any syndrome that causes decreased fetal movement, fetal hypotonia, or joint laxity can result in clubfoot due to positional deformation *in utero*.

- **Shprintzen–Goldberg syndrome** (MIM 182212)
  - ○ Autosomal dominant disorder, caused by heterozygous pathogenic variant in *SKI*
  - ○ Clinical features: craniosynostosis, ocular proptosis, hypertelorism, micrognathia, narrow palate with prominent palatine ridges, equinovarus clubfoot, joint hypermobility and laxity, contractures, pes planus, arachnodactyly, camptodactyly, pectus deformities (Figure 13.7)
    - ■ Mild ID
    - ■ Aortopathy is less severe than in Marfan and Loeys–Dietz syndromes, but the skeletal features are more extreme.

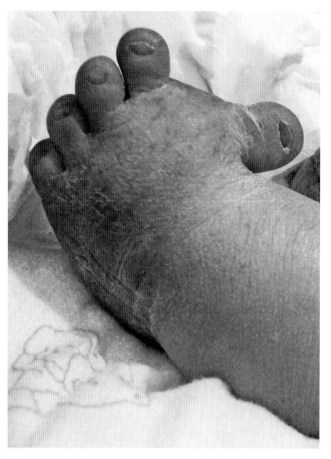

FIGURE 29.4  This baby with diastrophic dysplasia has clubfeet and a medially deviated great toe similar to the "hitchhiker" thumb that is characteristic of this disorder.

# Evaluation and Management

- Ask about pregnancy history: loss of a co-twin, CVS, early amniocentesis, bicornuate uterus or teratogens, including alcohol, seratonin reuptake inhibitors, tobacco, methotrexate.
- Document family history: consanguinity, clubfoot, musculoskeletal disorders.
- Evaluate parents: maternal obesity, seizure disorder, neurologic status, gait disturbance, calf muscle wasting, delayed grip release, myotonia.
- Examine the infant for other congenital anomalies: cleft palate; cardiac, renal, and CNS anomalies; and abnormalities of muscle and connective tissue.
- Genetic testing
  - ○ Microarray analysis: for both isolated and syndromic clubfoot
  - ○ Gene testing should be guided by phenotype.
- When clubfoot is syndromic or familial, obtain genetics evaluation.
- Treatment should be initiated as soon as possible.
  - ○ Radiographs are not usually needed for diagnosis, but they are used to follow treatment.
  - ○ Refer to pediatric orthopedics.

# Further Reading

Ahmad S, Bhatia K, Kannan A, Gangwani L. (2016) Molecular mechanisms of neurodegeneration in spinal muscular atrophy. J Exp Neurosci. 10:39–49. PMID 27042141

Alvarado DM, Buchan JG, Frick SL, et al. (2013) Copy number analysis of 413 isolated talipes equinovarus patients suggests role for transcriptional regulators of early limb development. Eur J Hum Genet. 21:373–80. PMID 22892537

Dietz, F. (2002) The genetics of idiopathic clubfoot. Clin Orthop Relat Res. 401:39–48. PMID 12151881

Chen C, Kaushal N, Scher DM, et al. (2018) Clubfoot Etiology: A meta-analysis and systematic review of observational and randomized Trials. J Pediatr Orthop. 38(8):e462–9. PMID 29917009

Dobbs MB, Gurnett CA. (2017) The 2017 ABJS Nicolas Andry Award: Advancing personalized medicine for clubfoot through translational research. Clin Orthop Relat Res. 475(6):1716–25. PMID 28236079

Johnston JJ, Sapp JC, Curry C, et al. (2014) Expansion of the TARP syndrome phenotype associated with de novo mutations and mosaicism. Am J Med Genet A. 164A:120–8. PMID 24259342

MacCarrick G, Black JH 3rd, Bowdin S, et al. (2014) Loeys–Dietz syndrome: A primer for diagnosis and management. Genet Med. 16:576–87. PMID 24577266

Nemec U, Nemec SF, Kasprian G, et al. (2012) Clubfeet and associated abnormalities on fetal magnetic resonance imaging. Prenat Diagn. 32:822–8. PMID 2267896

Sahin O, Yildirim C, Akgun RC, et al. (2013) Consanguineous marriage and increased risk of idiopathic congenital talipes equinovarus: A case–control study in a rural area. J Pediatr Orthop. 33:333–8. PMID 23482273

Werler MM, Yazdy MM, Kasser JR, et al. (2015) Maternal cigarette, alcohol, and coffee consumption in relation to risk of clubfoot. Paediatr Perinat Epidemiol. 29:3–10. PMID 25417917

# 30

# Upper Extremity Anomalies

## Clinical Consult

An otherwise healthy infant had a radial club hand, a contralateral triphalangeal thumb, and a "Swiss cheese" VSD. He had a small shoulder girdle and a nevus flammeus on the glabella. The family history was reported to be negative. Careful examination of the family revealed a hypoplastic thumb in the mother and a triphalangeal thumb in the maternal grandmother (Figure 30.1). These findings established the clinical diagnosis of **Holt–Oram syndrome** (MIM 142900).

This autosomal dominant syndrome, which is due to pathogenic variant in *TBX5*, can have reduced penetrance and variable (mild) expression. Involvement of the cardiac conduction system may complicate surgical repair of the heart.

## Definition

- Many classification systems have been proposed for congenital upper limb anomalies, but none are wholly satisfactory. Transverse, longitudinal (amelia, radial, and ulnar), central (split hand/foot), combined, and other defects are discussed in this chapter.
  - o Some upper limb anomalies are discussed in the chapters on overgrowth* (Chapter 3), arthrogryposis* (Chapter 28), syndactyly* (Chapter 33), and polydactyly* (Chapter 32).
  - o Upper limb (UL) anomalies often occur with lower limb (LL) anomalies, so some syndromes are mentioned in both this chapter and Chapter 31.
- Incidence 3.6/10,000 live births
- Long bone deficiencies are more common in UL (~65%) than in LL (25%).
  - o Usually involve the radius
  - o Ulnar defects are the rarest UL defects.
- Laterality
  - o Unilateral anomaly is more common than bilateral involvement.
  - o Bilateral UL defects have a higher likelihood of a genetic or chromosomal etiology.

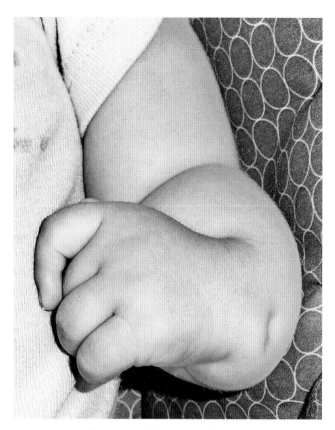

FIGURE 30.1 Holt–Oram syndrome in an infant with a radial club hand, triphalangeal thumb, and a VSD.

- o In the asymmetric group, males with an affected right arm predominate, especially for radial ray defects and Poland sequence.
- Associated anomalies 32%
  - o Uncommon among transverse terminal defects
  - o Mendelian disorder or other known condition 25–40%; chromosome anomaly 5%, teratogen <1%

# Differential Diagnosis

## Transverse Defects

### Isolated

- Isolated distal loss of the limb is usually unilateral.
  - o More common in UL than in LL
- Etiology
  - o Not considered to be a genetic condition
  - o Recurrence risk is low.
  - o Vascular insufficiency is hypothesized: placental emboli, hypovolemic hypoperfusion, early CVS.
  - o Several small studies suggest an association with maternal and/or child thrombophilia.

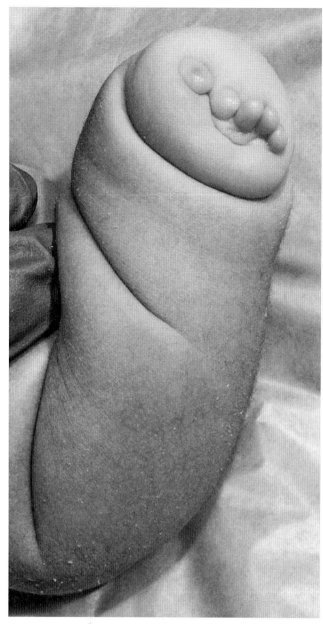

FIGURE 30.2 This infant has a transverse defect of the left hand, likely due to vascular insufficiency. There is a rudimentary hand with nubbins of tissue instead of fingers. Proximal elements are relatively spared.

- Clinical features
  - o Transverse terminal defect, most often at wrist
  - o Rudimentary digits ("nubbins") with occasional hypoplastic vestiges of nails may be present (Figure 30.2).
  - o No constriction rings or syndactyly

### Syndromic

- **Adams–Oliver syndrome** (MIM 100300)
  - o Autosomal dominant syndrome, caused by heterozygous pathogenic variant in *ARHGAP31* or *RBPJ*

- Autosomal recessive form, caused by biallelic pathogenic variants in *EOGT* and *DOCK6*
  - Clinical features are highly variable: cutis aplasia at the vertex or extensive symmetric areas of cutis aplasia on the scalp, limbs, and abdomen; cutis marmorata, skull defects, exencephaly, brachydactyly, terminal transverse defects of the limbs (Figure 30.3), microcephaly, cleft lip, congenital heart defects, pulmonary vein stenosis and pulmonary hypertension.

## Longitudinal Defects

### Amelia

- Complete absence of one or more limbs is rare.
- Incidence 1.4/100,000 births
  - More common in the offspring of mothers younger than age 20 years
- Isolated amelia is usually unilateral and sporadic. It occurs in one-third of affected patients.
- Amelia can occur with other anomalies after vascular disruption (see Figure 7.2) or maternal hyperthermia (Figure 30.4).
- Syndromic amelia
  - **Tetra-amelia** (Zimmer tetraphocomelia, MIM 273395)
    - Lethal autosomal recessive trait, caused by biallelic pathogenic variants in *WNT3*
    - Clinical features: absence of all limbs, cleft lip, hydrocephalus, agenesis of the corpus callosum, lung aplasia, absent kidney and spleen, imperforate anus
    - Usually stillborn or die soon after birth

### Radial Ray Defects

- Radial ray deficiencies may affect the radius, bones of the wrist, the thumb, and/or the thenar eminence. They can be isolated or syndromic.
- Chromosome anomalies: **trisomy 18\***
- Teratogens\*: valproic acid
- **Fanconi anemia** (MIM 227650)
  - A group of autosomal recessive chromosome fragility disorders that demonstrate an abnormal response to DNA damage, causing congenital anomalies and later, anemia and cancer
  - Clinical features are variable: small size for gestational age, microcephaly, IUGR, café au lait spots, radial defects, duplicated or hypoplastic thumb, VATER/VACTERL spectrum anomalies, deafness, genital anomalies.
    - Later: Aplastic anemia usually occurs in childhood.
  - Increased chromosome breakage with DEB is diagnostic but not universally present.
- **Holt–Oram syndrome** (MIM 142900; see Clinical Consult)

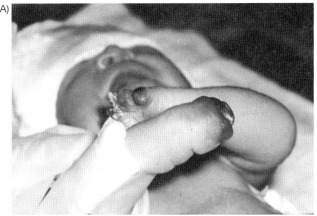

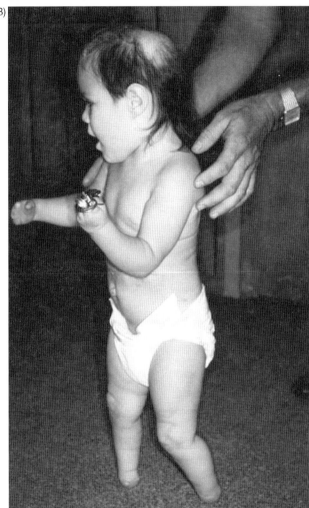

FIGURE 30.3 (A) Adams–Oliver syndrome in a newborn with symmetric transverse terminal defects of the hands and feet. Symmetric regions of cutis aplasia were present on the abdomen, knees, and scalp. The gauze dressing on her head covers a large full-thickness defect that penetrated through the skull. (B) The same child walking as a toddler. Note the healed areas of cutis aplasia and the prosthesis for her left hand.

- Autosomal dominant disorder, caused by a heterozygous pathogenic variant in *TBX5*; detection rate ~70%
- Positive family history common

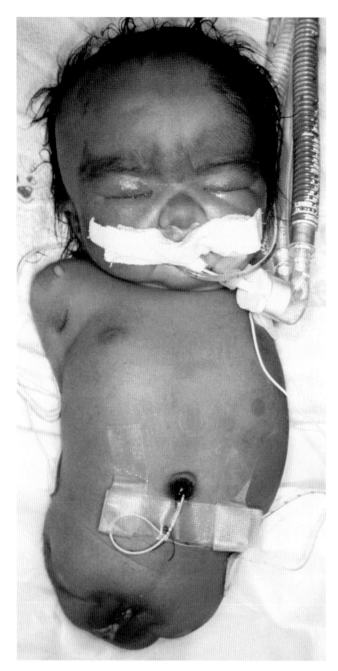

FIGURE 30.4 This infant with tetra-amelia and imperforate anus had respiratory insufficiency and died soon after birth. The mother had a prolonged episode of high fever during early gestation.

- **Lacrimoauriculodentaldigital syndrome** (LADD syndrome, Levy–Hollister syndrome, MIM 149730)
  - Variable autosomal dominant disorder, caused by a heterozygous pathogenic variant in *FGFR2*, *FGFR3*, or *FGF10*
  - Clinical features: severe lacrimal duct abnormalities, obstruction, chronic conjunctivitis, small cup-shaped ears; mixed hearing loss, duplication of the distal phalanx of the thumb, triphalangeal thumb, radial hypoplasia and syndactyly (Figure 30.5)
    - Later: Decreased salivation predisposes to dental caries, small peg-shaped lateral incisors and enamel hypoplasia, and occasional renal disease.

- **Thrombocytopenia absent radius syndrome** (TAR, MIM 274000)
  - Autosomal recessive disorder caused by a microdeletion in one copy of chromosome 1q21.1, detected by microarray, and a common polymorphism in *RBM8A* in the intact chromosome 1q21.1
    - Deletions of variable size are inherited from an unaffected parent in 80%.
  - 1 M:2 F; females predominate
  - Clinical features: Congenital or early onset megakaryocytic thrombocytopenia may resolve and later recur. Limb anomalies: bilateral radial aplasia or hypoplasia, thumbs present but may be hypoplastic, lower limb deficiencies, cystic hygroma, cleft palate
- **VATER/VACTERL\* association** (MIM 192350)
  - Sporadic nongenetic multiple congenital anomaly disorder
  - Clinical features: VSD or other cardiac defects, vertebral anomalies, anorectal malformation\*, imperforate

- Clinical features: Abnormal thumbs are triphalangeal, finger-like, short, or distally placed. Other fingers have short middle phalanges long metacarpals. Bilateral, bowed radius, dislocated radial head. Narrow shoulders.
  - Cardiac: septal or conduction defects, typically ASD or VSD
- **Okihiro syndrome** (MIM 607323), caused by alterations in *SALL4*, has an overlapping phenotype with the additional features of hearing loss, Duane anomaly, and kidney defects.

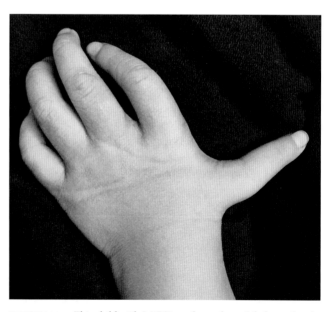

FIGURE 30.5 This child with LADD syndrome has triphalangeal and proximally placed thumbs.

anus, tracheo-esophageal fistula, radial ray defects (see Figure 18S.2), renal anomalies, single umbilical artery

### Ulnar Ray Defects

- Rarest of the limb deficiencies
- Isolated cases are often of unknown etiology.
- **Cornelia de Lange syndrome*** (CdLS, MIM 122470)
  - Autosomal and X-linked forms, caused by five or more genes involved in the cohesin ring that holds sister chromatids together
  - Clinical features: characteristic facial features, arched eyebrows, synophrys, hypertrichosis, ulnar ray defects and severe reduction defects in most severely affected infants (see Figure 11s.2). Lower limbs are not affected.
- **Fuhrmann syndrome** (fibular hypoplasia, femoral bowing, MIM 228930)
  - Autosomal recessive disorder, caused by biallelic pathogenic variants in *WNT7A*
  - Clinical features: primarily affects bones in the lower extremities with variable ulnar ray and finger deficiency
- **Goltz syndrome** (focal dermal hypoplasia, Goltz–Gorlin, MIM 305600)
  - X-linked trait, caused by hemizygous pathogenic variant in *PORCN* at Xp11.23
  - Most patients are females.
    - Affected females are functionally mosaic with varying severity due to random X-inactivation.
  - Usually lethal in males
    - The patchy pattern and varying percentage of abnormal cells in skin fibroblasts suggest somatic mosaicism in male survivors.
  - Clinical features: split hand (usually unilateral) or syndactyly or oligodactyly, focal dermal hypoplasia with herniation of fat through skin defects. Linear hypo- or hyperpigmentation. Ocular defects: coloboma, microphthalmia (Figure 33.4)
    - ID frequent
    - Affected mothers may have female infants affected with severe midline defects consistent with pentalogy of Cantrell or limb–body wall complex.
- **Ulnar–mammary syndrome** (MIM 181450)
  - Autosomal dominant disorder caused by heterozygous pathogenic variant in *TBX3*
  - Incidence 1/25,000 births
  - Clinical features: often asymmetric but may be bilateral, ulna is hypoplastic or absent, radioulnar synostosis, loss or hypoplasia of ulnar digits, small or absent nipples, absent axillary sweating, genital hypoplasia and delayed puberty in males
  - **Terminal deletion of chromosome 4q33** can produce a similar phenotype of ulnar agenesis and defects of middle, ring, and little fingers.

## Intercalary Defects

- Missing proximal or middle segment with preservation of distal elements (phocomelia)
- Thalidomide embryopathy
  - Anti-angiogenic drug, now used to treat leprosy and auto-immune disorders, induces limb malformations in 79–89%
  - Critical period: days 20–36 after conception
  - Clinical features: four limb phocomelia, shortening of proximal elements but relative preservation of distal elements. Variable phenotype: UL deficiency with normal lower limbs, LL only defects, absent thumb
    - Anomalies of ear, eye, GI, GU, and CNS increase mortality.
- **Absent ulna and fibula syndrome** (Al-Awadi/Raas–Rothschild phocomelia syndrome, AARRS syndrome, MIM 276820)
  - Autosomal recessive condition, caused by homozygous pathogenic variants in *WNT7A* leading to total lack of gene function
  - Clinical features: phocomelia, normal humerus and absent ulna, hypoplastic femurs, more severely affected or absent tibias and fibulas, absent post-axial digits, severe nails a/hypoplasia, often no toes, hypoplastic pelvis, sacrum
    - Genitalia: micropenis, cryptorchidism, Mullerian defects (absent vagina, uterus) in females with normal gonadal function
    - Imperforate anus, renal cysts, colonic stenosis, and other internal malformations
    - Occasional nonspecific craniofacial features, parietal–occipital skull defects (Schinzel phocomelia subtype)
    - Normal intelligence

## Central Defects

- **Split hand/foot malformation** (SH/SF, ectrodactyly, MIM 183600)
  - Heterogeneous group of autosomal dominant, recessive, and X-linked disorders, caused by at least five identifiable genes or microdeletions
    - Avoid disparaging terms ("lobster" or "claw hand")
  - Clinical features: highly variable absence of central digits of hands and/or feet, central metacarpal/metatarsal bones, syndactyly. Two main subtypes:
    - A: Typical cone-shaped cleft tapering and dividing the hand into two opposable parts
      - Mildest form: Third digit (middle finger or third toe) is absent/small, but the corresponding metacarpal/metatarsal bone is almost normal.
    - B: Monodactyly of the hand, usually sparing the little finger.
      - Deficiency of the central and radial rays but no cleft in the hand

## Combined Upper and Lower Limb Defects

- **Split hand/foot with long bone deficiency** (SHFLD1-3, MIM 119100, 6110685, 612576, 615416)
  - Markedly variable autosomal disorder with both dominant and recessive patterns of inheritance
    - At least 13 gene loci. Duplication of *BHLHA9* at 17p13.3 is necessary but not sufficient to produce phenotype in some dominant pedigrees.
  - Clinical features: variable intrafamilial penetrance and expression for SH/SF with or without absent tibias
  - **Split hand/foot with fibular hypoplasia** (MIM 113310) appears to be a separate entity.
- **Roberts syndrome** (pseudothalidomide syndrome, MIM 268300)
  - Autosomal recessive trait, caused by biallelic pathogenic variants in *ESCO2*, necessary for cohesion of sister chromatids
    - **SC phocomelia syndrome** (MIM 26900), a milder phenotype, is also caused by pathogenic variants in *ESCO2*.
  - Clinical features: UL more severely affected than LL; long bone deficiencies; brachydactyly; microcephaly; cardiac, renal, and other anomalies; penile enlargement. Corneal opacities are associated with intellectual disability.
  - Puffing and premature centromere separation is characteristic on routine chromosome analysis.

## Other Upper Extremity Disorders

- **Amniotic band disruption sequence** (MIM 217100)
  - A common, well-recognized sporadic cause of primarily distal limb defects
  - Incidence 1:5,000 births
  - Clinical features: asymmetric limb defects, circumferential constriction rings, distal swelling, terminal amputations and purse-string type of distal syndactyly (see Figure 33.3) with normal proximal limb development
    - Nubbins of digits distal to a constriction ring; those with a well-formed nail may be due to vascular insufficiency rather than terminal amputation.
    - Absence of a single limb bone (e.g., ulna) may be a consequence of early vascular insufficiency after amnion rupture.
    - Can accompany amyoplasia or gastroschisis

*Pearl*: Amniotic band disruption sequence rarely affects only one limb. A defect of a single limb, without a circumferential constriction ring, likely has another cause.

- **Limb–body wall complex**
  - Severe, lethal pattern of anomalies associated with early amnion rupture and abdominal wall defect

- Sporadic; early first trimester causation
  - Occasional history of blunt trauma, vaginal bleeding
  - Recurrence risk is low; familial cases are rare.
- Clinical features: placental–fetal adhesions, encephalocele, anencephaly, oblique facial clefts, UL and LL anomalies or normal limbs, severe scoliosis, skin tubes and tags, severe open body wall defect (Figure 22.1)
- **Moebius sequence** (MIM 157900)
  - Defects of multiple cranial nerve nuclei may be caused by vertebral or basilar artery insufficiency.
  - Usually sporadic; de novo mutations in *PLXND1* and *REV3L* have been reported. Can follow **misoprostol** exposure
  - Clinical features: expressionless face, bilateral or unilateral facial paralysis, lack of abduction of the eye (VI nerve paralysis) and vocal fold paralysis with stridor. Often seen with Poland sequence. (Figure 6.1)
  - Variable clinical course: Majority of children have significant feeding and language delays but normal intelligence.
- **Oromandibular–limb-hypogenesis spectrum** (Charlie M syndrome, Hanhart syndrome, MIM 103300)
  - Sporadic and broad spectrum of disorders; vascular etiology is suspected.
    - Early chorionic villous sampling (<10 weeks) has been associated with this disorder.

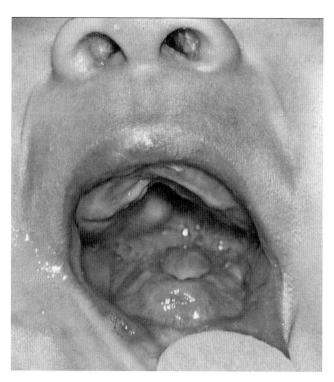

FIGURE 30.6  Microglossia, small mouth and mandible, and variable limb defects are characteristic of oromandibular–limb hypogenesis syndrome.

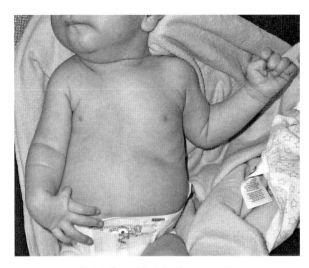

FIGURE 30.7 This infant with Poland sequence has an asymmetric chest wall. The right pectoralis major muscle is absent, and the nipple is hypoplastic. The right hand is radially deviated at the wrist.

○ Clinical features: microglossia (Figure 30.6), small mouth and mandible, variable limb defects: syndactyly, monodactyly, amelia
  ■ Significant overlap with Moebius sequence, which may share a common etiology
  ■ Variable outcome: can be lethal
- **Poland sequence** (MIM 173800)
  ○ Sporadic nongenetic disorder, may be caused by subclavian artery supply disruption sequence
  ○ Almost always unilateral, more often on the right side; 3 R:1 L
  ○ Males predominate
  ○ Clinical features: asymmetric chest wall, absence of the sternal head of pectoralis major muscle, loss of anterior axillary fold, ipsilateral radial and hand anomalies, brachydactyly, syndactyly or hypoplasia; can be subtle. Hypoplastic nipple on involved side (predicts later lack of breast development) (Figure 30.7)
    ■ Dextrocardia, missing or bifid ribs, lung agenesis
    ■ Often seen with facial palsy, Moebius sequence

## Evaluation and Management

- Document pregnancy history: trauma, hyperthermia, vasoactive and teratogenic agents, vaginal bleeding, threatened miscarriage, attempted abortion, chorionic villous sampling.
- Obtain a family history: similarly affected individuals, congenital anomalies, infant deaths, consanguinity.
- Examine parents and other relatives for subtle hand or upper limb anomalies, thenar hypoplasia, cutis aplasia.

- Placenta histology: vaso-occlusive lesions, infarctions, early amnion rupture
- Examine infant for nonskeletal anomalies: IUGR, microcephaly, facial movement, microglossia, scalp defects, asymmetry, absence of the pectoralis major, constriction rings, skin hyperpigmentation.
- Imaging studies
  ○ Obtain radiographs of both right and left upper extremities, even in apparently unilateral cases, and other affected limbs.
  ○ Abdominal US, echocardiogram, and ECG
- Laboratory studies: CBC with platelet count; consider thrombophilia evaluation in isolated transverse reduction defects.
- Genetic testing
  ○ Microarray especially for radial and ulnar agenesis or when TAR syndrome is suspected
  ○ Chromosome analysis for suspected aneuploidy or when Roberts syndrome is suspected (centromere puffing, premature separation)
  ○ Chromosome breakage studies with DEB whenever thumbs are abnormal to rule out Fanconi anemia
  ○ Targeted gene analysis for specific diagnoses
  ○ Consider exome sequencing or research studies in complex patients without a clear diagnosis.

## Further Reading

Al-Qattan MM. (2013) Molecular basis of the clinical features of Al-Awadi–Raas–Rothschild (limb/pelvis/uterus–hypoplasia/aplasia) syndrome (AARRS) and Fuhrmann syndrome. Am J Med Genet A. 161A:2274–80. PMID 23922166

Bedard T, Lowry RB, Sibbald B, et al. (2015) Congenital limb deficiencies in Alberta—A review of 33 years (1980–2012) from the Alberta Congenital Anomalies Surveillance System (ACASS). Am J Med Genet A. 167A:2599–609. PMID 26171959

Bermejo-Sánchez E, Cuevas L, et al. (2011) Amelia: A multi-center descriptive epidemiologic study in a large dataset from the International Clearinghouse for Birth Defects Surveillance and Research, and overview of the literature. Am J Med Genet C Semin Med Genet. 157C:288–304. PMID 22002956

Carli D, Fairplay T, Ferrari P, et al. (2013) Genetic basis of congenital upper limb anomalies: Analysis of 487 cases of a specialized clinic. Birth Defects Res A Clin Mol Teratol. 97:798–805. PMID 24343878

Elmakky A, Stanghellini I, Landi A, Percesepe A. (2015) Role of genetic factors in the pathogenesis of radial deficiencies in humans. Curr Genomics. 16:264–78. PMID 26962299

Gurrieri F, Everman DB. (2013) Clinical, genetic, and molecular aspects of split-hand/foot malformation: An update. Am J Med Genet A. 161A:2860–72. PMID 24115638

Houeijeh A, Andrieux J, Saugier-Veber P, et al. (2011) Thrombocytopenia-absent radius (TAR) syndrome: A clinical genetic series of 14 further cases. Impact of the associated 1q21.1

deletion on the genetic counseling. Eur J Med Genet. 54:e471–7. PMID 21635976

Koskimies E, Lindfors N, Gissler M, Peltonen J, Nietosvaara Y. (2011) Congenital upper limb deficiencies and associated malformations in Finland: A population-based study. J Hand Surg Am. 36:1058–65. PMID 21601997

Rohmann E, Brunner HG, Kayserili H, et al. (2006) Mutations in different components of FGF signaling in LADD syndrome. Nat Genet. 38:414–7. PMID 16501574

Shamseldin HE, Anazi S, Wakil SM, et al. (2016) Novel copy number variants and major limb reduction malformation: Report of three cases. Am J Med Genet A. 170:1245–50. PMID 26749485

# 31

# Lower Extremity Anomalies

## Clinical Consult

A term baby boy had severe, asymmetric lower extremity malformations with a negative family history. He had a deep dimple on the left lower leg, over a sharply angulated tibia and oligodactyly with three toes. On the right, he had a clubfoot and three toes (Figure 31.1). His hands were normal. Radiographs revealed bilateral absence of the fibulas and the two lateral (postaxial) toes and metatarsals. The baby's exam was otherwise normal without other associated anomalies.

This constellation of abnormalities is most consistent with the variable and rare **FATCO syndrome** (fibular aplasia, tibial campomelia, and oligosyndactyly, MIM 246570). The etiology is unknown, and all affected individuals, except one family with affected half-siblings, have been sporadic. This infant was enrolled in a research study, and genome sequencing is in progress. The baby was referred to a tertiary orthopedic center specializing in management of complex limb anomalies. At 4 months of age, his development was normal. Lower extremity defects are often complex and difficult to categorize.

## Definition

- Incidence varies regionally: ~3/10,000
  - Lower limb (LL) anomalies occur approximately half as often as upper limb (UL) anomalies
  - Approximately 10% of all limb anomalies involve both the upper and the lower limbs.
- The lower limbs begin development at approximately 4 embryonic weeks and are complete by approximately week 9.
- Males are more commonly affected: 55 M:45 F.
- The most common lower limb defects affect the femur; the next most common involve the fibula.
- When unilateral, lower limb anomalies occur more often on the left side (1.2 L:1 R).
- Associated anomalies
  - Isolated defect in 44%
  - Multiple congenital anomalies without a recognizable diagnosis 17%

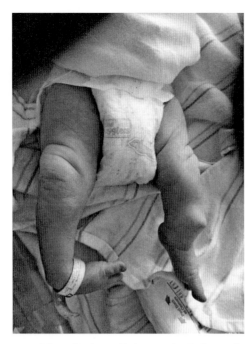

FIGURE 31.1 Bilaterally absent fibulae, angulated tibiae and oligodactyly in FATCO syndrome. The cause of this rare presentation is unknown.

- Diagnosed with a recognized condition 39%: including chromosome anomalies, teratogens, Mendelian disorders
- Lower limb defects are briefly reviewed in the following categories:
  - **Transverse defects**: terminal absence of distal parts (amputations)
    - The most common type of lower limb anomaly: 1.5/ 10,000
  - **Longitudinal defects**: deficiency of one of the distal long bones (tibia or fibular aplasia/hypoplasia) and their associated digital rays
  - **Intercalary defects**: loss of one segment of the limb (focal femoral agenesis)
  - **Central defects**: loss of central rays in the distal limb (spilt hand/foot)
  - Leg length overgrowth or undergrowth, clubfoot, arthrogryposis, polydactyly, and syndactyly are considered in other chapters.

# Differential Diagnosis

## Transverse Defects

- Isolated
  - Transverse defects occur less commonly in the lower extremity than in the upper extremity.
  - Mechanism is most likely vascular disruption.

- When isolated, very low recurrence risk
- Possible role of prothrombotic factors controversial and needs study
- Syndromic
  - **Adams–Oliver syndrome** (MIM 100300)
    - Autosomal dominant, highly variable disorder, caused by heterozygous variants in the *ARHGAP31, NOTCH1, DLL4, RBPJ* genes and others; autosomal recessive types reported
    - Clinical features: defects in scalp and skull at the vertex, cutis aplasia can occur elsewhere (knees and abdomen), symmetric transverse terminal defects of the hands and feet (Figure 30.3), congenital heart defects in 20%
  - **Amniotic band disruption sequence** (MIM 217100)
    - Sporadic disorder without a known or suspected genetic basis. Amniotic rupture in utero causes entrapment of fetal parts by amniotic strands and vascular compromise distal to the constrictions.
    - Clinical features: Usually asymmetric, but bilateral circumferential constriction rings, distal swelling and/or "purse-string" amputations, syndactyly; may involve any combination of limbs (Figure 31.2)
      - Can result in loss of an entire foot or lower leg but upper extremity involvement more common
      - Occasionally, visible amniotic strands are attached to the limbs at delivery.
      - Impression of umbilical cord wrapping may be evident on limbs (see Figure 28.3)
      - Rarely, oral or facial clefts, encephalocele/anencephaly/ exencephaly
    - Placental exam helps establish the diagnosis.

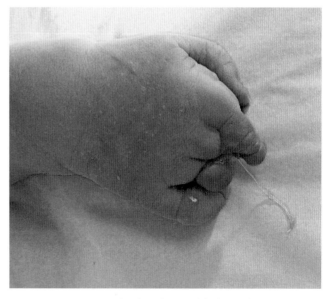

FIGURE 31.2 Amniotic bands with typical findings of distal amputations, constriction rings, and a visible strand of amnion.

## Longitudinal Defects

- Fibular deficiency
  - **FATCO syndrome** (*f*ibular *a*plasia, *t*ibial *c*ampomelia, and *o*ligosyndactyly syndrome, MIM 24657) (see Clinical Consult, Figure 31.1)
    - Sporadic disorder, no causative gene known
    - Clinical features: fibular aplasia, angulation of the tibia; oligosyndactyly primarily affects the lower extremity but upper extremity can also be involved. No other significant abnormalities
- Tibial deficiency
  - Tibial hemimelia characterized on the basis of radiologic findings into several types (Paley, 2016) may guide planning for surgical reconstruction.
  - Fibula is generally present, and polydactyly is frequent. Conditions are clinically variable, and an etiologic diagnosis can be challenging.

*Pearl*: When only one long bone is present in the lower leg, it may be difficult to identify based on expected fibular and tibial morphology. The absence of one of these bones affects the shape of the other.

- Isolated
  - May be recessive or dominant
- Syndromic
  - Chromosome disorders are reported with tibial deficiency, including del 8q23.2, del 7q21, and 10q distal trisomy.
  - **Tibial hypoplasia or aplasia with polydactyly and triphalangeal thumbs** (Werner mesomelic dysplasia, MIM 188740)
    - Autosomal dominant disorder due to heterozygous variants in the sonic hedgehog regulatory element region (*ZRS*) of the *LMBR1* gene.
    - Clinical features: tibial hypoplasia or agenesis; fibular duplication; non-opposable, triphalangeal thumb; variable pre- and postaxial polydactyly of the hands and feet (see Figure 32.1)
  - **Laurin–Sandrow syndrome** (MIM 135750)
    - Autosomal dominant disorder, due to pathogenic variant in *ZRS*
    - Complex syndrome with mirror-image duplication of hands and feet in a rosebud configuration, an unusual nasal configuration, and variable other tibial and ulnar deficiencies (see Figure 32.3)
  - **Gollop–Wolfgang complex** (MIM 228250)
    - Presumed autosomal recessive disorder without known genetic cause
    - Clinical features: unilateral bifurcation of the femur, ipsilateral absent tibia, oligodactyly

- **Acromelic frontonasal dysostosis** (MIM 603671)
  - Sporadic disorder but autosomal dominant inheritance reported in a mildly affected parent who was mosaic for the pathogenic variant
  - Caused by a single recurrent heterozygous missense variant in *ZSWIM6*
  - Clinical features: severe symmetric frontonasal dysplasia associated with median cleft face, bifid nose, unilateral or bilateral tibial hypoplasia or aplasia, talipes equinovarus, preaxial polydactyly of the feet
    - Severe ID
    - Other variable features: periventricular nodular heterotopia, aplastic or hypoplastic corpus callosum, hypopituitarism, patellar hypoplasia, cryptorchidism
- **Clubfoot, congenital, with or without deficiency of long bones and/or mirror-image polydactyly** (MIM 119800)
  - Autosomal dominant disorder, caused by *PITX1* deletions or pathogenic variants
  - Clinical features: Variable limb problems range from isolated clubfoot to tibial agenesis with mirror-image polydactyly. Upper extremities are normal.
  - Suspect this in families with more than one affected individual, especially when complex preaxial polydactyly is present.

## Intercalary Defects

- Femoral deficiency
  - **Femoral–facial syndrome** (MIM 134780)
    - Sporadic disorder without known genetic cause
      - One-third are infants of diabetic mothers.

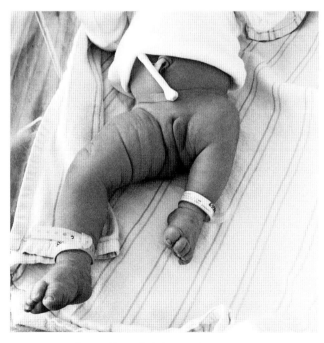

FIGURE 31.3 Femoral hypoplasia in a newborn.

- One of the most common lower extremity malformations
- Clinical features: femoral aplasia or hypoplasia; can be unilateral, bilateral, or asymmetric, often with involvement of the hip. Fibula may also be deficient (Figure 31.3 and 12S.1).
  - Facial features: small nose, long philtrum, thin upper lip, cleft palate, micrognathia
  - Variable upper limb, vertebral, rib; cardiac, renal, and GI anomalies

## Combined Defects

- Long bones of lower and upper extremities may both be involved in these syndromic conditions.
  - Limb anomalies due to variants in *GDF5*
    - The gene *GDF5* (growth/differentiation factor 5, also called cartilage-derived morphogenetic protein-1, *CDMP1*) plays a role in regulation of limb patterning, joint formation, and distal bone growth.
      - Homozygous or compound heterozygous variants in *GDF5* result in severe limb malformations. Heterozygous variants result in a variety of brachydactyly syndromes.
      - **Grebe type** of acromesomelic dysplasia (MIM 200700) severe; autosomal recessive
      - **Hunter–Thompson type** (MIM 201250) autosomal recessive and less severe
      - **Du Pan syndrome** (fibular hypoplasia and complex brachydactyly, MIM 228900) autosomal recessive
        - Clinical features: short stature, fibular hypoplasia, brachydactyly, short carpals and metacarpals, tibiotarsal dislocation (Volkmann deformity)
  - **Roberts syndrome** (MIM 268300)
    - Lethal autosomal recessive, caused by biallelic variants in *ESCO2*
    - Clinical features: severe tetraphocomelia of all four limbs with cleft lip/palate and craniofacial anomalies. Occasional survivors beyond neonatal period
      - Centromeric puffing is evident on routine cytogenetics (must request this analysis).
    - Variants in *ESCO2* also cause **SC phocomelia syndrome** (MIM 269000).
  - **Split hand/foot longitudinal deficiency** (SHFLD, MIM612576)
    - Autosomal dominant disorder with reduced penetrance
    - At least seven loci
    - Chromosomal rearrangements or abnormalities at 7q21.3, Xq26, dup 10q24, del 2q31, and dup17p13.3
    - The duplication syndrome at 17p13.3 involves the gene *BHLHA9*.
      - Duplications in this gene appear to be necessary but not sufficient to produce the SHFLD phenotype, suggesting that additional unknown regulatory genes play a role in this phenotype.

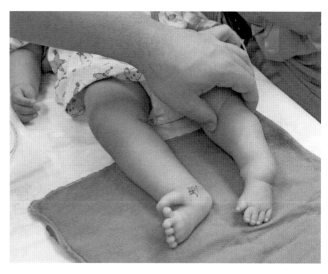

FIGURE 31.4 The rare SHFLD phenotype in an infant with a 17p13.3 duplication due in part to duplication of the gene *BHLHA9*.

- Clinical features: tibial hypoplasia and split hand/foot; minor manifestations in some affected individuals (Figure 31.4)
  - **Fuhrmann syndrome** (MIM 228930)
    - Autosomal recessive, caused by homozygous variants in *WNT7A* that result in partial decrease in gene function; not loss of function
    - Clinical features: fibular aplasia/hypoplasia, femoral bowing, polydactyly, syndactyly, oligodactyly, stick-like lower limbs, hypoplastic/aplastic nails, pelvic dysplasia, variable ulnar ray deficiency
  - **Femur–fibula–ulna complex** (FFU, MIM 228200)
    - Sporadic disorder without a known genetic cause; no known environmental or maternal causes
      - Recurrence risk is low. Out of ~500 published cases and 300 others, only one sib recurrence has been reported.
    - Clinical features: A unilaterally short femur is most common. A highly specific pattern of rare arm defects: amelia, humeroradial synostosis, and defects of the ulna and ulnar rays
      - No other associated malformations
  - **Mesomelic dysplasia, Savarirayan type** (MIM 605274)
    - A small chromosome deletion at 6p22.3 causes this phenotype.
    - Clinical features: Both the tibia and fibula are involved. The fibula is missing. The tibia is triangular and hypoplastic.
      - Amputation and prosthetics have been employed.
      - The upper extremities are mildly involved with widening of the ulna and decreased supination.
      - Intellectual disability is frequent.

## Central Defects

- **Split hand/split foot** (MIM 183600 and others)
  - Longitudinal deficiency of the central digits often involving the associated carpal/tarsal bones results in a split-hand or

split-foot appearance. These have been variously termed "ectrodactyly" and occasionally as a "lobster claw" (not a preferred term).

- The most severe form is monodactyly, when hand or foot has but a single digit.
- Syndactyly and hypoplasia can affect some remaining digits.

o Caused by single gene variants, chromosomal rearrangements, and sometimes by variants at more than one locus
- May be isolated or syndromic

o Isolated split hand/foot
- Autosomal dominant disorder, associated with one of at least six loci, most frequently 7q21.3
  - Many genes await discovery.
  - Striking variability in families and even between involved limbs in same individual
  - Germline mosaicism is responsible for some cases with more than one affected sibling and apparently unaffected parents.
- Autosomal recessive split hand/foot (MIM 220600) can be caused by variants in *DLX5*.

o Syndromic split hand/foot
- **Ectrodactyly, ectodermal dysplasia, and cleft lip/palate syndrome** (EEC, MIM 129900) most common syndrome associated with split hand/foot
  - Autosomal dominant, caused by a heterozygous variant in *TP63*—90% of EEC
  - Clinical features: cleft lip with or without cleft palate, split hand or foot (Figures 31.5 and 11.5), lacrimal duct problems, abnormal and missing teeth, sparse hair, decreased sweating
  - Wide variability in families

- *TP63* mutations also cause the closely related primarily ectodermal disorders that occasionally present with syndactyly or other limb defects **Rapp–Hodgkin syndrome** (MIM 129400) and **Hay–Wells syndrome** (AEC, MIM 106260)

## Evaluation and Management

- Assess family history and carefully examine relatives for minor expression of these variable malformations.
- Full radiographic assessment will help diagnose and plan orthopedic strategies.
- Options to preserve the limb and avoid amputation are being increasingly utilized.
- Genetic testing
  o Chromosome analysis to detect centromere puffing and chromosome rearrangements when considering Roberts syndrome or syndromes with split hand/foot
  o Chromosome microarray when there are multiple anomalies or ID
  o Limb deficiency gene panels are available, but appropriate selection may require a detailed phenotype and a clear differential diagnosis. Exome sequencing could be considered when no specific disorder is suspected.
  o A multidisciplinary approach in a tertiary referral center is needed for the management of these complex disorders

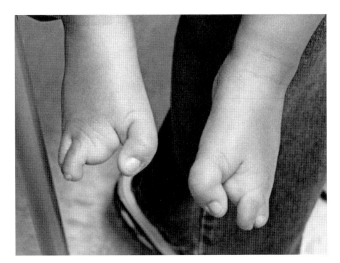

FIGURE 31.5 Split foot deformity in the ectrodactyly, ectodermal dysplasia, and clefting (EEC) syndrome.

## Further Reading

Bedoya MA, Chauvin NA, Jaramillo D, et al. (2015) Common patterns of congenital lower extremity shortening: Diagnosis, classification, and follow-up. Radiographics. 35:1191–207. PMID 26172360

Flöttmann R, Wagner J, Kobus K, et al. (2015) Microdeletions on 6p22.3 are associated with mesomelic dysplasia Savarirayan type. J Med Genet. 52:476–83. PMID 26032025

Lenz W, Zygulska M, Horst J. (1993) FFU complex: An analysis of 491 cases. Hum Genet. 91:347–56. PMID 8500790

Maas SM, Lombardi MP, van Essen AJ, et al. (2009) Phenotype and genotype in 17 patients with Goltz–Gorlin syndrome. J Med Genet. 46:716–20. PMID 19586929

Paley D. (2016) Tibial hemimelia: New classification and reconstructive options. J Child Orthop. 10:529–55. PMID 27909860

Petit F, Jourdain AS, Andrieux J, et al. (2014) Split hand/foot malformation with long-bone deficiency and BHLHA9 duplication: Report of 13 new families. Clin Genet. 85:464–9. PMID 23790188

Sowińska-Seidler A, Socha M, Jamsheer A. (2014) Split-hand/foot malformation—Molecular cause and implications in genetic counseling. J Appl Genet. 55:105–115. PMID 24163146

# 32

# Polydactyly

## Clinical Consult

A genetic consultation was requested for a term newborn male, with bilateral tibial aplasia and preaxial synpolydactyly of the hands and feet with seven digits on each extremity, who had not passed his first stool at several days of age (Figure 32.1). A rectal biopsy revealed aganglionosis. The father reported that he had Hirschsprung disease as an infant. On close examination, both the father and the son had triphalangeal thumbs, although the father did not have extra fingers. When the geneticist requested to see the father's feet, he admitted that his lower legs were similar to his son's at birth. He had undergone bilateral below the knee amputations and now wore prostheses. He had been told that his anomalies were caused by his mother's exposure to an anti-nausea drug during pregnancy. Until the birth of his son, he did not know that his anomalies had a genetic basis. The diagnosis of autosomal dominant tibial hypoplasia/aplasia with polydactyly syndrome and Hirschsprung disease (**Werner mesomelic syndrome**, MIM 188740) was made. Gene testing for *ZRS* was ordered.

## Definition

- Polydactyly is an extra digit, or part of a digit, that can be postaxial (on the ulnar/fibular side), preaxial (on the radial/tibial side), or mesoaxial (central; in the center of the hand or foot).
  - More than one type of polydactyly can occur in the same individual.
  - For complex and mirror-type polydactylies, see Malik (2014).
- Prevalence 0.3–3.6/1,000
- 2 M:1 F
- Isolated polydactyly
  - Usually sporadic and unilateral; mesoaxial polydactyly is rarely isolated.
  - When familial, it is usually bilateral and symmetric, with reduced penetrance and variants in ~20 genes can cause isolated polydactyly.
    - *ZRS* is a regulatory gene located close to *SHH* (Sonic Hedgehog) within *LIMBR1*, a limb patterning gene.

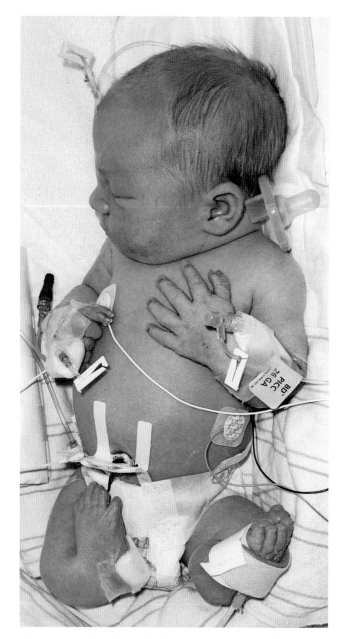

FIGURE 32.1 This infant with Hirschsprung disease has tibial agenesis, preaxial polydactyly of the hands, and synpolydactyly of the feet. His father was similarly affected with Werner mesomelic syndrome.

ZRS regulates the expression of *SHH* in the limb but not elsewhere.
   ■ *GLI3* and *PITX1* are critical genes in limb development.
   ○ Incidence varies by population.
      ■ Isolated postaxial polydactyly is a common autosomal dominant trait in African Americans.
      ■ Isolated preaxial polydactyly is more common in Native Americans and Asians than in Caucasians.
• Isolated postaxial polydactyly
   ○ Duplication of little finger or toe
      ■ The extra digit often does not always have a nail or a bony articulation (postminimus polydactyly).

   ○ Incidence 1–2/1,000 live births
      ■ Africans and African Americans: 1% have this common autosomal dominant trait.
      ■ Japanese: lowest rate of postaxial polydactyly
   ○ M > F
   ○ Bilateral > unilateral
   ○ Postaxial polydactyly predominates over preaxial 3:1.
      ■ Except among Japanese and Chinese, in whom preaxial polydactyly is more common than postaxial
   ○ Usually isolated: ~90% have no other anomalies.
      ■ When postaxial polydactyly involves all four extremities, ~8% have multiple congenital anomalies.
   ○ Recurrence risk ≤50%; nonpenetrance is common.
• Isolated preaxial polydactyly
   ○ Broad, bifid or duplicated thumb or great toe (Figure 32.2)
   ○ Primarily autosomal dominant traits
   ○ **Preaxial polydactyly types, I, II, and IV**
      ■ Autosomal dominant group of similar traits caused by heterozygous variants in *ZRS*
      ■ **Preaxial polydactyly type I** (MIM 174400, 601759)
         • Clinical features: triphalangeal or broad hallux or great toes

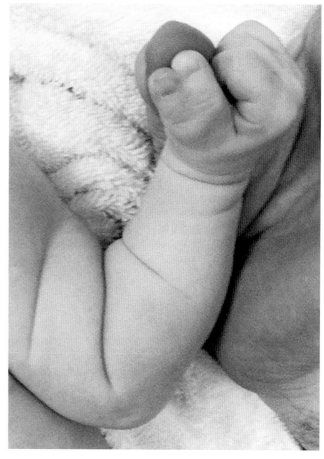

FIGURE 32.2 This infant has an isolated duplicated thumb.

- Preaxial polydactyly type II (MIM 174500)
  - Clinical features: triphalangeal thumb, decreased expression in females
- Preaxial polydactyly type IV (MIM 174700)
  - Clinical features: polysyndactyly, crossed preaxial and postaxial polydactyly
- Tibial hypoplasia/aplasia with polydactyly (Werner mesomelia syndrome, MIM 188740; see Clinical Consult)
- Laurin–Sandrow syndrome (MIM 135750)
  - Clinical features: mirror-image hands and feet (Figure 32.3); syndactylous fingers cupped in a rosebud manner, abnormal nasal configuration
- Preaxial polydactyly type III (MIM 174600)
  - Rare
  - Clinical features: index finger polydactyly
- Synpolydactyly (MIM 186000)
  - Clinical features: extra digit in a syndactylous web

## Differential Diagnosis

- Pathogenic variants in ~290 genes cause syndromic polydactyly. Verma and El-Harouni (2015) review syndromic postaxial polydactyly. Selected syndromes with polydactyly follow.
- Teratogens*
  - **Maternal diabetes***
    - Clinical features: duplicated proximally placed great toe, tibial hemimelia, femoral hypoplasia, clubfoot, vertebral segmentation defects; cardiac, renal, and ear anomalies
  - **Thalidomide embryopathy**
    - Clinical features: deficiency or polydactyly of thumbs or great toes, usually symmetric, bilateral. Phocomelia; skeletal anomalies; cranial nerve, ear, cardiac, and visceral malformations
- Chromosome anomalies
  - **Trisomy 13***
    - Clinical features: postaxial polydactyly; microphthalmia; scalp defects; malformations of brain, heart, oral clefts
  - **Microdeletion of chromosome 2q31.1**
    - Duplication of great toes, clinodactyly
- Polydactyly with craniosynostosis*
  - **Carpenter syndrome** (MIM 201000)
    - Autosomal recessive trait, caused by biallelic variants in *RAB23* and *MEGF8*
    - Clinical features: acrocephaly; variable craniosynostosis; brachydactyly; syndactyly; postaxial, central, and preaxial polydactyly

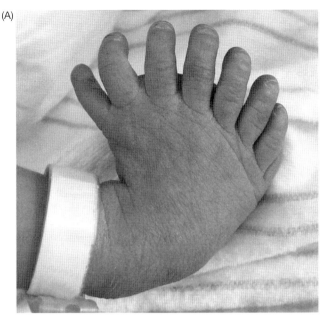

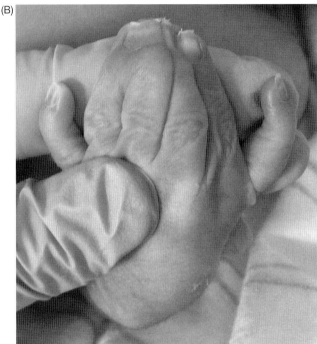

FIGURE 32.3 (A) This baby with Laurin–Sandrow syndrome has mirror-image feet: eight toes without a great toe. (B) The central fingers are joined in a polysyndactylous mass.

(Figure 13.5B); high birth weight; cardiac defects 50%; cryptorchidism
- **Greig cephalopolysyndactyly syndrome** (MIM 175700)
  - Autosomal dominant trait, due to heterozygous variant in *GLI3*
  - Clinical features: variable head shape, trigonocephaly, metopic craniosynostosis, frontal bossing, preaxial and postaxial polysyndactyly (Figure 32.4)

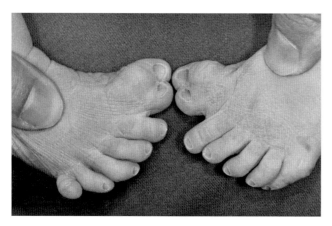

FIGURE 32.4 Preaxial and postaxial polydactyly with variable syndactyly is a pattern typical of Grieg cephalopolysyndactyly syndrome.

- Polydactyly with GI anomalies
  - **Tibial hypoplasia/aplasia with polydactyly and Hirschsprung disease** (Werner mesomelic syndrome, MIM 188740)
    - Autosomal dominant disorder, caused by heterozygous pathogenic variant in *ZRS*
    - Clinical features: tibial hypoplasia/agenesis, preaxial polydactyly of hands and feet, triphalangeal thumbs, variable Hirschsprung disease (Figure 32.1)
  - **Townes–Brocks syndrome** (MIM 107480)
    - Autosomal dominant trait, caused by a pathogenic variant in *SALL1*
    - Clinical features: triphalangeal and/or duplicated thumbs; anorectal atresia/stenosis; sensorineural hearing loss; small, dysplastic, or lop ears; colobomas; cataracts; renal, urogenital, cardiac defects (Figure 24.2)
- Polydactyly with macrocephaly*
  - **Basal cell nevus syndrome** (nevoid basal cell carcinoma syndrome, Gorlin syndrome, MIM 109400)
    - Autosomal dominant cancer predisposition syndrome caused by heterozygous pathogenic variant of *PTCH1* or microdeletion of 9q22.3 or, less commonly, *PTCH2* or *SUFU*
    - Clinical features: Various congenital anomalies, including macrocephaly, asymmetric or dilated ventricles, macrosomia, bifid ribs, oral clefts, vertebral anomalies, cardiac fibromas, and, less commonly, polydactyly of the feet (Figure 32.5A).
      - Medulloblastoma presents early, before age 3 years. Establishing the diagnosis prior to this time is important because radiation therapy should be avoided. Affected patients develop hundreds of basal cell carcinomas in the radiation field.
    - Examine parents for jaw cysts, palmar plantar pits (Figure 32.5B), calcification of falx cerebri, basal cell carcinoma, and ovarian fibroma.

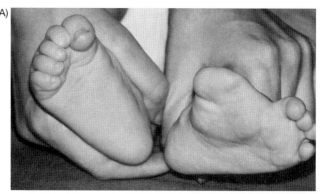

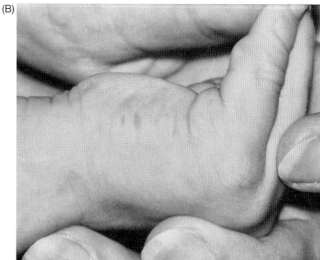

FIGURE 32.5 Polydactyly of the great toe (A) and palmar pits (B) are seen in Basal cell nevus syndrome, also known as Gorlin syndrome.

  - **Hydrolethalus syndrome** (MIM 236680)
    - Lethal autosomal recessive disorder, caused by biallelic pathogenic variants in *HYLS1*
    - Clinical features: hydrocephalus, midline CNS defects, agenesis of hypocampi, hypoplastic cerebellum and brainstem, hypothalamic hamartoma, micrognathia, polydactyly of hands and feet, abnormal lung lobation, stillbirth or neonatal death
  - **Pallister–Hall syndrome** (MIM 146510)
    - Autosomal recessive disorder, caused by biallelic pathogenic variants in *GLI3*
    - Clinical features: mexoaxial polydactyly of ring fingers, preaxial polydactyly of hands and feet, abnormal lung lobation, hypothalamic hamartoma, cleft lip and palate, cardiac defects
      - Usual neonatal lethality
    - Macrocephaly, small tongue, multiple oral frenulae, micrognathia
      - Phenotype overlaps with hydrolethalus syndrome
  - **Megalencephaly–polymicrogyria–polydactyly–hydrocephalus syndrome** (MPPH, MIM 603387) and **megalencephaly–capillary malformation** (MCAP, MIM 602501)

- Caused by heterozygous pathogenic variants, germ line (MPPH) and somatic and mosaic (MCAP), in genes in the PI3K-AKT-mTOR pathway: *PIK3CR2, AKT3* (MPPH), and *PIK3CA* (MCAP)
  - Pathogenic variant may be detectable only in affected tissue.
  - Clinical features: brain and body overgrowth, often asymmetric. Postaxial polydactyly in approximately half of the infants with MPPH and in many with MCAP (Figure 14.3)
- Polydactyly with microcephaly *
  - **Fanconi anemia** (MIM 227650)
    - Autosomal recessive disorders, caused by biallelic pathogenic variant in DNA repair genes
    - Increased chromosome breakage with DEB or mitomycin C is diagnostic.
    - Clinical features: hypoplastic or duplicated thumbs (see Figure 18S.3), prenatal and postnatal growth deficiency, microcephaly, café au lait spots, VATER/VACTERL spectrum anomalies
      - Later: red cell or pancytopenic anemia, cancer predisposition

*Pearl*: Mothers and other female relatives of infants with Fanconi anemia may be at increased risk for breast or ovarian cancer. *BRCA2*, one of the genes responsible for hereditary breast and ovarian cancer, causes Fanconi anemia type D1 in patients with biallelic pathogenic variants.

  - **Smith–Lemli–Opitz syndrome*** (SLOS, MIM 270400)
    - Autosomal recessive disorder of cholesterol biosynthesis, caused by biallelic pathogenic variants in *DHCR7A*
    - Clinical findings: postaxial polydactyly of hands/feet, short thumbs, thenar hypoplasia, Y-shaped syndactyly of toes 2–3. Upturned nose, ptosis, cataracts, micrognathia, cleft palate/bifid uvula. Microcephaly, holoprosencephaly 5%, hypotonia, CNS anomalies, poor suck. Cardiac, GI, and GU malformations (Figure 27.3)
    - Laboratory studies
      - Prenatal maternal serum screening: very low unconjugated estriol (uE3)
      - Increased 7-dehydrocholesterol
- Polydactyly syndromes with renal* cysts
  - Usually autosomal recessive traits, caused by pathogenic variants in genes associated with basal body and primary cilium. These ciliopathies share postaxial polydactyly, renal cysts, laterality defects, and CNS anomalies.
  - **Bardet–Biedl syndrome** (MIM 209900)
    - Clinical features: postaxial polydactyly 63–81%; may be the only sign in newborns. Hypogonadism 59–98%, large hyperechogenic kidneys or renal cysts
      - Later: obesity, pigmentary retinal dystrophy, ID
  - **Ellis van Creveld syndrome** (MIM 225500)
    - Biallelic pathogenic variants in *EVC* or *EVC2*

- Clinical features: disproportionate short stature, acromesomelia, postaxial polydactyly, dysplastic nails, multiple oral frenulae, natal teeth, heart defects, ASD, atrioventricular septal defect (AVSD)(Figure 36.8)
  - **Jeune syndrome** (MIM 208500, 611263)
    - Biallelic pathogenic variants in *IFT80, DYNC2H1, NEK1, TTC21B*, and others
    - Clinical features: narrow thorax, short ribs, respiratory insufficiency, postaxial polydactyly, cystic kidneys
  - **Joubert syndrome** (MIM 213300)
    - Clinical features: periodic or irregular breathing, cerebellar vermis hypoplasia, Dandy–Walker malformation, molar tooth sign on brain MRI (Figure 16.3), postaxial polydactyly, renal cysts, retinal dystrophy, hepatic fibrosis
  - **Meckel–Gruber syndrome** (MIM 249000)
    - Clinical features: usually lethal, occipital encephalocele, cystic kidney dysplasia, hepatobiliary ductal plate malformation, postaxial polydactyly (Figure 26.2)
  - **Oral–facial–digital syndrome type I** (MIM 300170)
    - X-linked dominant trait, caused by pathogenic variant in *OFD1*
      - Usually female; mostly lethal in males
    - Clinical features: renal cysts, midline cleft lip, cleft palate. Hypertelorism, hypertrophic oral frenulae, lobulated tongue, milia (Figure 11.6)

# Evaluation and Management

- Document family history: consanguinity, stillbirths, infant deaths, polydactyly, renal cysts, congenital anomalies, obesity, intellectual disability, poor vision.
- Examine parents: hands and feet for nubbins, scars from excision of extra digits, broad thumbs or great toes, triphalangeal thumbs.
- Record pregnancy history: abnormal maternal serum screening test, maternal diabetes mellitus, teratogens.
- Examine patient for other anomalies: multiple oral frenulae, lobulated tongue, abnormal breathing pattern, renal cysts.
- Brain imaging for macrocephaly, hypotonia, or unexplained poor feeding
- Genetic testing
  - Chromosome analysis for suspected aneuploidy
  - Chromosome microarray for polydactyly with multiple congenital anomalies
  - Chromosome breakage studies for thumb polydactyly with poor growth, microcephaly, or VATER/VACTERL-like anomalies
    - DEB is preferred over mitomycin C.
  - Gene or genomic testing as indicated by phenotype
- Order 7-dehydrocholesterol when suspecting SLOS.

# Further Reading

Adam MP, Hudgins L, Carey JC, et al. (2009) Preaxial hallucal polydactyly as a marker for diabetic embryopathy. Birth Defects Res A Clin Mol Teratol. 85:13–9. PMID 18798547

Al-Qattan MM, Shamseldin HE, Salih MA, Alkuraya FS. (2017) GLI3-related polydactyly: A review. Clin Genet. 92:457–466. PMID 28224613

Bergmann C. (2012) Educational paper: Ciliopathies. Eur J Pediatr. 171:1285–1300. PMID 21898032

Biesecker LG. (2011) Polydactyly: How many disorders and how many genes? 2010 update. Dev Dyn. 240:931–942. PMID 21445961

Deng H, Tan T, Yuan L. (2015) Advances in the molecular genetics of nonsyndromic polydactyly. Expert Rev Mol Med. 17:e18. PMID 26515020

Farrugia MC, Calleja-Agius J. (2016) Polydactyly: A review. Neonatal Netw. 35(3):135–42. PMID 27194607

Holmes LB. (2002) Teratogen-induced limb defects. Am J Med Genet. 112:297–303. PMID 12357474

Malik S. (2014) Polydactyly: Phenotypes, genetics and classification. Clin Genet. 85:203–212. PMID 24020795

Norbnop P, Srichomthong C, Suphapeetiporn K, Shotelersuk V. (2014) ZRS 406A>G mutation in patients with tibial hypoplasia, polydactyly and triphalangeal first fingers. J Hum Genet. 59:467–70. PMID 24965254

Verma PK, El-Harouni AA. (2015) Review of literature: Genes related to postaxial polydactyly. Front Pediatr. 3:8.PMID 25717468

# 33

## Syndactyly

## Clinical Consult

A genetic consultation was requested for a full-term male, who was rooming in with his mother after an unremarkable pregnancy and delivery. He had cutaneous syndactyly of the ring and little fingers, microphthalmia, and hypoplastic alae nasi (Figure 33.1). He was otherwise healthy, and he fed well. The parents were unaffected and denied consanguinity. Based on the clinical features, the geneticist diagnosed **oculo-dento-digital dysplasia** (ODDD) and arranged for *GJA1* gene analysis to be done at a follow-up visit. The next day, he was discharged with his mother. While sleeping in his car seat on the way home, he became unresponsive and asystolic. Despite emergency services, he could not be resuscitated. Gene testing, arranged by the coroner on postmortem tissue, revealed a heterozygous de novo pathogenic variant in *GJA1*. This gene codes for the gap junction channel protein connexin43, which is prevalent in the cardiac conduction system. The likely cause of death was a lethal arrhythmia, which has been reported, rarely, in this syndrome.

ODDD is a channelopathy that is recognized by syndactyly and characteristic facial features. Lethal arrhythmia is a rare complication. Channelopathies cause 10–15% of deaths attributed to SIDS.

## Definition

- Syndactyly is a cutaneous or bony connection between two or more contiguous digits. It can affect just the fingers or the toes or both, in various combinations.
- Incidence 1/2,500 births
- 7 M:3 F
- Simple syndactyly 60%, has cutaneous fusion only
- Complex syndactyly 40%, has bony fusion
- Unilateral syndactyly 64%, right > left
- Isolated syndactyly 25%
  - Monogenic syndactyly occurs as an isolated trait in at least nine recognizable patterns (Malik, 2012).
    - Most are autosomal dominant traits with incomplete penetrance and variable expression.

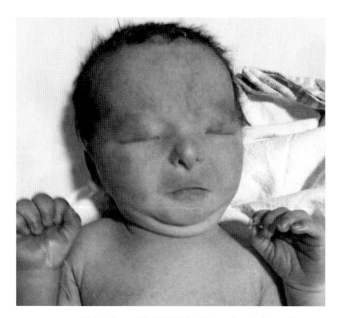

FIGURE 33.1 This infant with ODDD had hypoplastic alae nasi, microphthalmia, and cutaneous syndactyly of the ring and little fingers.

- Syndromic syndactyly 34%
  - More than 300 syndromes include syndactyly of the fingers or toes.
  - Some of the more common multiple congenital anomalies syndromes that include syndactyly are reviewed next.

## Differential Diagnosis

- Chromosome anomalies
  - **Down syndrome***
  - **Triploidy**: 69,XXX (or 69,XYY, 69,XXY) or triploid mosaicism
    - Clinical features: IUGR, hydrocephalus, cleft palate, syndactyly of fingers (3–4) (Figure 33.2)
- **Amniotic band disruption sequence** (MIM 217100)
  - Usually a sporadic disruption event that follows early amnion rupture with subsequent entanglement of fetal parts
  - Clinical features: circumferential constriction bands, asymmetric distal amputations, syndactyly can be fenestrated,

- Syndactyly type 1 accounts for 70% of nonsyndromic syndactyly.
  - Clinical features: partial or complete syndactyly of middle and ring fingers and/or the second and third toes
  - There are four subtypes.
    - Subtype 1, or **zygodactyly** (MIM 609815), is the mildest and most common subtype, in which cutaneous syndactyly affects only toes 2 and 3, without hand involvement. It is of no clinical significance.
    - Subtype 2 is an autosomal dominant form (MIM 185900) caused by **microduplication of chr 2q35**.
      - A larger microduplication of 2q35 causes craniosynostosis, Philadelphia type.

*Pearl*: Skin syndactyly of the second and third toes that is less than one-third the length of the toe is considered a normal variant.

- Syndactyly associated with other digital malformations 40%
  - Syndactyly with brachydactyly: e.g. **brachysyndactyly syndrome** (MIM 610713)
  - Syndactyly with oligodactyly: e.g. split hand/foot syndromes
  - **Synpolydactyly** (syndactyly type II, MIM 186000): An extra set of phalanges is present in the syndactylous web between the middle and ring fingers.
  - Polysyndactyly: In **Haas-type syndactyly** (MIM 186200), the hands are cupped with complete cutaneous syndactyly of six digits, without bony fusion.

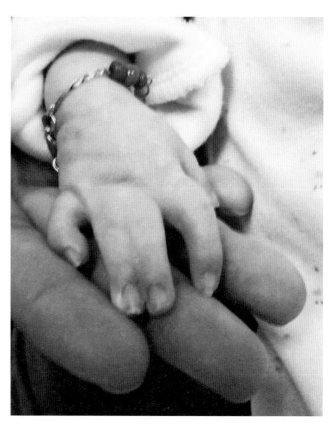

FIGURE 33.2 The classic pattern of syndactyly of the middle and ring fingers in an infant with triploidy.
SOURCE: Courtesy of Carlos Ferreira, MD, National Children's Medical Center, Washington, DC.

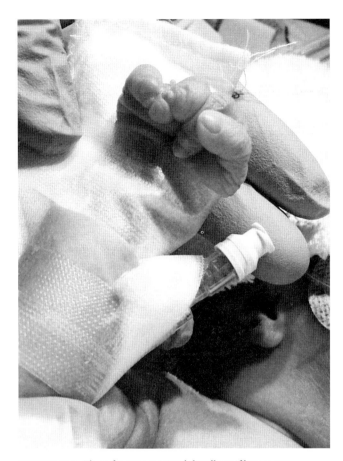

FIGURE 33.3 These fingers are joined distally as if by a purse-string closure in amniotic band sequence. Note the circumferential constriction rings, terminal amputation, distal swelling, and the unaffected fingers nearby.

or digits can be joined more tightly distally as if by a purse string (Figure 33.3)

- **Apert syndrome** (MIM 101200)
  - Autosomal dominant trait, caused by heterozygous, usually de novo pathogenic variant in *FGFR2*
  - Clinical features: acrocephaly, craniosynostos (see Figure 13.3), bony syndactyly of all fingers and toes, sometimes including fusion of the nails. Other bony fusions can include cervical vertebrae and tarsal bones.
- **Carpenter syndrome** (MIM 201000)
  - Autosomal recessive trait, caused by biallelic pathogenic variants in *RAB23*
  - Clinical features: acrocephaly, variable suture craniosynostosis, brachydactyly and syndactyly of hands, preaxial polydactyly and syndactyly of toes (see Figure 13.5), cardiac defects, poor growth
- **Curry–Jones syndrome** (MIM 601707)
  - Recurrent somatic mosaicism for missense pathogenic variant in *SMO*, causes activation of Sonic hedgehog signaling pathway

- Gene alteration more likely to be detected in saliva, skin, affected tissue
  - Clinical features: preaxial polydactyly of feet, cutaneous syndactyly, streaky skin lesions, unicoronal craniosynostosis (see Figure 13.6), iris colobomas, microphthalmia, CNS malformations, intestinal malrotation, trichoblastoma, medulloblastoma, mild ID
- **Filippi syndrome** (MIM 272440)
  - Autosomal recessive disorder, caused by pathogenic variants in *CKAP2L*
  - Clinical features: low birth weight, poor growth, microcephaly, cleft palate, cryptorchidism, soft tissue syndactyly of fingers (3–4) and toes (2–4), clinodactyly of little finger, prominent forehead, high nasal bridge, hypoplastic alae nasi
    - Later: ID, seizures
- **Fraser syndrome** (MIM 219000)
  - Autosomal recessive trait, caused by biallelic pathogenic variants in *FRAS1, FREM2, GRIP1*
  - Clinical features: cryptophthalmos (Figure 24.1), syndactyly, laryngeal stenosis, renal and genital anomalies
- **Goltz syndrome** (focal dermal hypoplasia, MIM 305600)
  - X-linked dominant trait that affects primarily females due to in utero lethality in affected males, caused by a pathogenic variant in *PORCN* on Xp11.23
  - Clinical features: focal atrophy and linear hypopigmentation, syndactyly (Figure 33.4), polydactyly, ocular anomalies
- **Greig cephalopolysyndactyly syndrome** (MIM 175700)
  - Autosomal dominant trait, caused by heterozygous pathogenic variant in *GLI3*
  - Clinical features: unusual head shape, hypertelorism, frontal bossing, pre- and postaxial polydactyly, variable syndactyly (Figure 32.4)
- **Oculo-dento-digital dysplasia** (ODDD, MIM 164200, 25780)
  - Autosomal dominant disorder, caused by heterozygous pathogenic variant in *GJA1*, which encodes connexin43, a major component of the gap junction apparatus that allows intercellular communication in the heart and other organs
  - Clinical features: microphthalmia, cataract, coloboma, short palpebral fissures, hypoplasia of the alae nasi giving the nose a pinched appearance, characteristic syndactyly of the ring and little fingers (Figure 33.1)
  - Pathogenic variants in this gene have been identified in samples from infants who died of SIDS.
    - Arrhythmias may be underrecognized.
- **Poland sequence** (MIM 173800)
  - Usuallly sporadic, asymmetric disorder of chest wall and ipsilateral upper limb
  - Most have no known genetic cause but a de novo heterozygous variant in *REV3L* has been reported in a patient with both Poland and Moebius sequences.

(A)

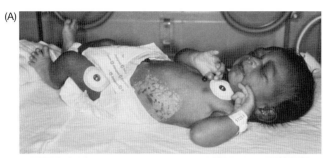

(B)

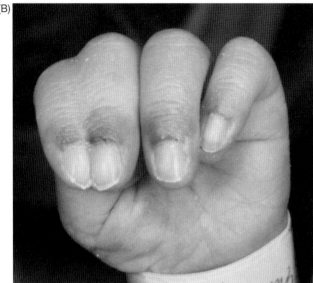

FIGURE 33.4 (A) This female infant with Goltz syndrome has focal areas of dermal hypoplasia on her ear and face, patchy skin depigmentation, and polydactyly of the right thumb. (B) The same infant has syndactyly of the left index and middle fingers.

o Clinical features: unilateral absent sternal head of pectoralis major muscle (Figure 30.7), ipsilateral hand and finger anomalies including symbrachydactyly, absent nipple, pulmonary and cardiac defects. Can occur with Moebius sequence.
  ■ Males predominate.
• **Smith–Lemli–Opitz syndrome\*** (MIM 270400)
  o Autosomal recessive multiple congenital anomaly syndrome, caused by biallelic pathogenic variants in *DHCR7*
  o Clinical features: Y-shaped syndactyly of toes (2–3) is a characteristic feature (Figure 17S.2). Low birth weight, microcephaly, ptosis, broad nasal tip, anteverted nares, long philtrum, proximally placed thumbs, postaxial polydactyly of the hands and less commonly of the feet, cleft palate, congenital heart defects (50%), undervirilized male genitalia. Elevated 7-dehydrocholesrol is diagnostic.
• **STAR syndrome** (MIM 300707)
  o X-linked dominant disorder, reported in females, caused by a loss-of-function pathogenic variant in *FAM58A*

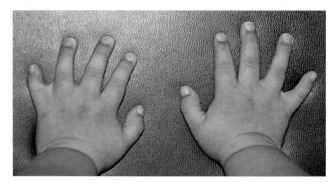

FIGURE 33.5 Syndactyly of the little, ring, and middle fingers in Timothy syndrome.

o Clinical features: STAR is an acronym for the cardinal features of *s*yndactyly of toes 2–5, *t*elecanthus, *a*nogenital, and *r*enal malformation. Hypoplastic labia, lop ears, clinodactyly of the little finger, radial ray anomalies, congenital heart defects, craniosynostosis
  ■ Later: normal intellectual development
• **Timothy syndrome** (MIM 601005)
  o Autosomal dominant long QT syndrome, caused by heterozygous missense and recurrent pathogenic variants in exon 8 of *CACNA1C*
    ■ Somatic mosaicism can cause mild expression in parents.
  o Clinical features: cutaneous webbing in 100%, involving fingers (2–5) and toes (2–3) (Figure 33.5); congenital heart disease 61% (hypertrophic cardiomyopathy, PDA, VSD, TOF), long QTc interval, 2:1 AV block, bradycardia or other arrhythmias, cardiac arrest, SIDS, depressed nasal bridge, thin upper lip, round face 85%, hypoglycemia
    ■ Anesthesia or medications can trigger arrhythmias.
    ■ Later: syncope, seizures, ID, autism; average age of death 2.5 years
  o Most patients require an implantable cardioverter defibrillator.

## Evaluation and Management

• Obtain family history: consanguinity, SIDS, unexplained death, eye anomalies, arrhythmia.
• Examine the parents: short palpebral fissures, hypoplastic alae nasi, syndactyly, chest wall asymmetry.
• Examine infant for other anomalies: IUGR, dysmorphic features, craniosynostosis, absent pectoralis muscle, constriction rings, cardiac defects, eye anomalies.
• ECG for long QT syndrome
• Chromosome analysis for suspected aneuploidy
• Chromosome microarray followed by gene testing as appropriate for patients with associated congenital anomalies

# Further Reading

Deng H, Tan T. (2015) Advances in the molecular genetics of non-syndromic syndactyly. Curr Genomics. 16:183–93. PMID 26069458

Malik, S. (2012) Syndactyly: Phenotypes, genetics and current classification. Eur J Hum Genet. 20:817–24. PMID 22333904

Tomas-Roca, L, Tsaalbi-Shtylik A, Jansen JG, et al. (2015) De novo mutations in **PLXND1** and REV3L cause Möbius syndrome. Nat Commun. 6:7199. PMID 26068067

Van Norstrand DW, Asimaki A, Rubinos C, et al. (2012) Connexin43 mutation causes heterogeneous gap junction loss and sudden infant death. Circulation. 125:474–81. PMID 22179534

# Part VIII

## Skeletal Dysplasias

# 34

# Skeletal Dysplasias

## Overview

## Clinical Consult

A female infant was born at 37 week's gestation to non-consanguineous parents after a pregnancy marked by polyhydramnios and preterm labor. Because the infant was 46 cm long and had mild total body edema, the initial diagnostic impression was possible Turner syndrome. However, she had a cleft palate and rhizomelic shortening of her long bones. Her face was mildly flat but otherwise non-dysmorphic (Figure 34.1). Radiographs revealed a small chest, poor vertebral ossification, epiphyseal ossification defects and a defect in the ossification of the skull base, consistent with a skeletal dysplasia, most likely a type II collagenopathy.

Respiratory management required immediate ventilatory support and, eventually, a tracheostomy. Her chest remained small; her partial pressure of carbon dioxide ($pCO_2$) rose and oxygen requirements increased consistent with pulmonary hypoplasia. She smiled and was very responsive. At 4 weeks of life, gene analysis revealed a de novo pathogenic variant in *COL2A2*. Although exact clinical predictions are not possible based only on molecular information, her clinical course and her phenotype were most consistent with **hypochondrogenesis** (MIM 200610) and a life-limiting outcome.

The medical staff was divided about continuing with full support. Following extensive discussion, the family chose palliative care, and she was transferred to a hospice facility. Four days later, she died peacefully, several hours after the ventilator was discontinued.

This case illustrates the complicated issues that arise as management proceeds in the absence of adequate information about the diagnosis and prognosis. The lack of a prenatal diagnosis, the long turnaround time for molecular results, and this child's appealing personality complicated medical decision-making and resulted in divergent opinions on end-of-life care among nursing and medical staff. When the diagnosis and prognosis are unclear, as in this case, invasive procedures such as tracheostomy should be deferred, if possible, to await molecular information and further delineation of the clinical course.

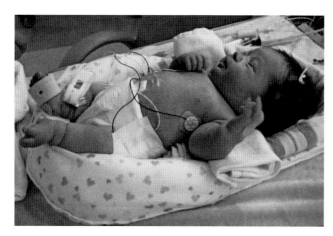

FIGURE 34.1 Hypochondrogenesis in a one month-old with rhizomelic shortening of extremities, cleft palate, and respiratory insufficiency due to a *COL2A2* de novo variant.

# Definition

- Skeletal dysplasias comprise a widely diverse group of more than 450 conditions, of which more than 100 are identifiable prenatally.
- The initial assessment centers on making a diagnosis and determining whether or not the condition is viable or life-limiting.
  - Multidisciplinary management that includes radiology and clinical genetics improves outcomes for infants and families in these complex situations.
  - Lethality is most often determined by the presence or absence of pulmonary hypoplasia, but the presence of other anomalies such as CNS or cardiac defects also impacts prognosis.
- Establishing the diagnosis is critical for accurate counseling for recurrence risk.
- Skeletal dysplasias are caused, most commonly, by de novo dominant variants, but autosomal recessive conditions also occur, even in the absence of a positive family history.
- Among the viable skeletal dysplasias, **achondroplasia*** is the most common and most easily recognizable after birth but can seldom be diagnosed by US until the late second trimester.
- Among the life-limiting skeletal dysplasias, death due to pulmonary hypoplasia may not occur immediately after birth. Affected babies may survive a few weeks, months or even years with maximal support. In addition, as therapeutic options emerge for some disorders, such as hypophosphatasia, the distinctions increasingly blur between life-limiting conditions and ones that may be compatible with long-term survival.
- When the diagnosis is compatible with life, evaluation for associated abnormalities, anticipatory guidance, and appropriate referrals for information and support will help families achieve an optimal quality of life for their child.

# Evaluation and Management

## Prenatal Evaluation

- Among the >100 skeletal dysplasias that present prenatally, many are life-limiting in the perinatal period due usually to a small chest and secondary pulmonary hypoplasia.
- An accurate diagnosis, or a close approximation, can be achieved with prenatal US in ~60% of fetal cases.
  - Assessment of viability versus lethality should be possible in almost 100% of the disorders recognized in the fetus.
- Prenatal imaging can guide the differential diagnosis.
  - Note the gestational age (based on first trimester scan) at which discrepant growth was first noted.
  - Long bone measurements >3 SD below the mean for gestational age strongly suggest a skeletal dysplasia, especially when head circumference is >75th percentile.
  - Assess bone mineralization of long bones and cranium. Rule out fractures.
  - Assess shape and size of fingers and scapula.
  - Evaluate amniotic fluid volume and any evidence of hydrops.
  - Compare relative head, abdomen, and chest circumferences.
    - Assess pulmonary hypoplasia, the most critical step in determining viability.
    - Lethality can be most reliably determined by the ratio of fetal chest circumference to fetal abdominal circumference. If <0.6, this is most likely a perinatally life-limiting disorder.
    - A femur length to abdominal circumference ratio of < 0.16 also suggests a lethal outcome.
  - Low-dose CT with 3D reconstruction may offer a more definitive diagnosis than US.
- Prenatal genetic testing
  - May be limited by time required to culture cells following amniocentesis and the turnaround time in the molecular lab (several weeks)
    - Direct DNA analysis utilizing skeletal dysplasia panels or a "rapid" exome may be possible on uncultured amniocytes allowing a specific diagnosis with within a short turn around time.
    - New testing options will likely become available, allowing rapid diagnoses, with cell-free DNA technology.
  - When a previous child was affected
    - Expedite molecular testing of any banked DNA; contact the laboratory for rapid turnaround time.
    - Review previous child's US findings and clinical phenotype.
    - Consider targeted molecular testing from CVS or amniocentesis if diagnosis known or can be established before prenatal testing.
  - When a parent is affected
    - Establish the molecular basis of their disorder early to allow rapid, targeted prenatal testing if the family desires

this. Note that full gene sequencing takes longer than variant-specific targeted testing.

o When both parents are affected with the same or different skeletal dysplasias
- Recurrence risks and prognosis depend on the diagnosis.
- Establish a molecular diagnosis for parents if not known.
- Homozygous or compound heterozygous mutations in the fetus may be life limiting.
- In conjunction with parents, plan a prenatal strategy.

## Postnatal Evaluation

- **Clinical assessment**
  o Measurements: length; span, chest, head circumference, upper to lower segment (US:LS) ratio
    - Lower segment: measure from top of pubic symphysis to heel. Subtract LS from height for US.
    - The normal US: LS ratio is 1.7 in term infants. A higher ratio suggests limb shortening.

*Pearl*: Arm span should approximately equal length in infants and children.

  - Chest circumference should approximately equal head circumference.
  - Hand length; middle finger length
  o Assess body part with greatest shortening clinically. All combinations of the following are possible:
    - Rhizomelia—proximal segments short (humerus, femur)
    - Mesomelia—middle segments short (radius, tibia)
    - Acromelia—hands and feet short
    - Spondylo—vertebrae short
  o Document other clinical findings: cleft palate, oral frenulae, cataracts, small corneas, nail hypoplasia, genital abnormalities, polydactyly, and so on.
  o Photographs: whole body, face, hands (dorsum and palmar side), feet, and close up of any notable features
- **Radiographic assessment**
  o Skeletal survey
    - Anteroposterior (AP) of long bones (one side is sufficient), AP and lateral of skull, AP and lateral of spine, AP of pelvis, AP of hands with fingers straightened as much as possible, AP feet
    - Cervical spine films can be deferred in most viable newborns until mid-infancy because this region is difficult to interpret in neonates.

*Pearl*: A "babygram," AP and lateral, may offer quick and useful diagnostic information for immediate neonatal management, but it is not a substitute for a full set of radiographs which can be done slightly later.

- **Molecular testing**
  o If a clinical and radiologic diagnosis cannot be readily determined, obtaining DNA for further study is advisable. DNA may be useful even when the clinical diagnosis is clear but the disorder has multiple possible molecular causes (e.g., **osteogenesis imperfecta II** [MIM 166210]).
  o Use cord blood in (EDTA) lavender-top tube if available. Otherwise, obtain another source of DNA (blood or tissue)
  o Choose gene tests, a sequencing panel or exomes based on careful clinical and radiologic phenotyping, preferably in conjunction with a geneticist and/or consulting pediatric radiologist.
  o Utilize the Genetic Test Registry (GTR) to locate laboratories that perform desired testing.
    - https://www.ncbi.nlm.nih.gov/gtr
  o Consider saving DNA (from cord blood, amniotic fluid, placental biopsy, cheek brush DNA) when the diagnosis is not clear on clinical or radiographic grounds or there are financial constraints. This will allow for later clinical or research molecular testing.

*Pearl*: Obtain blood in lavender-top tubes from umbilical cord at delivery in both lethal and nonlethal disorders to avoid the need for phlebotomy or skin biopsy after delivery.

- If needed, take a full-thickness skin biopsy from an area cleaned well with alcohol wipes and covered by the diaper. Place the biopsy sample in sterile culture media for immediate transport to lab (do not freeze).
  o Alternatively, biopsy the fetal side of the placenta using sterile procedure.
- Other assessments in viable infants
  o Ophthalmology—almost all
  o Cardiology—many
  o Immunology—metaphyseal disorders
  o Audiology—all
  o Orthopedics for casting, braces, monitoring, and so on
- Consult with outside experts when local experience with these rare disorders is limited or diagnosis unclear.
  o International Skeletal Dysplasia Registry: http://ortho.ucla.edu/isdr
  o European Skeletal Dysplasia Network: http://www.esdn.org
- Refer for genetic follow-up in both viable and lethal conditions
  o For known common conditions- management, surveillance, anticipatory guidance, and recurrence risk counseling
  o For rare or unknown conditions- interpretation of molecular testing, genetic counseling, and planning surveillance in subsequent pregnancies
  o For referral to relevant support groups and resources

# General Guidelines

- Establish a prenatal management plan whenever possible.
  - For a lethal or life-limiting skeletal dysplasias
    - Counsel the family early in pregnancy and discuss all options including pregnancy termination.
    - For continuing pregnancies, support vaginal delivery over cesarean section when possible. Obtain cord blood. Perform all necessary testing postnatally to facilitate diagnosis (see the previously presented clinical evaluation).
    - At delivery or termination, obtain fetal radiographs, photographs, molecular studies.
    - Offer bereavement and culturally appropriate pastoral support. Hospice and palliative care services may be needed.
    - Autopsy is important if diagnosis is unclear.
      - Biopsy proliferative zone from metaphysis; include margins of cartilage and calcified bone for pathologic examination.
  - For viable skeletal dysplasias
    - Develop, discuss, and document the delivery and resuscitation plan with full participation and agreement of the family and clinical care team: obstetrician, geneticist, neonatologist, and nursing.
    - Plan cesarean section delivery when relative macrocephaly precludes vaginal delivery. This is especially common in achondroplasia.
    - Immediately after delivery, examine the infant and reaffirm or modify the plan based on findings.
    - Evaluate and manage pulmonary function.
    - Assess as in the previously presented clinical evaluation.
      - Identify additional abnormalities; obtain measurements, photographs, and radiographs; and order molecular panel or targeted testing.
      - Consult relevant specialists (Genetics, Pulmonary, ENT, Ophthalmology).

- Refer to genetics for further evaluation, surveillance, management, and later subspecialty referrals as well as counseling for recurrence and referral to relevant support groups.

# Further Reading

Bonafe L, Cormier-Daire V, Hall C, et al. (2015) Nosology and classification of genetic skeletal disorders: 2015 revision. Am J Med Genet A. 167A:2869–92. PMID 26394607

Chandler N, Best S, Hayward J, et al. (2018) Rapid prenatal diagnosis using targeted exome sequencing: a cohort study to assess feasibility and potential impact on prenatal counseling and pregnancy management. Genet Med. [Epub ahead of print] PMID 29595812

Forman MR, Zhu Y, Hernandez LM, et al. (2014) Arm span and ulnar length are reliable and accurate estimates of recumbent length and height in a multiethnic population of infants and children under 6 years of age. J Nutr. 144:1480–7. PMID 25031329

Kumar M, Thakur S, Haldar A, Anand R. (2016) Approach to the diagnosis of skeletal dysplasias: Experience at a center with limited resources. J Clin Ultrasound. 44:529–39. PMID 27218215

Milks KS, Hill LM, Hosseinzadeh K. (2017) Evaluating skeletal dysplasias on prenatal ultrasound: An emphasis on predicting lethality. Pediatr Radiol. 47:134–45. PMID 27904917

Nikkel SM (2018) Skeletal Dysplasias: What Every Bone Health Clinician Needs to Know. Curr Osteoporos Rep. 15(5):419–24. PMID 28808977

Panda A, Gamanagatti S, Jana M, Gupta AK. (2014) Skeletal dysplasias: A radiographic approach and review of common non-lethal skeletal dysplasias. World J Radiol. 6:808–25. PMID 25349664

Toru HS, Nur BG, Sanhal CY, et al. (2015) Perinatal diagnostic approach to fetal skeletal dysplasias: Six years' experience of a tertiary center. Fetal Pediatr Pathol. 34:287–306. PMID 26376227

Zhou X, Chandler N, Deng L, et al. (2018) Prenatal diagnosis of skeletal dysplasias using a targeted skeletal gene panel. Prenat Diagn. 38(9):692–99. PMID 29907962

# 35

## Skeletal Dysplasias

## Life-Limiting

## Clinical Consult

A 26-year-old mother, recently arrived from Honduras, presented in labor at term in a small rural hospital. An US for fetal position showed severely shortened limbs and a relatively large head. Because the diagnosis was unknown, an emergency cesarean section was performed. A 1800-g, 45-cm baby boy with an obvious skeletal dysplasia and small chest had Apgar scores of $2^1$ and $6^5$. He was immediately placed on a ventilator, requiring maximal settings. He was transported to a tertiary care NICU. Radiographs were obtained, and neonatology requested a STAT genetics consult. He had multiple rolls of skin on the arms and legs and distally tapering fingers. Chest circumference was 39 cm (Figure 35.1A). Radiographs revealed a restricted small chest, bowed femurs with a "French telephone receiver" appearance, and wafer-like vertebral bodies with relatively normal ossification (Figure 35.1B). The geneticist made a clinical diagnosis of **Thanatophoric dysplasia**.

The lethal prognosis for this disorder was conveyed via an interpreter to both parents. The baby's father was able to travel to see and hold the baby. After additional discussion and hospice involvement, the parents agreed to discontinue support. DNA was saved for future testing. After an experienced pediatric radiologist confirmed the diagnosis, further studies were deemed unnecessary. The parents were given a very low risk for recurrence and offered ongoing bereavement support.

This vignette illustrates the clinical management issues that inevitably arise in the absence of prenatal diagnosis. Thanatophoric dysplasia can almost always be diagnosed in utero with reasonable certainty in an experienced perinatal center. This allows the parents, neonatologist, geneticist, and obstetrician to make a thoughtful delivery plan. When this lethal diagnosis is made early in pregnancy, it is appropriate to offer interruption of pregnancy. If possible, cesarean section should be avoided for fetal indications. If transport to a regional NICU had not been available in this case, consultation with radiology experts online or via telemedicine would have also allowed an accurate diagnosis and assisted in management.

(A)

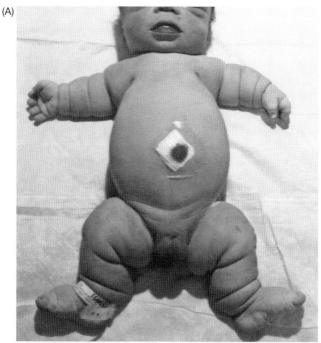

(B)

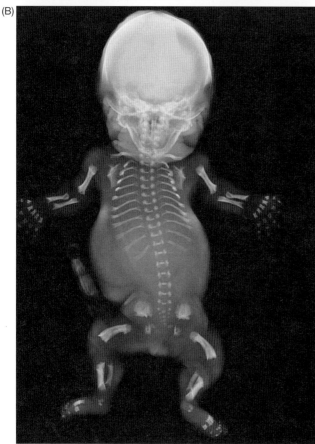

FIGURE 35.1  (A) Physical findings in Thanatophoric dysplasia. Note rolls of redundant skin, marked limb shortening, and the very small chest. (B) Anteroposterior radiograph in Thanatophoric dysplasia. Note "French telephone receiver" femurs; restricted chest; and severely small, wafer-like vertebrae.
SOURCE: Shiela Unger, MD. Centre Hospitalier Universitaire Vaudois, Lausanne Switzerland.

# Definition

- Of the more than 450 types of skeletal dysplasia, approximately 200 are lethal or life-limiting. This is a diverse group, and most have an early US presentation. Death occurs from severe pulmonary hypoplasia due to a small and constricted thorax as well as associated major congenital anomalies.
- Occasional long-term survivors are seen in several dysplasias that are considered lethal. Variable phenotypes are increasingly seen in conditions once thought to have a uniform clinical presentation, and some have an unexpectedly longer survival.
- New therapies may alter the course of previously lethal disorders such as perinatal **hypophosphatasia**.
- Some of the more common lethal dysplasias are discussed in this chapter. Many others are obscure or rare and are not discussed here. **Osteogenesis imperfecta\*** is discussed in Chapter 37.
- Determining the mode of inheritance is critical for recurrence risks. Absence of a positive family history may be consistent with autosomal recessive, autosomal dominant, or X-linked inheritance.
- Radiographic findings have been the mainstay of diagnosis. Molecular testing is playing an increasingly important role in diagnosis, prognosis, and management. Sequencing panels and rapid exome sequencing are clinically available. Careful phenotypic assessment will assist in choosing the most appropriate molecular test or panel.

# Differential Diagnosis

- **Thanatophoric dysplasia** (MIM 187600, 187601)
  - Autosomal dominant, sporadic disorder, caused by de novo mutation in *FGFR3*, often associated with increased paternal age
  - Rare: 0.24–0.69/10,000 births
  - The most common of the lethal disorders
    - Survival usually brief
    - Long-term ventilatory support not advisable in view of lethal prognosis
  - Recurrence risk is low.
  - Prenatal US findings include severe long bone shortening and sometimes bowing seen as early as 13 weeks, small chest, frontal forehead prominence, and polyhydramnios. Occasionally, cloverleaf skull is seen.
    - Characteristic fetal MRI findings after 20 weeks include small chest, disproportionately enlarged head with prominent forehead, and recognizable changes in the temporal lobes.

- Clinical features at birth: micromelic limbs, upper arms are more severely shortened (rhizomelia) than lower limbs. Small thorax, relative macrocephaly. Type 1, the more common type, has frontal bossing; type 2 has a cloverleaf skull. Small hands; distally tapering fingers have "trident" appearance. Rolls of redundant skin over extremities
  - Radiographic features include typical short, often bent femurs like a "French telephone receiver" and platyspondyly (Figure 35.1B).
- **Short rib polydactyly ciliopathy syndromes** (SRP, MIM 208500 and others)
  - At least 16 different SRPs, generally autosomal recessive disorders, are caused by pathogenic changes in multiple genes affecting ciliary function, including *WDR34, IFT172, IFT52, NEK1.*
  - Nonskeletal manifestations: cleft palate, midline cleft lip, pre- and postaxial polydactyly, microglossia, lobulated tongue, cystic kidneys, hypoplasia of epiglottis/larynx, genital ambiguity, fetal hydrops.
    - Syndromes differ in their involvement of other organs and by the appearance of the metaphyses.
  - Radiologic features: constricted thoracic cage, short ribs, short tubular bones, a "trident" appearance of the acetabular roof
  - Several forms of SRP are perinatally lethal, but two, **Jeune asphyxiating thoracic dystrophy** (MIM 208500) and **Ellis–van Creveld syndrome** (MIM 225500), are compatible with life beyond the newborn period.
- **Campomelic dysplasia** (MIM 114290)
  - Autosomal dominant disorder, due to de novo heterozygous variants in *SOX9*
  - Prenatal findings: severe limb shortening with tibial bowing, relative macrocephaly, abnormal scapulae
  - Clinical features: usually life-limiting severe dysplasia, flat face with high forehead, cleft palate, short palpebral fissures, anterior bowing of tibia with skin dimples over convexity of leg (Figure 35.2A), clubfeet, sex reversal in two-thirds of XY males
  - Radiographic findings include short flat vertebrae, hypoplastic scapulae, bowing especially of tibia, small iliac wings (Figure 35.2B)
  - Most die in the neonatal period.
  - Order regular chromosomes to rule out translocation disrupting *SOX9*
    - Tracheobronchial hypoplasia and small chest size contribute to early lethality.
  - In long-term survivors: progressive kyphoscoliosis, myopia, conductive hearing loss, dental caries, sleep apnea, frequent respiratory complications, the need for tracheostomy and multiple orthopedic procedures.
    - In the absence of CNS abnormalities, IQ may be normal.
- **Achondrogenesis IA** (MIM 200600)
  - Autosomal recessive disorder, due to homozygous or compound heterozygous variants in *TRIP11*

- Clinical features: extremely short limbs, flat face; hydrops frequent
- Radiographic features: decreased ossification of skull and vertebral bodies; pubic bones and cervical and upper thoracic pedicles ossified
- Infants stillborn or lethal in perinatal period
- **Achondrogenesis IB** (MIM 600972)
  - Lethal autosomal recessive disorder, due to homozygous or compound heterozygous variants in *DTDST (SLC26A2)*
  - Absent ossification of pubic bones, sacrum, and ischial bones
  - Allelic to **diastrophic dysplasia** (MIM 222600), which is a much milder condition
- **Achondrogenesis II/hypochondrogenesis** (MIM 200610)
  - A spectrum of severe disorders due to heterozygous de novo dominant variants in *COL2A1,* which encodes type II collagen
    - The severity of type II collagenopathies ranges from lethal disorders such as hypochondrogenesis (MIM 200610) to relatively mild **spondyloepiphyseal dysplasia congenita** (MIM 183900) and **Stickler syndrome type I** (MIM 108300), which is a much milder arthropathy.
  - Prenatal features: Severe short stature is evident in utero in severe Type II collagenopathies.
  - Clinical findings: hydrops, cardiac disease, cleft palate, myopia, microtia, foot polydactyly
  - Radiologic findings: large calvarium; very small short ribs; small iliac wings with absent ischia, pubic bones, and sacrum; failure of ossification of spine; severely short limbs with relative sparing of hands
  - Severe forms are lethal in the perinatal period. A few survivors may live several months or years with intensive support (see Clinical Consult in Chapter 34).
- **Atelosteogenesis I** (MIM108720)
  - Autosomal dominant disorder, due to de novo heterozygous variant in *FLNB*, that encodes filamin B
    - Stillborn or death in the days after birth; rarely a longer survivor
  - May be in the same spectrum as a similar disorder, **Boomerang dysplasia** (MIM 112310)
  - Clinical findings: Hydrops, frontal bossing, micrognathia, midface hypoplasia, prominent eyes, hypoplastic nose, occasional cleft palate (Figure 35.3)
  - Radiographic features: severe shortening of limbs; distal hypoplasia of the humeri and femurs; hypoplasia of the midthoracic spine; occasionally complete lack of ossification of single hand bones; hypoplasia/absence of fibula; dislocated elbows, hips, and knees
- **Atelosteogenesis II** (MIM 256050)
  - Autosomal recessive disorder, due to biallelic variants in *SLC26A2*
    - Stillborn or death soon after birth
  - Allelic to **diastrophic dysplasia** and **achondrogenesis 1B**
  - Clinical findings: abducted thumbs and great toes, cleft palate, talipes equinovarus

(A)

(B)

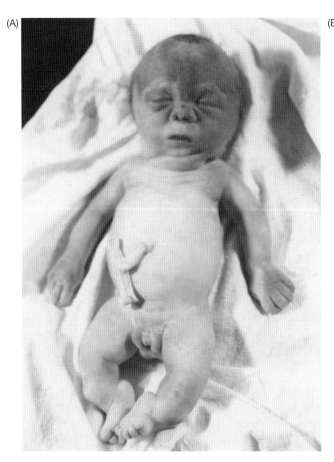
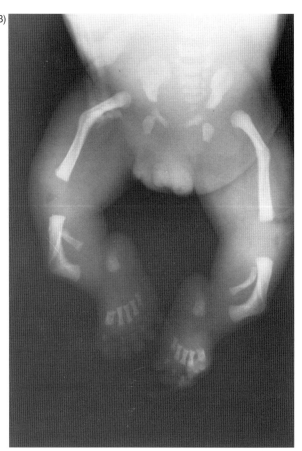

FIGURE 35.2 (A) Campomelic dysplasia. Note the sharply angulated tibias where pretibial dimples are usually seen. Note the undervirilized male genitalia in this infant with 46,XY (B) Note the angulated short femurs and tibiae and the clubfeet.

o Radiologic features: severe micromelia; bifid distal humerus; short, dumbbell-shaped femur
• **Hypophosphatasia, perinatal form** (MIM 241500)
  o Autosomal recessive disorder, caused by variants in *ALPL*, coding for tissue-nonspecific isoenzyme of alkaline phosphatase (TNSALP)

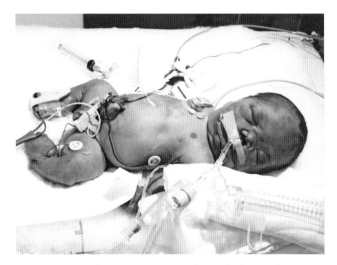

FIGURE 35.3 Ateleosteogenesis I. Note the notched nares, short limbs, small chest, very short fingers, and clubfeet.

  ▪ Carrier parents have low alkaline phosphatase levels.
  o Clinical features: hypercalcemia, fractures, bowing, small chest, blue sclera (Figure 35.4A)
  o Prenatal and radiographic findings: severe limb shortening and hypomineralization of fetal skeleton, clavicles relatively spared (Figure 35.4B)
  o Neonatal death from respiratory insufficiency is usual, but rapid treatment with asofostase alfa (recombinant TNSALP) (Strensiq) may change the course of this disease.

*Pearl*: Hypophosphatasia can confused with osteogenesis imperfecta (OI) because both can have fractures and blue sclera. Spurs on long bones at the knees and elbows, when they occur, are diagnostic for the perinatal lethal form of hypophosphatasia.

• **Hypophosphatasia, infantile form** (MIM 241500)
  o Autosomal recessive disorder, caused by milder allelic variants in the same gene, *ALPL*
    ▪ Parental levels of alkaline phosphatase are low, and urinary phosphoethanolamine levels are high.
  o Clinical features: failure to thrive, irritability, hypotonia, rachitic skeletal changes, increased intracranial pressure, large fontanels
  o Mortality 50%

(A)    (B)

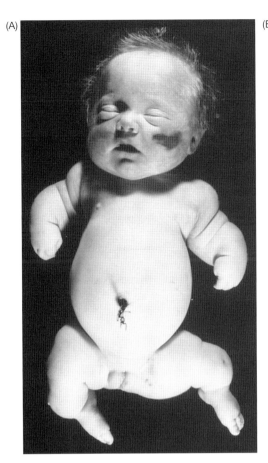
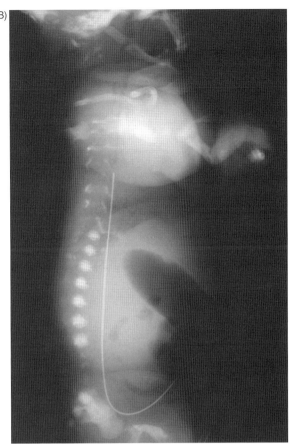

FIGURE 35.4  (A) Perinatal lethal hypophosphatasia. Note the bowing, marked shortening, and angulation of long bones, in addition to the small chest. (B) Lateral radiographs of perinatal hypophosphatasia. Markedly reduced ossification is apparent.

- o In survivors with milder forms, early enzyme replacement therapy with recombinant TNSALP (asfotase alfa) ameliorates symptoms.
- **Rhizomelic chondrodysplasia punctata I** (MIM 215100)
  - o Autosomal recessive peroxisome biogenesis disorder caused by homozygous or compound heterozygous variants in *PEX7*
    - ■ Distinct from the nonlethal X-linked recessive, X-linked dominant, and teratogenic causes. (See Clinical Consult in Chapter 36)
  - o Clinical findings: rhizomelic shortening; asymmetry, cataracts and flat face with low nasal bridge. Severe ID; most have seizures. Ichthyosis in approximately one-third
    - ■ Other structural defects (e.g., heart and cleft palate)
    - ■ Survival beyond infancy can occur, but disabilities are significant and most affected children do not live beyond age 10 years.
  - o Radiologic features: distinctive metaphyseal flaring, epiphyseal and extra-epiphyseal stippling and foci of calcification (Figure 35.5). Coronal clefts on lateral films of spine
  - o Order biochemical tests of peroxisome function: red blood cell concentration of plasmalogens (deficient), plasma concentration of phytanic acid (elevated), plasma VLCFA (normal)

- o Utilize gene panel testing for chondrodysplasia punctata that will include genes for type 2 and 3 as well. Distinction of these types is difficult in the neonate.
- **Rhizomelic chondrodysplasia punctata 2 and 3** (MIM 222765, 600121)
  - o Autosomal recessive, caused by variants in *GNPAT* and *AGPS*
  - o Clinical features: milder clinical course with longer survival
  - o Other syndromes that cause epiphyseal stippling include **trisomies 13\*** and **18\***, peroxisomal disorders such as Zellweger syndrome, and some lysosomal storage diseases.

## Evaluation and Management

- Formulate a birth and postnatal plan when a life-limiting skeletal dysplasia is prenatally detected.
  - o See Chapter 34 for a review of fetal US findings that are associated with lethality.
- Take a complete set of anteroposterior (AP) and lateral radiographs: skull, chest, vertebrae, pelvis, long bones, hands

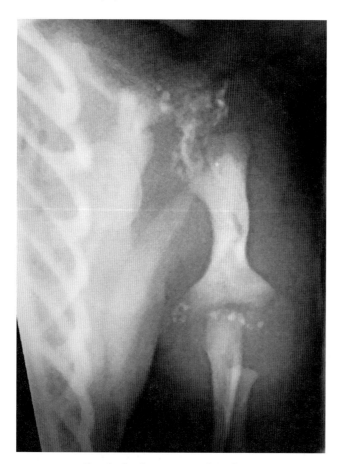

FIGURE 35.5 Chondrodysplasia punctata due to homozygous variants in *GNPAT*. Note striking epiphyseal stippling.

and feet. AP and Lateral "babygrams" can be useful for immediate management decisions.

- Take clinical photographs.
- Consult experts—a clinical geneticist and/or a skeletal dysplasia registry—early in the evaluation (http://ortho.ucla.edu/isdr and http://www.esdn.org).
- Genetic testing

○ Molecular confirmation is almost always indicated to confirm a clinical diagnosis.

■ **Thanatophoric dysplasia** may be an exception, when the clinical presentation and radiographs are definitive, because it is invariably caused by a new dominant pathogenic variant in *FGFR3* and the recurrence risk is low.

○ Utilize skeletal dysplasia sequencing gene panels, which are increasingly diagnostic as new genes are discovered and added. Pick panels after careful clinical and radiologic characterization.

○ Choose exome sequencing if diagnosis unclear or after a negative targeted sequencing panel.

○ Consider banking DNA or freezing tissue for possible later study if testing is not possible.

- Refer parents for supportive genetic consultation and interpretation of sequencing panel results.

## Further Reading

Bams-Mengerink AM, Koelman JH, Waterham H, et al. (2013) The neurology of rhizomelic chondrodysplasia punctata. Orphanet J Rare Dis. 8:174. PMID 24172221

Bonafé L, Mittaz-Crettol L, Ballhausen D, Superti-Furga A. (2014) Atelosteogenesis type 2. In: Pagon RA, Adam MP, Ardinger HH, et al., editors. GeneReviews [Internet]. Seattle, WA: University of Washington, Seattle; 1993–2017. PMID 20301493

Karczeski B, Cutting GR. (2013) Thanatophoric dysplasia. In: Pagon RA, Adam MP, Ardinger HH, et al. editors. GeneReviews [Internet]. Seattle, WA: University of Washington, Seattle; 1993–2017. PMID 20301540

Krakow, D. (2015) Skeletal dysplasias. Clin Perinatol. 42:301–319. PMID 26042906

Offiah AC. (2015) Skeletal dysplasias: An overview. Endocr Dev. 28:259–76. PMID 26138847

Parnell SE, Phillips GS. (2012) Neonatal skeletal dysplasias. Pediatr Radiol. 42 Suppl 1:S150–7. PMID 22395727

Schmidts M. (2014) Clinical genetics and pathobiology of ciliary chondrodysplasias. J Pediatr Genet. 3:46–94. PMID 25506500

# 36

## Skeletal Dysplasias

### Viable

## Clinical Consult

An infant girl was born spontaneously at 32 weeks to a 26-year-old African American G3 mother, whose previous children were normal. Two years prior to this pregnancy, she was diagnosed with mixed connective tissue disease. She had high titers of anti-U1 nRNP (U1 small nuclear ribonucleoprotein) and anti-SSA and anti-SSB antibodies. During the pregnancy, she did well with low-dose prednisone treatment. The infant, whose birth weight was 1,300 g, had nasal hypoplasia, mild rhizomelic shortening of the upper extremities, hypoplasia of the distal phalanges, and radial deviation of the index fingers (Figure 36.1). Radiographs revealed stippling of the proximal femoral epiphyses, metacarpals, and calcanei, with faint stippling of the vertebral bodies. She did not have heart block. Developmentally, she did well. She had short stature. At age 9 years, unilateral sensorineural hearing loss and bilateral small cortical cataracts were noted.

This baby had **chondrodysplasia punctata** (CDP), due to transplacental passage of maternal antibodies, most likely anti-U1 nRNP, although this is not certain. The mechanism by which **maternal collagen vascular disease** causes CDP remains unclear. Antibodies may interfere with vitamin K metabolism and/or be directed at important signaling molecules in bone development. This condition is probably underascertained.

*Pearl*: Nasal hypoplasia in the context of any maternal collagen vascular disease should prompt radiographs for epiphyseal stippling that may disappear by ~1 year of age. Subtle bony changes remain.

## Definition

Many skeletal dysplasias identifiable in neonates are compatible with life, although severe short stature and other medical complications often ensue. Quality of life may be variably impacted. After ruling out **achondroplasia***, the most common viable skeletal dysplasia, other skeletal disorders that present in the newborn period should be considered. More than 400 skeletal dysplasias have been described, but others remain poorly delineated. The most common disorders are listed in this chapter,

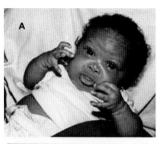
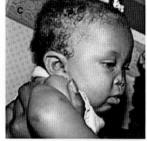
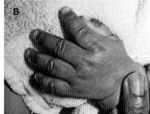
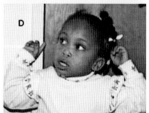

FIGURE 36.1 Chondrodysplasia punctata due to maternal collagen vascular disease. Note hypoplastic nose and small distal phalanges. *Source*: Courtesy of the American Journal of Medical Genetics (2008) 146A(23):3038–53.

grouped by cardinal findings: cleft palate, epiphyseal stippling, immune deficiency, and so on. Achondroplasia, fractures, and life-limiting skeletal dysplasias are reviewed in separate chapters.

- **SHORT STATURE WITH MYOPIA, CLEFT PALATE, AND FREQUENT HEARING LOSS**
  - The type II collagenopathies are a heterogeneous group of disorders ranging from lethal conditions, such as achondrogenesis/hypochondrogenesis, to much milder disorders, such as Stickler syndrome. Those discussed here are of intermediate severity.
    - **Spondyloepiphyseal dysplasia congenita** (SEDC, MIM 183900)
      - Usually de novo and sporadic, this is an autosomal dominant disorder, caused by heterozygous variant in *COL2A1*.
        - Recurrence in siblings is attributed to germline mosaicism in a parent, but autosomal recessive cases have been documented.
      - Clinical features: short stature, 44.5 cm (mean birth length ≥36 weeks' gestation), occasionally recognized prenatally. Cleft palate 22% (of these, 50% have Pierre Robin sequence)
        - Severe myopia 45%, retinal detachment 12%, conductive hearing loss 32%
        - Odontoid hypoplasia 56%, atlantoaxial instability 28%
        - Some characteristic skeletal features may not be evident in early infancy.
      - Natural history
        - Late walking with waddling gait
        - Protuberant abdomen (Figure 36.2)
        - Normal intelligence

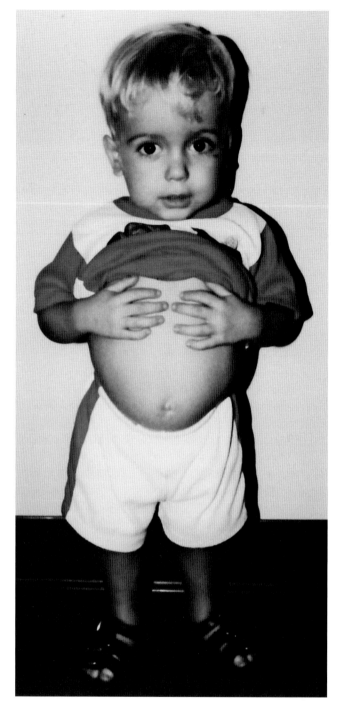

FIGURE 36.2 Spondyloepiphyseal dysplasia in a short non-dysmorphic child. He has a short trunk and lordosis contributing to his protuberant abdomen.

- Significant joint pain is unusual.
- Advise against contact sports or gymnastics due to risk of retinal detachment and cervical spine abnormalities
  - **Kniest dysplasia** (MIM 156550)
    - Autosomal dominant, usually sporadic, due to a heterozygous variants in *COL2A1*

- Clinical features: short stature, depressed midface, prominent eyes, congenital severe myopia, cataracts, retinal detachment, cleft palate, joint contractures, hearing loss

- **SKELETAL DYSPLASIAS WITH STIPPLED EPIPHYSES (CHONDRODYSPLASIA PUNCTATA—CDP)**
  - Heterogeneous group of disorders with epiphyseal stippling in infancy, short stature, skin disease (ichthyosis), cataracts, hearing loss, and normal to mild intellectual impairment
    - Many are caused by abnormalities in the cholesterol metabolic pathway.
  - Teratogens
    - Diphenylhydantoin, alcohol, rubella, CMV, warfarin, maternal collagen vascular disease (see Clinical Consult)
  - Chromosomal disorders
    - Aneuploidy: **Down syndrome\***, **trisomies 13\* and 18\***
    - Deletion of Xp22.3
  - Metabolic disorders
    - Peroxisomal disorders
    - Lysosomal storage diseases: **I cell disease** (MIM 252500)
    - Diseases of cholesterol metabolism: **Smith–Lemli–Opitz syndrome** (MIM 270400), **sterol delta 8 isomerase deficiency** (MIM 302960), **CHILD syndrome** (MIM 308050), **Greenberg dysplasia** (MIM 215140)
  - Deficiency or disorders of vitamin K metabolism
    - **Keutel syndrome** (MIM 245150)
      - Autosomal recessive disorder, due to biallelic variants in *MGP*, which causes deficiency of human matrix Gla protein
      - Clinical features: peripheral pulmonary artery stenosis, hearing loss, calcification of larynx and ear pinna
  - Single gene disorders
    - **Conradi–Hünermann–Happle syndrome** (MIM 302960)
      - Mosaic X-linked dominant disorder seen in females, due to variants in *EBP* at Xp11.22-23
        - Lethal in most males; surviving males are somatic mosaics.
      - Clinical features: short stature, cataracts, coarse lusterless hair, skeletal asymmetry. Mosaic skin changes: swirly pigmentation, atrophic orange peel, ichthyotic changes following the lines of Blaschko (Figure 36.3)
      - Abnormal sterol profile
    - **Chondrodysplasia punctata** (brachytelephalangic CDP, MIM 302950)
      - X-linked recessive disorder, caused by pathogenic variants in *ARSE* (arylsulfatase E) at Xp22.33
        - May occur as a contiguous gene deletion syndrome that includes steroid sulfatase deficiency and X-linked Kallman syndrome

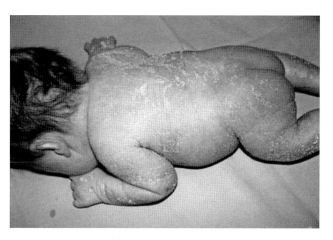

FIGURE 36.3  X-linked dominant Conradi–Hünerman–Happle syndrome with patchy icthyotic skin changes following the lines of Blaschko.
SOURCE: Courtesy of Javier Canueto Alvarez, MD, Hospital Universitario de Salamanca, Salamanca, Spain.

- Clinical features: short stature, cataracts, hearing loss, nasal hypoplasia, distal phalangeal hypoplasia, mild ID (Figure 36.4)
  - Ichthyosis reflects the involvement of the steroid sulfatase locus at Xp22.3.
- Chondrodysplasia punctata due to maternal conditions
  - Nongenetic condition associated with maternal collagen vascular disease (lupus, mixed connective tissue disease, scleroderma, hyperemesis gravidarum, and gastric bypass surgery with inadequate nutrition). Antibodies to proteins in early bone development (e.g., matrix GLA protein or proteins in vitamin K metabolism) may be causative.
  - Findings consistent with other forms of CDP, including nasal hypoplasia, distal digital hypoplasia, cataracts, hearing loss, and short stature, are common.

- **VERTEBRAL MALFORMATIONS WITH OR WITHOUT SKELETAL DYSPLASIA**
  - May be isolated or syndromic, due to a single gene disorder or to a chromosome abnormality
  - Severity ranges from asymptomatic to severe, often lethal, recessive disorders with respiratory insufficiency.
    - Hemivertebrae, wedge-shaped vertebrae, vertebral bars, and other segmentation abnormalities
    - Associated rib abnormalities may cause respiratory compromise and a poor prognosis.
  - Teratogens
    - Maternal pregestational diabetes, twins, valproic acid, alcohol
  - Common syndromes with vertebral anomalies
    - **Alagille syndrome** (MIM 118450)
    - **Goldenhar syndrome** (MIM 164210)
    - **VATER/VACTERL association** (MIM 192350)
    - **Spondylothoracic dysostosis** (STD, Jarcho–Levin syndrome, spondylocostal dysostosis, MIM 277300)

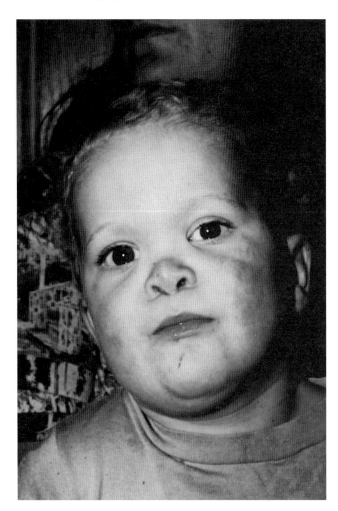

FIGURE 36.4  X-linked recessive chondrodysplasia punctata due to a terminal deletion at Xp22.3. Note the hypoplastic nose.

- A range of usually autosomal recessive disorders of vertebral segmentation, most commonly caused by variants in *DLL3*, in the Notch signaling pathway
  - Variants in *MESP2, LFNG, HES7*, other Notch signaling genes, cause similar phenotypes
  - Biallelic variants in *TBX6* (MIM 122600), which can include a deletion at 16p11.2, cause vertebral anomalies from scoliosis to severe spondylocostal dysostosis.
  - Autosomal dominant transmission also occurs.
  - **Jarcho–Levin syndrome** refers to most severe phenotype, frequently lethal
- Clinical features: short stature, increased thoracic anterior posterior diameter, characteristic posterior rib fusion, causing a "crab-like" appearance on radiographs
- Significant inter- and intrafamilial variability
- Later respiratory compromise may be severe. Reduced lung volumes and chest wall stiffness lead to thoracic insufficiency.

- Only 25% survive to adolescence. New orthopedic interventions may improve outcome in surviving children.

- **SKELETAL DISORDERS WITH IMMUNE DYSFUNCTION**
  - **Cartilage-hair hypoplasia** (CHH, MIM 250250)
    - Autosomal recessive disorder, due to variants in *RMRP* that impair ribosomal assembly and affect cyclin-dependent cell cycle regulation
    - Clinical features: severe disproportionate short stature, recognized prenatally in ~75%. Short fingers and toes, bowed femurs and tibias >75% (Figure 36.5). Fine, often blond, sparse silky hair
      - Complete alopecia with loss of eyebrows, eyelashes, and body hair, 15%
    - Medical complications can be life-threatening.
      - Immune: impaired lymphocyte proliferation and T cell function 88%
        - Newborn screening for severe combined immunodeficiency syndrome (SCID) may identify some infants prior to clinical recognition
        - With SCID, may require bone marrow transplant
        - Severe varicella infection 11%

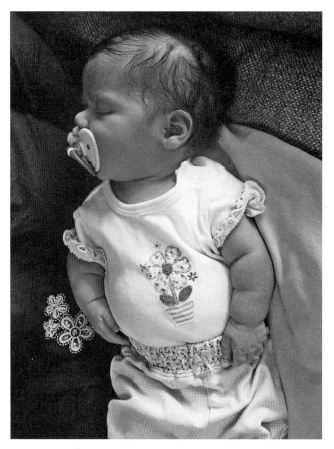

FIGURE 36.5  Cartilage-hair hypoplasia in infant with generalized limb shortening and fine sparse hair. Identifying this condition early is critical due to severe immune deficiencies requiring bone marrow transplantation. Newborn screening may identify infants in some states.

- Hematologic: macrocytic, hypoplastic anemia ~80%; may require transfusions
- GI: Hirschsprung disease 7–8%, intestinal malabsorption, failure to thrive
- Cutaneous and visceral granulomas
  - Differential diagnosis includes other metaphyseal dysplasias: **Schwachman–Diamond syndrome** (MIM 260400), **Omenn syndrome** (MIM 603554), **Schimke immunoosseous dysplasia** (MIM 242900).
- **Metaphyseal dysplasia without hypotrichosis** (MIM 250460)
  - Allelic autosomal recessive disorder, also caused by biallelic variants in *RMRP*
  - Clinical features: similar to CHH but normal hair and no immunodeficiency, anemia, or gastrointestinal issues
- **Anauxetic dysplasia** (MIM 607095)
  - Autosomal recessive disorder, caused by biallelic variants in *RMRP*
  - Clinical features: extreme short stature of prenatal onset, midface hypoplasia, relative macroglossia, dislocated hips
    - Later: dental anomalies, mild intellectual disability
  - Atlantoaxial instability may lead to cord compression.

- **OTHER SKELETAL DYSPLASIAS**
  - **Diastrophic dysplasia** (MIM 222600)
    - Autosomal recessive disorder, caused by biallelic variants in *SLC26A2*
    - Clinical features: cystic ear swelling, cleft palate >40%, submucous cleft palate or microform in additional 30%. "Hitchhiker thumbs" (Figure 36.6), ulnar deviation of the fingers, gap between the first and second toes. Clubfeet, contractures and deformities of large joints
      - Occasionally lethal at birth
      - Later: early onset osteoarthritis, normal intelligence

*Pearl*: The cystic ear in diastrophic dysplasia is not improved by surgery. Treat it conservatively.

  - **Three M syndrome** (MIM 273750)
    - Underascertained autosomal recessive disorder, due to biallelic variants in *CUL7* in >75% or, less commonly, *OBSL1* (MIM 610991) and *CCDC8* (MIM 614145)
    - Clinical features: low birth weight, severe pre- and postnatal growth restriction, relative macrocephaly, triangular face, prominent forehead, flat midface, anteverted nares, full lips, protuberant abdomen, lordotic posture, flat feet, scapular winging, normal intelligence (Figure 36.7)
    - Radiographic features: long slender tubular bones, reduced bone age, tall vertebral bodies, joint hypermobility
  - **Jeune asphyxiating thoracic dystrophy** (MIM 208500)

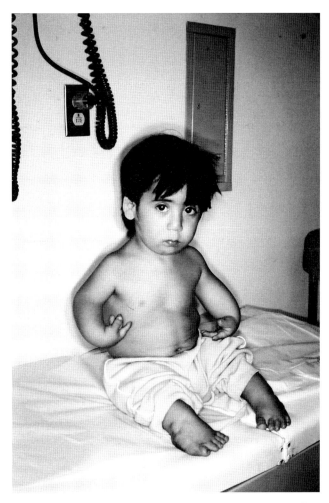

FIGURE 36.6 Diastrophic dysplasia. Note the "hitchhiker thumbs," repaired clubfeet, and cystic distortion of the ear pinna.

- Autosomal recessive short rib polydactyly syndrome, caused by pathogenic variants in ciliary genes, most commonly *DYNC2H1*, 59%
- Clinical features: small narrow chest; polydactyly; renal, liver, and retinal involvement
  - Pulmonary insufficiency 60%, occasionally requires tracheostomy
  - Baujat et al. (2013) found retinal abnormalities (older than age 5 years) 50%, renal disease 17%, and liver disease 22%.
- Radiographs: narrow thorax, short long bones, trident-shaped acetabular roof
- Advances in surgical management offer treatment options for the small chest.
  - **Ellis–van Creveld syndrome** (MIM 225500)
    - Autosomal recessive ciliopathy, due to biallelic variants in *EVC* or *EVC2*, an adjacent gene at 4p16
    - Clinical features: postaxial polydactyly, hypoplastic nails (Figure 36.8), natal teeth. Congenital cardiac defects 60%, most commonly a common atrium
    - Radiographic features: short limbs, short ribs

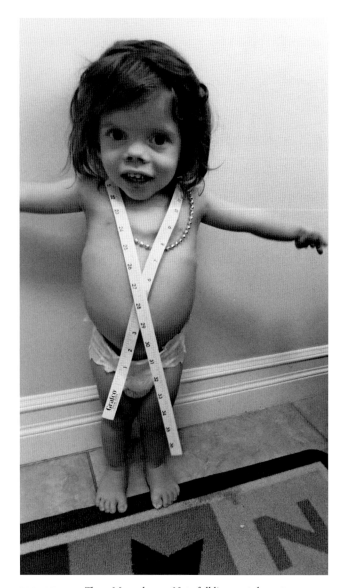

FIGURE 36.7 Three M syndrome. Note full lips, protuberant abdomen, and flat feet.

## Evaluation and Management

- Review pregnancy history: teratogen exposures, maternal diabetes, autoimmune disorder.
- Document family history: consanguinity, short stature in relatives, fetal and neonatal deaths.
- Examine parents: disproportionate short stature, high myopia, cleft palate.
- See general guidelines in Chapter 34.
- Examine body proportions, and measure upper to lower segment ratios.
- Assess for other anomalies and consult with specialists as needed.
  - Evaluate the palate.

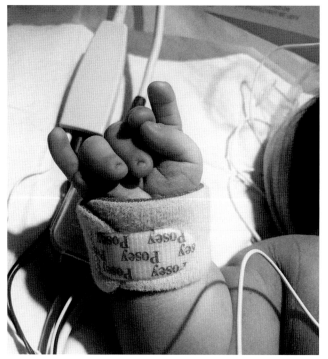

FIGURE 36.8 Hands in infant with Ellis–van Creveld syndrome. Note postaxial polydactyly and marked nail hypoplasia.

  - Ophthalmology assessment: SEDC, CDP, OI
  - Dermatology: CDP
  - Orthopedics, monitoring, bracing, casts, surgery
  - Immunology: complete evaluation for CHH
    - Serial CBC: CHH
    - Avoid live vaccines: CHH
  - Audiology screening: CDP, SEDC
  - Consider maternal disease as a possible cause, and order appropriate diagnostic tests on mother if indicated.
- Order a complete skeletal survey. Review it with an experienced pediatric radiologist.
- Utilize skeletal dysplasia experts.
  - International Skeletal Dysplasia Registry: http://ortho.ucla.edu/isdr
  - European Skeletal Dysplasia Network: http://www.esdn.org
- Order genetic testing *after* radiologic and clinical phenotyping.
  - Microarray when the clinical presentation is atypical or when associated with nonskeletal congenital anomalies
  - Locate labs that offer specific gene panels or single gene tests: https://www.ncbi.nlm.nih.gov/gtr.
  - Exome sequencing may be cost-effective in atypical cases or those with negative gene panel results.
- Offer families information on support groups.
  - Little People of America: http://www.lpaonline.org
- Consider participation in research protocols or clinical trials: https://www.clinicaltrials.gov.
- Refer for genetic consultation and follow-up.

# Further Reading

Al-Dosari MS, Al-Shammari M, Shaheen R, et al. (2012) 3M syndrome: An easily recognizable yet underdiagnosed cause of proportionate short stature. J Pediatr. 161:139–45. PMID 22325252

Alrukban H, Chitayat D. (2018) Fetal chondrodysplasia punctata associated with maternal autoimmune diseases: a review. Appl Clin Genet. 11:31–44. PMID 29720879

Baujat G, Huber C, El Hokayem J, et al. (2013) Asphyxiating thoracic dysplasia: Clinical and molecular review of 39 families. J Med Genet. 50:91–8. PMID 23339108

Cañueto J, Girós M, González-Sarmiento R. (2014) The role of the abnormalities in the distal pathway of cholesterol biosynthesis in the Conradi–Hünermann-Happle syndrome. Biochim Biophys Acta. 1841:336–44. PMID

Giampietro PF, Raggio CL, Blank RD, et al. (2013) Clinical, genetic and environmental factors associated with congenital vertebral malformations. Mol Syndromol. 4:94–105. PMID 23653580

Schmidts M. (2014) Clinical genetics and pathobiology of ciliary chondrodysplasias. J Pediatr Genet. 3:46–94. PMID 25506500

Terhal PA, Nievelstein RJ, Verver EJ, et al. (2015) A study of the clinical and radiological features in a cohort of 93 patients with a *COL2A1* mutation causing spondyloepiphyseal dysplasia congenita or a related phenotype. Am J Med Genet A. 167A:461–75. PMID 25604898

# Skeletal Dysplasias

# Fractures in Infancy

## Clinical Consult

A genetic consultation was requested for a 1-day-old female with a large fontanel and hypotonia who appeared to have short arms and legs. The family history was negative, and the mother had no fetal US exams after 16 weeks. She was a non-dysmorphic baby with a large fontanel extending onto the metopic suture and a split sagittal suture. Exam confirmed mild rhizomelic shortening of the arms and legs and mild tibial bowing (Figure 37.1). She cried when her L leg was manipulated. Skeletal X-rays revealed bowing, fractures, osteopenia, and Wormian bones consistent with **osteogenesis imperfecta** (OI). Molecular studies revealed a de novo heterozygous variant in *COL1A1* most consistent with OI type III or IV. She has sustained multiple fractures, and her clinical course is most consistent with **OI type IV**. At 4 months, she started treatment with IV pamidronate (bisphosphonate), and her fracture rate stabilized. Her parents travel to a distant regional OI clinic for her follow-up visits and orthopedic procedures. They are pursuing enrollment in clinical trials.

This child illustrates the variable presentation of OI in the newborn. Her diagnosis was prompted by nonspecific findings of large fontanels and hypotonia. Early molecular diagnosis allowed institution of pamidronate therapy at a young age. New treatments for OI are likely to emerge during the next few years, and parents should be encouraged to consider clinical trials.

## Definition

Neonatal fractures occur in a number of disorders, most commonly in OI. Other conditions that cause bone fragility and predispose to fractures are discussed here.

- Osteogenesis imperfecta encompasses a growing group of disorders that cause an increased fracture rate, ranging from a few to thousands in a lifetime.
- The morbidity and mortality of OI range from perinatal lethality to progressively deforming bony changes to a normal life span with relatively normal stature.

*Pearl*: The clinical severity of OI can vary greatly, even within families whose members share a common variant.

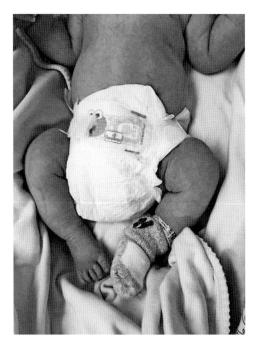

FIGURE 37.1 A diagnosis of type IV osteogenesis imperfecta was established on molecular testing in this

newborn with very mild limb shortening, pain on movement of the leg, and tibial bowing. Radiographs showed Wormian bones.

- OI is a group of generalized connective tissue disorders that affect bones, sclera, teeth, and hearing.
- Distinguishing lethal from nonlethal types is important for optimal management of all OI subtypes.
- Combined prevalence for all types of OI is 6–7/100,000.
- Molecular genetics
  - OI types I–IV are caused by variants in *COL1A1* and *COL1A2*.
  - 90% of affected patients have an autosomal dominant pathogenic variants in type I collagen.
    - The mildest forms of the disease are caused by nonsense variants.
    - Missense variants produce more severe, progressively deforming types of OI.
    - Approximately 60% of patients with mild types of OI have a de novo variant.
  - Most of the remaining 10% have autosomal recessive disorders in genes primarily involved in the processing and trafficking of type I collagen or in bone homeostasis.
  - In severe forms of OI, early treatment with biphosphonates appears to stabilize fracture rate.

## Differential Diagnosis

The more common types of OI, which comprises types I–XVIII, and other fracture-causing syndromes are summarized here.

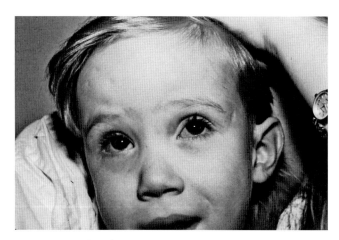

FIGURE 37.2   Blue sclera in type I osteogenesis imperfecta.

- **Osteogenesis imperfecta type I** (MIM 166200)
  - Classic autosomal dominant OI, caused by heterozygous variants in *COL1A1* or *COL1A2*
  - Prevalence 3–4/100,000; the most common form of OI
  - Clinical features: highly variable fracture rate, non-deforming fractures
    - Fracture onset ~1 year; rate of fractures diminishes after puberty and increases after menopause. Low bone density. Prenatal fractures are uncommon but do occur.

*Pearl*: Low bone density on a dual-energy X-ray absorptiometry (DEXA) scan can identify an apparently unaffected carrier parent.

    - Blue sclerae 100% (Figure 37.2). age dependent hearing loss, 50%. Dentinogenesis imperfecta common but may also be absent or occur as isolated finding without OI.
    - Hypermobility, poor wound healing, easy bruising
    - Mitral valve prolapse ~18%; occasional mild aortic root dilation
    - Stature normal or near normal; intelligence normal
- **Osteogenesis imperfecta type II** (MIM 166210)
  - Usually autosomal dominant, perinatal lethal form of OI
    - Variants in several genes cause autosomal recessive perinatal lethal OI with similar appearance.
  - Typically caused by a heterozygous variants in *COL1A1* or *COL1A2*
  - Prevalence 1–2/100,000
  - Recurrence risk is low. Recurrences documented due to germline mosaicism in one parent
  - Prenatal findings
    - Fetal US in the early second trimester, at 13 or 14 weeks' gestation, may detect soft, unossified calvarium; beaded ribs; short crumpled long bones; and platyspondyly.
    - Decreased viability in utero: hydrops fetalis, intrauterine death, premature onset of labor
  - Clinical features: blue sclerae, thin skin, marked long bone shortening and bowing (Figure 37.3)

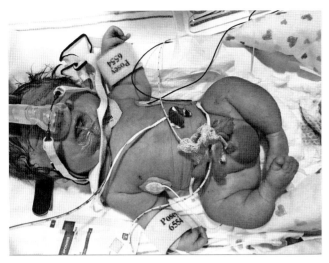

FIGURE 37.3 Infant with lethal type II osteogenesis imperfecta. Note extreme bone shortening and bowing.

○ Radiologic findings: underossified calvarium, short limb dwarfism, decreased bone density, multiple pre-natal fractures affecting ribs ("beaded" appearance) and long bones ("crumpled" appearance). Small chest and rib fractures cause respiratory insufficiency.

○ More than 60% of infants die on the first day; 85% die in the first week. Survival beyond the first year is rare and usually requires continuous ventilator support.

■ Save cord blood for molecular testing or obtain skin sample (using sterile technique) postmortem for DNA testing.

*Pearl*: Delivery by cesarean section does not reduce fracture risk.

- **Osteogenesis imperfecta type III** (MIM 259420)
  ○ Usually an autosomal dominant disorder, this is a progressive deforming type of OI that is caused by heterozygous variants in *COL1A1* or *COL1A2*.
    ■ Autosomal recessive trait in some families
  ○ Prenatal findings
    ■ Limb length begins to fall below the normal curve at 17 or 18 weeks gestation.
  ○ Clinical features
    ■ Sclerae are light blue at birth but may normalize with age.
    ■ Bone deformity and bowing ("saber" shins)
    ■ Severe short stature
    ■ Severe dentinogenesis imperfecta
  ○ Early bisphosphonate therapy can be beneficial.
- **Osteogenesis imperfecta type IV** (MIM 166220)
  ○ Autosomal dominant disorder causing a common but variable type of OI, due to heterozygous variants in *COL1A1* or *COL1A2*

○ Clinical features: normal sclerae, variable fractures, tibial and femoral bowing at birth, short stature
  ■ Variable dentinogenesis imperfecta
○ Benefit from bisphosphonate therapy
- **Osteogenesis imperfecta type V** (MIM 610967)
  ○ Autosomal dominant disorder, caused by heterozygous variants in *IFITM5*
  ○ Clinical features: long bones moderately deformed; moderate to severe bone fragility of long bones and vertebral bodies
    ■ Frequent fractures, $3.2 \pm 2.3$ fractures/year
    ■ No blue sclerae or dentinogenesis imperfecta
    ■ Radiographs show hyperplastic callus formation at fracture sites, calcification of the interosseous membrane between the radius and ulna, and the presence of a radio-opaque metaphyseal band adjacent to the growth plates.
- **Osteogenesis imperfecta types VI–XVII**
  ○ Autosomal recessive disorders, caused by biallelic mutations in *SERPINF1, CRTAP, TMEM38B*, and several others
  ○ Homozygous or compound heterozygous mutations in *WNT1* (MIM 615220) cause severe **OI type XV** (MIM 615220) and variable intellectual deficiency with unilateral hypoplasia of the cerebellum and frequent ptosis (Figure 37.4).
- **Bruck syndrome** (OI type XI, MIM 259450, 609220, 610968)
  ○ Autosomal recessive disorder, caused by biallelic variants in *FKBP10* or *PLOD2*
  ○ Clinical features: arthrogryposis, pterygia, osteopenia, scoliosis, progressive deformity, fractures. Contractures not invariable
  ○ Zolendronic acid is beneficial: a newer bisphosphonate with a longer half-life and greater potency.

**Non-Genetic Causes of Fractures**

- Nonaccidental injury (NAI)
  ○ Not often a consideration in the newborn but becomes a greater concern in the re-hospitalization of a preterm infant
  ○ Clinical features: bruises follow the pattern of an object or hand; posterior rib fractures, transverse fractures of several digits, metacarpals, or metatarsals, and metaphyseal chip fractures suggest NAI.
    ■ Each of these fracture types can be seen in infants and children with OI, but they occur less commonly than in the context of trauma.
  ○ *COL1A1* and *COL1A2* sequencing is increasingly used as a first-tier test in such patients. Variants of unknown significance complicate interpretation of test results.

*Pearl*: The diagnoses of OI or X-linked hypophosphatemic rickets is commonly offered as a legal defense in cases of child abuse in infancy, but the diagnostic yield for a molecular abnormality in such cases is only ~5%.

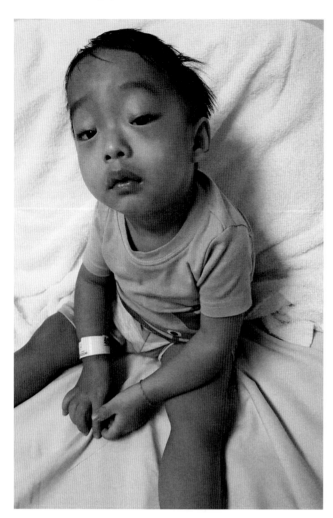

FIGURE 37.4 OI XV due to homozygous mutations in *WNT1*. Intellectual disability is common and ptosis is frequent in this condition.

### Metabolic bone disease of prematurity (MBDP)

- Causes bone pain, rickets, decreased bone mineral density, and fractures. An iatrogenic disorder.
  - Risk factors: chronic illness in severely premature infants, very low birth weight (<1,000 g), prolonged total parenteral nutrition (>4 weeks), bronchopulmonary dysplasia, diuretic, glucocorticoids, and caffeine use.
  - Affects infants with birth weight <1,000 g: new NICU management protocols have reduced the frequency.
  - Presents at 6–12 weeks of age.
  - Laboratory findings: low phosphorous (<2 mmol/L, 6.1 mg/dL) and elevated alkaline phosphatase (>500 IU/L).
- Treatment includes vitamin D, calcium, and phosphorous.

*Pearl*: Metabolic bone disease of prematurity can be distinguished from OI by normal bone morphology on early routine radiographs.

### Other Genetic Causes of Fractures

- **Cole–Carpenter syndrome** (MIM 112240)
  - Autosomal dominant disorder, due to heterozygous pathogenic variants in *P4HB* or *SEC24D*
  - Clinical features: bone fragility, craniosynostosis, hydrocephalus, proptosis, hypertelorism
    - Both lethal and nonlethal forms exist.
    - Cognitive outcome variable
- **Hypophosphatasia**
  - Autosomal dominant or recessive types, of varying severity
  - All types are caused by mutations in *ALPL*.
  - Low or absent serum alkaline phosphatase activity; increased urinary excretion of phosphoethanolamine
  - Variants of hypophosphatasia are classified by the age of onset.
    - **Hypophosphatasia, prenatal/infantile form** (MIM 241500)
      - Clinical features: severe skeletal changes; major portions of the skull, ribs, and tubular bones not ossified; hypercalcemia
      - Usually death occurs in the first years of life.
      - Mildly affected neonates may have congenital bowing of the long bones with osseous spurs.
      - Prenatal diagnosis and immediate implementation of treatment with asfotase alfa improve survival in some reports.
    - **Hypophosphatasia, childhood/juvenile form** (MIM 241510)
      - Clinical features: later onset and slower progression with skeletal changes and early loss of teeth
    - **Hypophosphatasia, adult form** (MIM 146300)
      - Clinical features: may shed primary teeth early but no overt manifestation of bone disease

*Pearl*: Adult-type autosomal hypophosphatasia may occasionally present in utero with significant bowing and be confused with OI type II.

- **Spondyloepimetaphyseal dysplasia with joint laxity** (MIM 271640, 615291)
  - Autosomal recessive disorder, caused by biallelic loss-of-function variants in *B3GALT6*
  - Clinical features: blue sclera, digital hypermobility, joint dislocations, scoliosis, clubfeet and hip dislocation, dislocated radial head, progressive scoliosis, platyspondyly
    - Oval face, prominent eyes, long philtrum
    - Resembles severe Ehlers–Danlos syndrome
- **Stuve–Wiedemann syndrome (Schwartz–Jampel syndrome type 2)** (MIM 601559)
  - Autosomal recessive condition, caused by loss-of-function variants in *LIFR*

- Clinical features: pursed lips, bowed limbs, corneal ulcers, fractures, contractures of elbows, and camptodactyly of digits
  - Bowing of long bones with wide flared metaphyses of decreased density
- Most infants have feeding and respiratory difficulties, often with hyperthermia, leading to death within first months or years of life.
- **Fetal akinesia deformation sequence** (FADS;MIM 208150, 300073)
  - Heterogeneous, usually autosomal recessive lethal disorders (see Arthrogryposis chapter)
  - Clinical features: ribs and tubular bones are slender and straight. Bone structure is normal, but muscle mass is reduced. Prenatal and postnatal fractures probably due to lack of movement
- Rickets
  - At least nine different genetic forms of rickets (autosomal dominant, autosomal recessive, and X-linked) exist, as well as dietary and environmental causes
    - **X-linked hypophosphatemic rickets** (MIM 307800)
      - X-linked dominant disorder, due to variants in *PHEX*
      - Most common heritable form of rickets
      - Clinical diagnosis is challenging in the newborn without a family history because clinical and biochemical features often develop later.
      - Clinical features: genu varum, splayed and cupped metaphyses, decreased bone density, loss of the zone of provisional calcification at the metaphyses, craniosynostosis of coronal and sagittal sutures
      - Laboratory findings: hypophosphatemia, normal parathyroid hormone, hypocalciuria, increased alkaline phosphatase
      - Treat with supraphysiologic doses of calcitriol, $1,25(OH)_2$ vitamin D, and oral phosphate replacement.
    - **Vitamin D-dependent rickets 2A** (MIM 277440)
      - Autosomal recessive condition, caused by biallelic variants in *VDR*, which encodes the vitamin D receptor, leads to decreased end-organ sensitivity to vitamin D
      - Clinical features: onset within first 6 mos. Common radiographic findings of rickets include, decreased bone density, abnormal bone morphology, metaphyseal fraying, cupping and flaring. Long bones may be bowed.
        - With or without alopecia
      - Laboratory findings:
        - hypocalcemia, increased alkaline phosphatase, increased 1,25 dihydroxyvitamin D3.
        - Resistant to Vitamin D treatment
    - **Autosomal Dominant Hypophosphatemic Rickets** (MIM 193100)
      - Caused by variants in *FGF23* and others

- Bone pain, rickets, tooth abscesses; highly variable onset- age 1- adult.
- Laboratory findings: hypophosphatemia, normal 1,25 dihydroxyvitamin D, n normal calcium and PTH.
- Responds to Vitamin D and phosphate

# Evaluation and Management

- Document family history: short stature, blue sclerae, and fracture history in relatives; hearing loss; dentinogenesis imperfecta; fetal losses; document previous affected individuals.
- Examine parents: blue sclerae, enamel abnormalities, short stature, hypermobility, bone deformities.
- Examine infant for associated features: scleral hue, hyperextensibility, bruising, contractures, craniosynostosis.
- Obtain complete skeletal survey: AP and lateral skull and spine, AP chest, pelvis, long bones, hands and feet.
  - A "babygram" can be helpful in immediate newborn management.
  - Note degree of ossification, Wormian bones, bowing, vertebral changes.
  - Early consultation with experts at a skeletal dysplasia registry if diagnosis not apparent
- Order gene panels consistent with the differential diagnosis.
  - If OI is likely, start by sequencing *COL1A1* and *COL1A2*.
  - In severe or lethal perinatal OI, when *COL1A1* and *COL1A2* sequencing is negative, reflex to a gene panel for recessive forms of OI.
- Panels and targeted single gene testing for hypophosphatasia and hypophosphatemic rickets depending on clinical phenotype
- Handle patients with bone fragility disorders carefully to minimize trauma.
  - Fractures occur with diaper changing. Lift the baby by raising the buttocks from below, not by holding the legs up.
  - Use egg crate foam bedding for support.
- Treatment
  - Severe OI, types III or IV: Consider bisphosphonate therapy early in infancy.
    - Early treatment can decrease bone pain and irritability; reduce fracture incidence; increase bone mineral density, muscle strength, and mobility; and improve feeding.
  - Hypophosphatasia: The FDA approved asfotase alfa (Strensiq) in 2015.
    - Asfotase alfa improves overall survival and ventilator-free survival in patients with perinatal or infant onset. Immediate treatment may change course in severe perinatal disease.
    - 97% of treated patients were alive at 1 year versus 42% of controls.
- Recommend comprehensive, multidisciplinary care for infants with severe bone fragility to optimize outcome.

- Include dentist, endocrinologist, geneticist, orthopedic surgeon, pediatrician, physical and occupational therapist, rehabilitation specialist, and social worker.
- Refer families to support groups for information and advocacy.
  - OI Foundation: http://www.oif.org.
  - Hypophosphatasia: https://www.magicfoundation.org
- Consider enrollment in research .
  - For gene discovery (genomic or exomic testing): available through international skeletal dysplasia registries
  - For new therapies: https://clinicaltrials.gov

## Further Reading

Bronicki LM, Stevenson RE, Spranger JW. (2015) Beyond osteogenesis imperfecta: Causes of fractures during infancy and childhood. Am J Med Genet C Semin Med Genet. 169:314–27. PMID 26531771

Dwan K, Phillipi CA, Steiner RD, Basel D. (2016) Bisphosphonate therapy for osteogenesis imperfecta. Cochrane Database Syst Rev. 19;10:CD005088. PMID 27760454

Forlino A, Marini JC. (2016) Osteogenesis imperfecta. Lancet. 387:1657–71. PMID 26542481

Lambert AS, Linglart A. (2018) Hypocalaemic and hypophosphatemic rickets. Best Pract Res Clin Endocrinol Metab. 32(4):455–476. PMID 30086869

Mornet E. (2018) Hypophosphatasia. Metabolism. 82:142–55. PMID 28939177

Pepin MG, Byers PH. (2015) What every clinical geneticist should know about testing for osteogenesis imperfecta in suspected child abuse cases. Am J Med Genet C Semin Med Genet. 169:307–13. PMID 2656659

Thomas IH, DiMeglio LA. (2016) Advances in the classification and treatment of osteogenesis imperfecta. Curr Osteoporos Rep.14:1–9. PMID 26861807

# Part IX

## Skin System

# 38

## Skin

## Ectodermal Dysplasias

## Clinical Consult

A term Hispanic female had severe erythema, scaling skin, and sparse hair. The genetic consultant initially suspected an ichthyosis syndrome. When re-evaluated at several months of age, she had dry skin without scales, dark circles under her eyes, and mild midface underdevelopment (Figure 38.1). She had one peg-shaped tooth, consistent with an ectodermal dysplasia. When her fingertips were examined with an ophthalmoscope, she had decreased numbers of sweat pores. A chromosome microarray revealed a region of homozygosity at 2q13, the locus of the gene *EDAR*. Confirmatory testing identified a homozygous variant in *EDAR*, establishing the diagnosis of **autosomal recessive hypohidrotic ectodermal dysplasia** (ED). The family was informed that oligodontia was likely and counseled about the 25% recurrence risk.

The parents were advised to apply cool wet cloths and to mist with cool water to prevent overheating in warm weather. They were cautioned to seek prompt evaluation and treatment for fevers.

Neonates with ED may present with erythema and scaling that suggest ichthyosis rather than an ED. Chronologic follow-up will usually narrow the differential diagnosis.

## Definition

- Ectodermal dysplasias are inherited skin disorders that involve at least two ectodermal appendages: hair, nails, teeth; sweat, sebaceous, and mucous glands.
- More than 170 ED conditions exist, with at least 77 causative genes.
  - Exome sequencing has contributed to the rapid increase in the understanding of these disorders.
- ED phenotypes evolve with time.
  - A positive family history of ED may be the only clue in newborns.
  - Scaling, erythema or a collodion membrane in the neonate may initially suggest an ichthyosis.
  - Later, decreased sweating can cause unexplained fever.

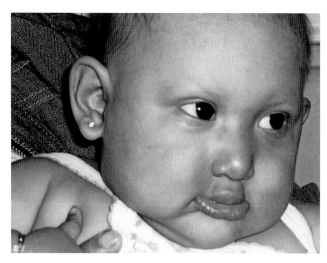

FIGURE 38.1 Autosomal recessive ectodermal dysplasia. Note midface underdevelopment and sparse eyebrows and eyelashes.

■ Dentists may be the first to identify ED in the older child.

# Differential Diagnosis

## Hypohidrotic Ectodermal Dysplasia

- **X-linked hypohydrotic ectodermal dysplasia** (XLHED, MIM 305100)
  ○ This X-linked form is caused by variants in *EDA*.
  ○ Accounts for 65–75% of ED
  ○ Girls may sometimes be as severely affected as boys.
  ○ Clinical features: sparse lightly pigmented hair, dark circles under eyes, midface underdevelopment, prominent forehead and depressed nasal bridge decreased sweating, normal nails (Figure 38.2)

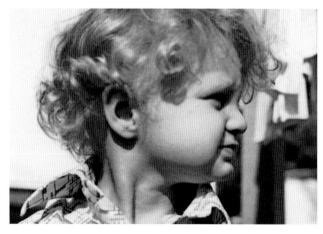

FIGURE 38.2 X-linked recessive ectodermal dysplasia. This child had very few permanent teeth, midface underdevelopment, depressed nasal bridge, and prominent forehead.

○ Later: oligodontia, abnormally shaped teeth, eczema, atopic dermatitis, chronic sinusitis, asthma, nosebleeds, dry eyes

- **HED with immunodeficiency** (MIM 300291)
  ○ X-linked disorder, due to variants in *IKBKG*
  ○ Clinical features: dysgammaglobulinemia with recurrent infections, decreased sweating, normal hair
- HED with T-cell deficiency (MIM 612132)
  ○ Autosomal dominant disorder, due to mutation in *NFKB1A*
  ○ Clinical features: recurrent infections, FTT, sparse scalp hair
- Pathogenic variants in these genes also cause autosomal recessive (AR) and autosomal dominant (AD) types of HED
  ○ *EDAR* (AR, MIM 224900) 10–15%
  ○ *WNT10A* (AR, MIM 257980) 5–6%
  ○ *EDARADD* (AD, MIM 614940; AR, MIM 614940) 1–2%

*Pearl*: Estimate numbers of sweat pores by examining fingertips with an ophthalmoscope. Look for glints of sweat in pores. Compare patient to similar-aged controls.

## Syndromic Ectodermal Dysplasias

- **Ectrodactyly, ectodermal dysplasia, clefting syndrome, type 3** (EEC3, MIM 604292)
  ○ Autosomal dominant disorder, due to heterozygous variants in *TP63* (Figure 11.5, and 31.5)
  ○ Clinical features: coarse hair, lacrimal duct abnormalities, hypodontia, thickened palms and soles. Split hand/split foot (ectrodactyly), GU anomalies. Normal sweating
  ○ Allelic forms of ED have overlapping phenotypes.
    ■ **Acro–dermo–ungual–lacrimal–tooth syndrome** (ADULT, MIM 103285)
      • Ectrodactyly, syndactyly, finger- and toenail dysplasia, frontal alopecia, lacrimal duct atresia, primary hypodontia
    ■ **Limb–mammary syndrome** (MIM 603543)
      • Limb anomalies similar to EEC, hypoplasia/aplasia of the breast and nipple. Occasional lacrimal duct atresia, nail dysplasia, decreased sweating, missing teeth, cleft palate
    ■ **Rapp–Hodgkin syndrome** (MIM 129400)
      • Sparse wiry hair, hypodontia, cleft lip/palate, decreased sweating, ridged pitted nails, hypospadias
    ■ **Ankyloblepharon, ectodermal defects, cleft lip/palate syndrome** (AEC, MIM 106260)
      • Wiry hair, alopecia, ankyloblepharon, lacrimal duct abnormalities, cleft lip/palate, hypodontia, limb abnormalities, syndactyly. Thick, absent, or hyperconvex nails (Figure 38.3). Severe open erosions on scalp and other sites. Normal sweating
- **Clouston syndrome** (MIM 129500)
  ○ Autosomal dominant disorder, due to heterozygous variants in *GJB6*

(A)

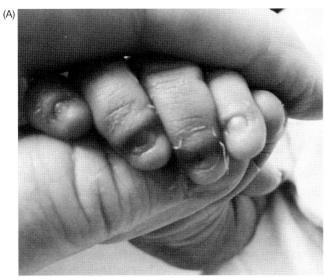

(B)

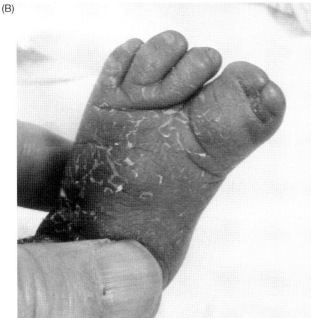

FIGURE 38.3  (A) AEC syndrome (ankyloblepharon, ectodermal dysplasia and clefting) with severe nail underdevelopment (B) Syndactyly in AEC syndrome is a variable finding.

 

   o Clinical features: brittle, slow-growing hair; occasional alopecia, sparse eyebrows and lashes; cataracts, strabismus, severe nail dystrophy and hypoplasia, palmoplantar hyperkeratosis
      ■ Normal sweating
- **Witkop syndrome** (tooth/nail syndrome, MIM 189500)
   o Autosomal dominant ED, due to heterozygous variants in *MSX1*
   o Clinical features: variable congenitally missing permanent and/or primary teeth. Nails are thin, brittle, and spoon-shaped. Toenails are more affected than fingernails. Nail findings improve with age.

# Evaluation and Management

- Document family history: consanguinity, identify key phenotypic features in older affected relatives.
- Examine parents: missing or abnormally shaped teeth, abnormal nails, wooly or sparse hair, decreased or patchy areas of sweating.
- Genetic testing
   o When family history is not diagnostic, consider delaying testing for a few months to allow phenotype to evolve.
      ■ Early dentition and hair growth provide important clues.
   o Single gene testing is appropriate for X-linked HED, and for *TP63* when ED occurs with cleft lip or split hand/foot.
   o Gene panels for nonsyndromic HED are useful in the absence of an X-linked family history. Include common genes: *EDA1, EDAR, EDARRAD, WNT10A*.
   o Exome sequencing is useful for atypical ED or when initial gene panel testing is nondiagnostic.
- Counsel families about the consequences of decreased sweating, and recommend ways to prevent hyperthermia.
   o Use air conditioning; limit outside activities in warm weather.
   o Mist infants and young children with a squirt bottle, and monitor body temperature.
- Anesthetic risks are increased. Inform anesthesiologist before procedures.
- Anticipate complications. Refer to dermatology, dentistry, otolaryngology, pulmonary, ophthalmology, and gastroenterology.
   o Eczema in hypohidrotic ED can be challenging.
   o Decreased salivation increases risk for caries; treat dry mouth.
   o Oligodontia requires early dental prostheses and later implants.
   o Sinusitis, asthma, dry eyes, nosebleeds, recurrent upper respiratory infections, reflux, and failure to thrive
   o Oral clefts and limb defects need specialty care.
- Enroll in research protocols: https://www.clinicaltrials.gov.
   o Treatment of the scalp lesions in AEC is a research goal.
   o Successful in-utero treatment of XLHED recently reported (Schneider H, 2018)
   o Refer families to the National Foundation for Ectodermal Dysplasias: https://www.nfed.org.

# Further Reading

D'Assante R, Fusco A, Palamaro L, et al. (2015) Unraveling the link between ectodermal disorders and primary immunodeficiencies. Int Rev Immunol. 35:25–38. PMID 25774666

Fete M, Hermann J, Behrens J, Huttner KM. (2014) X-linked hypohidrotic ectodermal dysplasia (XLHED): clinical and diagnostic insights from an international patient registry. Am J Med Genet A. 164A(10):2437–42. PMID 24664614

Itin PH. (2014) Etiology and pathogenesis of ectodermal dysplasias. Am J Med Genet A. 164A:2472–7. PMID 24715647

Koch PJ, Dinella J, Fete M. (2014) Modeling AEC—New approaches to study rare genetic disorders. Am J Med Genet A. 164A:2443–54. PMID 24665072

Pagnan NA, Visinoni ÁF. (2014) Update on ectodermal dysplasias clinical classification. Am J Med Genet A. 164A:2415–23. PMID 25098893

Schneider H, Faschingbauer F, Schuepbach-Mallepell S, et al. (2018) Prenatal correction of X-linked hypohidrotic ectodermal dysplasia. N Engl J Med. 378(17):1604–1610. PMID 29694819

Trzeciak WH, Koczorowski R. (2016) Molecular basis of hypohidrotic ectodermal dysplasia: An update. J Appl Genet. 57:51–61. PMID 26294279

Wright JT, Grange DK, Fete M. (2017) Hypohidrotic ectodermal dysplasia. In: Pagon RA, Adam MP, Ardinger HH, et al. editors. GeneReviews [Internet]. Seattle, WA: University of Washington, Seattle; 1993–2017. PMID 20301291

# 39

## Skin

## Epidermolysis Bullosa

## Clinical Consult

A 36-week-gestation male was followed in utero for IUGR, mild cardiac hypertrophy, and debris-filled amniotic fluid. The parents were first cousins of Yemeni descent. Three years previously, their first daughter died at 3 days of age from widespread blistering and denuded skin. At birth, this baby boy had total alopecia with absent nails. He had a scalded appearance, and more than 50% of his skin was eroded (Figure 39.1). An echocardiogram revealed cardiomyopathy. His condition deteriorated, and the family decided to discontinue support. **Autosomal recessive lethal acantholytic epidermolysis bullosa,** a subtype of epidermolysis bullosa simplex, was the suspected diagnosis. Electron microscopy of skin showed acantholysis and subsequent gene sequencing in the Netherlands revealed a homozygous deletion in *DSP*, the gene that encodes desmoplakin, the major linker in desmosomes in epithelia and myocardium (Bolling et al., 2010). Unfortunately, the family could not be located for follow-up genetic counseling.

Cardiomyopathy, a distinctive feature of this rare condition, aided in the diagnosis. Interestingly, mutations in the same gene cause autosomal dominant arrhythmogenic right ventricular cardiomyopathy as well as several other syndromes involving the skin, hair, and heart.

## Definition

- Epidermolysis bullosa (EB) is characterized by skin fragility and blisters following minimal friction or abrasion.
- More than 30 distinct clinical disorders and at least 18 genes cause EB.
  - Subtypes differ in mode of inheritance, the presence or absence of associated abnormalities, the distribution of lesions, and clinical severity.
- Classification: four main EB groups
  - According to a 2013 consensus report, classify EB first by level of skin cleavage and then subclassify by laboratory and genetic testing.
  - **EB simplex** (EBS): Blisters occur within the epidermis.
  - **Junctional EB** (JEB): Blisters form below the basal keratinocytes.

261

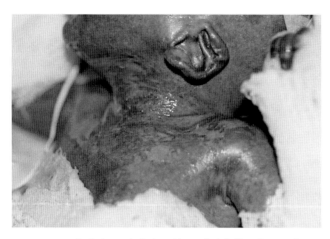

FIGURE 39.1 Lethal acantholytic epidermolysis bullosa in a newborn with extensive denudation of his skin.

○ **Dystrophic EB** (DEB): Cleavage plane occurs below the lamina densa, at the anchoring fibrils located below the basement membrane in the upper dermis.

○ **Kindler syndrome**: Multiple cleavage planes are intraepidermal, intralamina lucida, or sublamina densa.

## Differential Diagnosis

• **Epidermolysis bullosa simplex** (EBS)
  ○ Most common, 75–85% of EBS
  ○ Autosomal dominant disorder, caused by heterozygous variants in *KRT5* and *KRT14* in ~75% of the many types
  ○ Rare variants in genes encoding other structural proteins, including desmoplakin, plakophilin-1, plakoglobin, integrins A6 and B4, type XVII collagen, plectin, transglutaminase 5, and dystonin

*Pearl*: The simplex forms of EB generally heal without scarring, but secondary infection is a common complication that can result in significant scarring.

○ **Main types of EBS**
  ■ **EBS, localized** (MIM 131800), formerly EBS Weber–Cockayne type
    • Clinical features: mildest form, affects mostly hands and feet, palmoplantar hyperhidrosis
      • Blistering or ulceration of the oral mucosa in infants
      • Hair and teeth are normal; nail dystrophy is rare. Blisters heal without scarring or milia.
  ■ **EBS, generalized severe** (MIM 131760), formerly EBS Dowling–Meara type
    • Clinical features: trauma or friction-induced blistering in infancy, nail dystrophy, nail shedding, hair loss

    • Blisters heal without scarring, but hypopigmentation is common.
  ■ **EBS, generalized intermediate** (MIM 131900), formerly EBS Koebner type
    • Clinical features: blistering at birth or early infancy, generally mild involving hands, feet, and extremities. Hair, teeth, and nails normal
      • Lesions often heal with post-inflammatory dyspigmentation (Figure 39.2).

○ **Rare lethal forms of EBS are autosomal recessive**
  ■ **Acantholytic EBS** (MIM 609638) due to variants in *DSP*, distinguished by the presence of cardiomyopathy (see Clinical Consult)
  ■ **EBS with muscular dystrophy** (MIM 226670) and **EBS with pyloric atresia** (MIM 612318) both due to mutations in *PLEC1*
• **Junctional epidermolysis bullosa** (JEB)
  ■ **JEB generalized severe** (MIM 226700), formerly JEB Herlitz type
    • Autosomal recessive disease, due to pathogenic variants in *LAMC2, LAMB3, LAMA3*, has complete absence of laminin 332.
    • Clinical features: extensive mucocutaneous blistering at birth with early lethality, atrophic scarring, webbing, contractures, milia
      • Exuberant granulation tissue around mouth, nose, face
      • Airway involvement 25%
      • Eyes, GU, GI involvement
      • Onychodystrophy (thickened, yellow), absent nails
  ■ **JEB generalized intermediate** (MIM 226650), formerly JEB non-Herlitz type
    • Autosomal recessive disorder, due to mutations in several genes, including: *COL17A1, LAMA3, LAMB3, LAMC2*

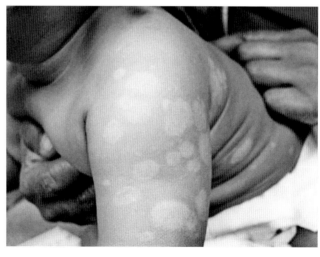

FIGURE 39.2 Depigmentation of healing lesions in epidermolysis bullosa simplex, generalized intermediate.

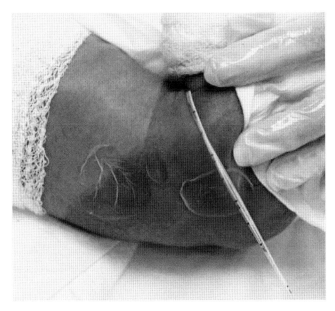

FIGURE 39.3  A newborn with junctional epidermolysis bullosa, generalized intermediate and extensive blistering.

- Clinical features: indistinguishable from other forms of generalized EB but variable. Blisters heal with scarring. Chronic hand involvement results in syndactyly, and mitten deformities. Involvement of the hair, nails and teeth (Figure 39.3)
  - Multiple organ involvement: heart, kidneys, GI and GU tracts
  - Glomerulonephritis, renal amyloidosis, IgA nephropathy and cardiomyopathy

- **JEB with pyloric atresia** (MIM 226730)
  - Autosomal recessive disorder, due to mutations in *ITGB4* or *ITGA6*
  - Clinical features: severe disorder with frequent neonatal lethality. Renal anomalies: dysplastic kidneys, hydronephrosis, absent bladder
- **Dystrophic epidermolysis bullosa** (DEB)
  - All are caused by pathogenic variants in *COL7A1*: one major dominant form and two major recessive forms; many subtypes
    - **Dominant DEB** (MIM 131750)
      - Clinical features: blisters at birth or soon after, primarily affecting skin overlying bony prominences: knees, ankles, and dorsa of the hands and feet. Blisters heal with scarring and milia but less with age.
        - Nail dystrophy the most important diagnostic feature
        - Mucosal involvement rare; teeth normal
    - **Generalized severe recessive DEB** (MIM 226600)
      - Clinical features: blisters at birth, spontaneously or after mild trauma, affect knees, elbows, hands, feet, back of the neck, shoulders, and over spine. Occasional

congenital absence of the skin. Healing occurs with scarring and milia. Scarring alopecia common
  - Oral, esophageal, anal, and ocular mucosae have erosions and scarring.
  - Dystrophic teeth, restricted mouth opening and tongue mobility cause severe caries
  - Pseudosyndactyly due to repeated blistering and scarring is hallmark of recessive DEB. Mitten deformities. Contractures of hands and feet begin in first year and progress (Figure 39.4)
  - Esophageal strictures lead to reduced food intake and nutritional deficiency.
  - Later: high risk of squamous cell carcinomas; the leading cause of death in this group
  - **Generalized recessive DEB—intermediate** (MIM 120120)
    - Clinical features: blistering less severe, absence of mutilating deformities. Skin lesions heal with scars and milia. Oral, dental, nail, and hair findings similar to severe recessive DEB but less extensive
      - Variable phenotype: widespread disease in some; in others, limited to extremities. Increased squamous cell cancer risk
- **Kindler syndrome** (MIM 173650)
  - Autosomal recessive disorder, caused by loss-of-function mutations in *FERMT1*. Distinct from other forms of DEB
    - Clinical features: trauma-induced skin blistering at birth, severe photosensitivity, progressive poikiloderma (a combination of skin atrophy, telangiectasia, and dyspigmentation), extensive skin atrophy
      - Life span normal

### Other Causes of Neonatal Blisters
- **Peeling Skin syndrome** (PSS, MIM 270300; 609796)
  - Heterogeneous group of autosomal recessive disorders causing superficial painless peeling and blistering without

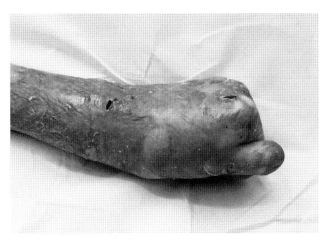

FIGURE 39.4  Recessive dystrophic epidermolysis bullosa causes severe extensive blistering in the newborn period, followed by scarring, contractures, and digital fusion as seen in this adult. SOURCE: Courtesy of Anna Bruckner, MD, University of Colorado, Denver, CO.

mucosal fragility. Two forms: acral PSS involves hands and fee and generalized PSS causes widespread peeling with erythema and severe pruritus.

- ○ Acral PSS caused by homozygous or compound heterozygous variants in TMG5; carriers common in European populations. Generalized PSS caused by variants in CHST8 (Type A) or loss of function variants in CSDN (Type B)
- ○ Heals without scarring. May have residual itching and atopic symptoms

- **Miscellaneous causes**
  - ○ Trauma: benign sucking blisters
  - ○ Infection: herpes simplex, bullous impetigo, staphylococcal scalded skin syndrome, neonatal candidiasis, neonatal varicella
  - ○ Maternal autoimmune disease: bullous pemphigus, pemphigoid gestationis, pemphigus vulgaris
  - ○ Genetic disorders: incontinentia pigmenti, ectodermal dysplasia, bullous congenital ichthyosiform erythroderma, pachyonychia congenita

## Evaluation and Management

- Obtain family history: consanguinity, other affected individuals.
- Examine lesions for distribution, depth, oral lesions, GI manifestations. Document with photographs.
- Consult genetic, dermatology, and distant EB experts early.
- Genetic testing
  - ○ Targeted single gene testing or extensive gene panels (>30 genes) facilitates rapid diagnosis, counseling, and determination of natural history, and prognosis.

*Pearl*: Panel testing should now be the first choice for diagnosis as it avoids delays in accurate diagnosis and can evaluate all of the various forms of EB in one test. It is increasingly replacing the need for detailed dermatopathology studies—careful clinical descriptions remain essential.

- Biopsy, including dermis (when necessary)
  - ○ Immunofluorescence mapping (IFM) in a freshly created blister is a method to diagnose the type of EB.
    - ■ Routine microscopy cannot reliably determine subtypes because both JEB and DEB show subepidermal blistering.
  - ○ To preserve antigens, the biopsy has to be transported in normal saline to the testing dermatopathology laboratory within 24 hours. Use Michel's media if transport will take longer.
  - ○ Electron microscopy is useful but not widely available
- Management
  - ○ Avoid skin trauma to prevent new blisters.

- ■ Loose clothing, gentle handling, padding of bony prominences. Avoid rubbing; pat skin instead.
- ■ Avoid adhesives. Use nonstick dressings around ECG probes, pulse oximeter probes, and IVs.
- ○ Meticulous wound care promotes healing and lowers risk for infection.
  - ■ Lubricate skin with Vaseline or other bland ointment.
  - ■ Keep in cool, air-conditioned environment. Overheating increases skin fragility.
  - ■ In older infants, prophylactic wrapping may reduce new blister formation.
  - ■ Limit use of topical antibiotics and antimicrobial dressings to cases with significant infection, not just colonization.
- ○ Maintain nutrition.
  - ■ Nutritional needs are similar to those of a burn patient.
  - ■ Supplemental gastrostomy feeding may be needed.
- ○ Monitor and treat noncutaneous complications: renal, eye, gastrointestinal, syndactyly from scarring.
- ○ Consider participating in research protocols for EB therapy that is cell based, gene based, or protein based: https://www.clinicaltrials.gov.
- ○ Psychosocial support
  - ■ Utilize resources for families with regard to clothing, diapers, and videos for parents and care providers: http://www.debra.org.
  - ■ A nurse educator is available through debRA International.
  - ■ Multidisciplinary teams including mental health professionals help manage these devastating disorders.

## Further Reading

Bolling MC, Veenstra MJ, Jonkman MF, et al. (2010) Lethal acantholytic epidermolysis bullosa due to a novel homozygous deletion in DSP: Expanding the phenotype and implications for desmoplakin function in skin and heart. Br J Dermatol. 162:1388–94. PMID 20302578

Cohn HI, Teng JM. (2016) Advancement in management of epidermolysis bullosa. Curr Opin Pediatr. 28:507–16. PMID 27386970

Fine JD, Bruckner-Tuderman L, Eady RA, et al. (2014) Inherited epidermolysis bullosa: Updated recommendations on diagnosis and classification. J Am Acad Dermatol. 70:1103–26. PMID 24690439

Gonzalez, ME. (2013) Evaluation and treatment of the newborn with epidermolysis bullosa. Semin Perinatol. 37:32–9. PMID 23419761

Has C, Fischer J. (2018) Inherited epidermolysis bullosa: New diagnostics and clinical phenotypes Exp Dermatol. 00:1–7. PMID 29679399

Ma JE, Hand JL. (2017) What's new with common genetic skin disorders? Minerva Pediatr. 69:288–97. PMID 28425690

Pfendner EG, Lucky AW. (2018) Dystrophic epidermolysis bullosa. In: Pagon RA, Adam MP, Ardinger HH, et al. editors. GeneReviews

[Internet]. Seattle, WA: University of Washington, Seattle; 1993–2017. PMID 20301481

Samuelov L, Sprecher E. (2014) Peeling off the genetics of atopic dermatitis-like congenital disorders. J Allergy Clin Immunol. 134(4):808–15. PMID 25282561

Uitto J, Bruckner-Tuderman L, Christiano AM, et al. (2016) Progress toward treatment and cure of epidermolysis bullosa: Summary of the DEBRA International Research Symposium EB2015. J Invest Dermatol. 136:352–8. PMID 26802230

Youssefian L, Vahidnezhad H, Uitto J. (2016) Kindler syndrome. In: Pagon RA, Adam MP, Ardinger HH, et al. editors. GeneReviews [Internet]. Seattle, WA: University of Washington, Seattle; 1993–2017. PMID 26937547

# 40

## Skin

## Ichthyoses

## Clinical Consult

A primigravida teenage mother presented at term in labor. At delivery, the amniotic fluid was milky. The infant had severe respiratory distress due to pulmonary hypertension that was the focus of intensive care management. The skin was red, with generalized fine scales and hyperkeratosis. There were fissures in the flexion creases. The hair was fine and wispy (Figure 40.1A). Under the microscope, a hair sample revealed the typical "bamboo hair" pattern consistent with trichorrhexis invaginata (Figure 40.1B). The diagnosis of **Netherton syndrome** was confirmed by the detection of homozygous mutations in *SPINK5*.

Microscopic examination of hair shafts can facilitate a diagnosis and should be considered in conditions with scaling and erythroderma. Netherton syndrome is a diagnostic challenge due to the broad differential diagnosis. In this case, the pulmonary hypertension may have been induced by the exfoliated cells in an effect similar to that of meconium: inducing a pulmonary inflammatory reaction and increasing pulmonary vascular resistance.

## Definition

- The congenital ichthyoses are a heterogeneous group of disorders characterized by generalized skin scaling.
- More than 50 genes encode structural proteins or enzymes that cause scaling, confirming marked genetic heterogeneity.
- Erythroderma can be the presenting feature in the newborn, with scales more evident over time.
- Neonatal erythroderma is a common presenting sign for various disorders.
  - Seborrheic dermatitis, erythrodermic psoriasis
  - Bullous and nonbullous congenital ichthyosiform erythroderma
  - Staphylococcal scalded-skin syndrome
  - Severe atopic dermatitis
  - Immunodeficiency syndromes: **Omenn syndrome** (MIM 603554), a type of severe combined immunodeficiency
  - Metabolic disorders: holocarboxylase synthetase deficiency, essential fatty acid deficiency, and others

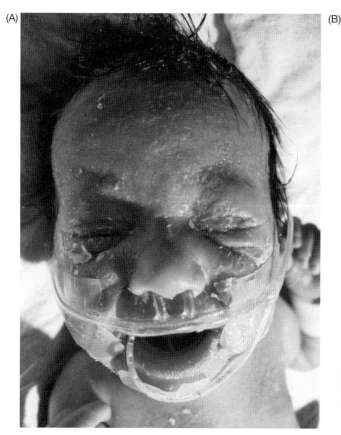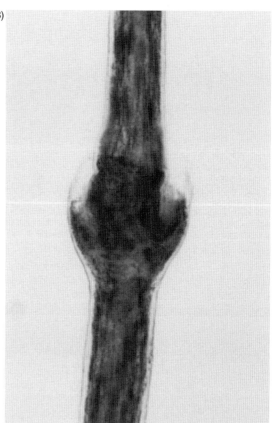

FIGURE 40.1  (A) A newborn with Netherton syndrome. Note extensive scaling and erythema (B) associated trichorrhexis invaginata (bamboo hair).

## Differential Diagnosis

### Nonsyndromic Ichthyoses

- **Ichthyosis vulgaris** (MIM 146700), most common form of ichthyosis
  - Autosomal dominant or recessive disorder, caused by pathogenic variants in the filaggrin gene, *FLG*, important in formation of the skin barrier
    - Mildly affected patients have heterozygous variants.
    - Severe patients have homozygous or compound heterozygous variants.
  - Incidence 1 in 250 births
  - Clinical features: Ichthyosis is evident after 3 months of age.
    - Predisposes to atopic disorders: eczema, allergic rhinitis
- **X-linked ichthyosis** (MIM 308100)
  - X-linked disorder affects males, relatively common and fairly mild
  - Caused by mutation or deletion in the steroid sulfatase gene, *STS*, at Xp22.3
  - Family history: X-linked distribution of affected males
  - Prenatal diagnosis is common.
    - Maternal serum estriol is very *low*.
    - Positive maternal serum screening test for **Smith–Lemli–Opitz syndrome\*** or **trisomy 18\*** syndrome
  - Clinical features: may be symptomatic or asymptomatic in the newborn. Affected males have dry, centrally adherent scale, especially around the neck, back, and legs.
  - Less commonly, large deletions include other genes in this gene-rich area, causing ichthyosis with complex contiguous gene syndromes.
    - **X-linked recessive chondrodysplasia punctata** (MIM 302950; Figure 40.2)
      - Deletion or pathogenic variant of *ARSE* at Xp22.33
      - Clinical features: nasal hypoplasia, epiphyseal stippling, developmental delay, hearing loss
    - **Kallmann syndrome** (MIM 308700)
      - Deletion of or variant in *KAL1*
      - Clinical features: anosmia, hypogonadotrophic hypogonadism

*Pearl*: Pregnant *STS* mutation carriers can fail to enter labor spontaneously and may require induction at term.

- **Harlequin ichthyosis** (MIM 242500)
  - Rare autosomal recessive disorder caused by homozygous or compound heterozygous loss-of-function variants in the gene *ABCA12*
  - A clinically distinct and genetically homogeneous entity

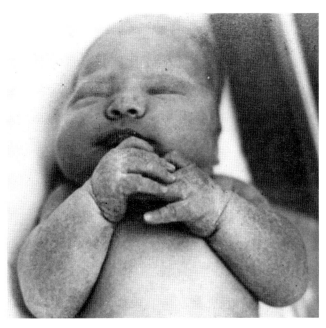

FIGURE 40.2  X-linked chondrodysplasia punctata due to a terminal deletion on Xp resulting in generalized ichthyosis in this newborn.

- Clinical features: thick plate-like scales, ectropion (eversion of eyelids), eclabium (eversion of lips) (Figure 40.3)
  - Deep fissures are red and oozing.
- Usually lethal disorder in the first days and weeks of life due to respiratory compromise, sepsis, dehydration
- Some infants have survived with early treatment.
  - Oral etretinate or 13-*cis*-retinoic acid started in the first few days of life
    - Plaques may disappear over weeks.
    - Phenotype changes to a severe congenital ichthyosiform erythroderma
    - Variable neurologic outcome
  - Carefully evaluate the decision to treat with each family.

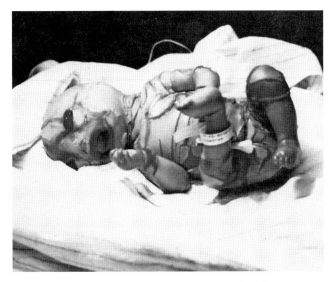

FIGURE 40.3  Thick plate-like scales, ectropion, and eclabium in Harlequin ichthyosis, usually lethal in the newborn period.

- **Lamellar ichthyosis** (LI, MIM 612281) and **congenital ichthyosiform erythroderma** (CIE, MIM 242100) now generally considered a spectrum of disorders
  - Autosomal recessive disorders with overlapping phenotypes and genotypes
  - Caused by variants in one of several genes, including *TGM1, ALOXE3, ALOX12B, NIPAL4, CYP4F22,* and *ABCA12*
    - Mutations in *TGM1* account for approximately one-third of the recessive ichthyoses.
  - Clinical features: ectropion, palmoplantar keratoderma, thickening of the palms and soles, of varying severity
    - A collodion membrane—a tight, shiny, translucent membrane—covers the entire body (Figure 40.4). It sheds after repeated applications of emollient.
      - In LI, collodion membrane is replaced by thick plate-like, adherent scales.
      - In CIE, scaling tends to be milder than in LI, with variable erythroderma and ectropion.
    - Sweat gland function may be impaired.

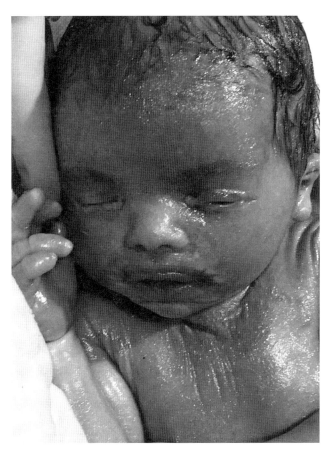

FIGURE 40.4  Lamellar ichthyosis with collodion membrane and underlying erythema due to compound heterozygous mutations in *ALOX12B*.
SOURCE: Courtesy of Maries Joseph, MD, Valley Children's Hospital, Madera, CA.

- **Epidermolytic ichthyosis** (MIM 113800)
  - Also called epidermolytic hyperkeratosis or bullous congenital ichthyosiform erythroderma
  - Autosomal dominant disorder of keratinization caused by variants in the keratin 1 and 10 genes: *KRT1* and *KRT10*
  - Clinical features: marked skin fragility, blistering, erythroderma
    - Can be confused with epidermolysis bullosa
    - Symptoms tend to improve in older children and adults. Hyperkeratosis is prominent over the flexion creases.
  - Dermatopathology is characteristic.

## Syndromic Ichthyoses

- The majority of these autosomal recessive disorders are due to deficiency in lipid transport or secretion or other impairments of the normal lipid composition of the epidermis.
- **Sjögren–Larsson syndrome** (MIM 270200)
  - Rare autosomal recessive condition, caused by variants in *ALDH3A2*
  - Clinical features: significant erythema, pruritus, ocular abnormalities. Photophobia and macular degeneration are evident early.
    - Later: ichthyosis with brownish scales, spasticity before age 2 years, involves primarily lower extremities
      - Pruritis distinguishes this from all other ichthyoses.
      - ID
  - Brain MRI: markedly decreased myelin
- **Trichothiodystrophy** (MIM 126340)
  - Severe autosomal recessive disorder caused by variants in *ERCC2*, involved in nucleotide excision repair
  - Clinical features: microcephaly, brittle, sulfur-deficient hair with a diagnostic "tiger tail" banding pattern. Early skin findings can be similar to an exfoliative erythroderma (Figure 40.5).
    - Later: ID
  - Brain MRI: decreased myelin

- **Gaucher disease type 2** (MIM 230900)
  - Rare autosomal recessive lysosomal storage disease caused by variants in *GBA*, the gene encoding acid β-glucosidase
    - Gaucher syndrome, type 2, is the severe infantile neuronopathic type, the rarest type of Gaucher syndrome.
  - Clinical features: may have collodion membrane
    - Infants may initially appear normal but eventually develop hepatosplenomegaly and progressive neurologic signs: opisthotonus, swallowing impairment, seizures.
  - Bone marrow shows lipid-laden macrophages.
  - Progressive and lethal
    - Enzyme replacement therapy under investigation
- **Netherton syndrome** (MIM 256500); (see Clinical Consult)
  - Autosomal recessive disorder caused by biallelic variants in *SPINK5*

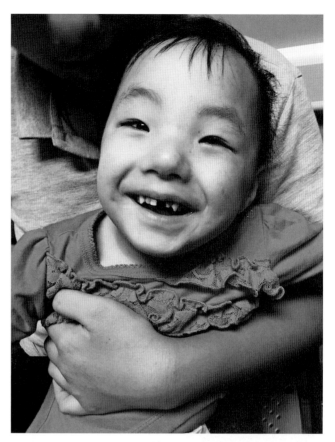

FIGURE 40.5 Homozygous variants in *ERCC2* on exomes were consistent with the clinical diagnosis of trichothiodystrophy. This child presented as a newborn with generalized erythema and scaling. She had ID, sparse easily broken hair, abnormal nails, and decreased myelin on MRI.

  - Prenatal findings: Exfoliation of fetal skin in utero may lead to milky amniotic fluid and rarely to pulmonary sequelae after delivery.
  - Clinical features: generalized exfoliative erythroderma, fine scales, abnormal "bamboo" hair, trichorrhexis invaginata (see Figure 40.1B)
    - Later: atopic dermatitis, elevated IgE, failure to thrive, recurrent infections, similar to an immune deficiency
- **Neu–Laxova syndrome** (MIM 256520, 616038)
  - Autosomal recessive lethal disorder caused by variants in *PHGDH* and *PSAT1*, in the L-serine biosynthetic pathway
    - The extreme end of the spectrum of serine biosynthetic errors
  - Prenatal findings: severe IUGR, microcephaly, contractures, lens opacification on US, hydrops, decreased fetal movement
  - Clinical features: severe ichthyosis with ectropion, eclabium and proptosis, generalized edema, microcephaly, lissencephaly, hypoplastic lungs, short limbs and digits (see Figure 5.4)
- **Restrictive dermopathy** (MIM 275210)
  - Rare lethal skin disorder, likely laminopathy. Two types exist in the same genetic pathway.

- Autosomal recessive type caused by null mutations in *ZMPSTE24*
- Autosomal dominant type caused by de novo variants in *LMNA*
  - Prenatal findings: polyhydramnios, severe IUGR
  - Clinical features: thin, tightly adherent translucent skin with erosions at flexure sites, visible superficial vessels. Often premature
    - Pinched nose with tiny "O"-shaped mouth (Figure 40.6)
    - Generalized joint contractures
  - Death usually occurs in several days.

- **Neutral lipid storage disease** (MIM 275630)
  - Also called Chanarin–Dorfman syndrome
  - Autosomal recessive disorder caused by variants in *ABHD5*
    - Encodes an enzyme involved in long-chain fatty acid oxidation

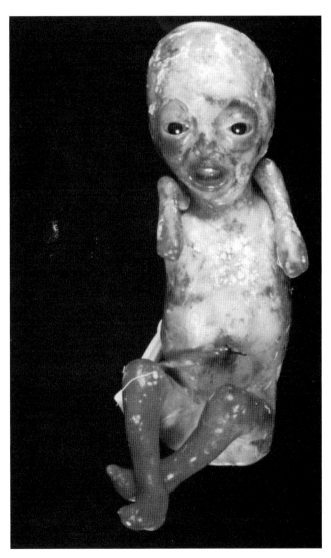

FIGURE 40.6 Lethal restrictive dermopathy: deceased infant with severe IUGR, "O"-shaped mouth, and shiny adherent ichthyotic skin with erosions.

- Triglycerides accumulate in the cytoplasm of leukocytes, muscle, liver, fibroblasts, and other tissues.
- Clinical features: collodion membrane or erythroderma that improves over time, mild to moderate fine white scale on an erythematous background, lamellar scaling on the trunk. Hepatosplenomegaly, myopathy

- **Ichthyosis prematurity syndrome** (MIM 608649)
  - Autosomal recessive disorder, caused by biallelic variants in *FATP4*
    - Encodes a fatty acid transporter protein
  - Prenatal findings: separation of amnion and chorion, polyhydramnios
    - Pregnancy complications are common in midgestation.
  - Clinical features: prematurity; thick skin; erythroderma covered by a greasy, thick vernix-like scale
    - Respiratory compromise, tracheal obstruction due to amniotic fluid debris, pneumothorax, aspiration pneumonia, asphyxia
    - Later: mild chronic pruritic ichthyosis

- **Keratitis–ichthyosis–deafness syndrome** (KID, MIM 148210)
  - Rare, typically autosomal dominant disorder, caused by heterozygous variant in *GJB2*, encoding connexin 26
  - Clinical features: generalized erythroderma, variable degree of scaling and leathery skin, progressive corneal involvement. Constriction of fingers and toes. Sensorineural deafness, generally severe and bilateral
    - Later: corneal transplantation
  - An autosomal recessive form (MIM 242150) has no causative gene.
    - Clinical features as above and short stature, progressive cirrhosis
      - Later: ID

- ***Congenital hemidysplasia with ichthyosiform erythroderma and limb defects syndrome*** (CHILD syndrome, MIM 308050)
  - Rare X-linked dominant disorder, caused by pathogenic variants in genes involved in cholesterol synthesis: *NSDHL* and, less commonly, *EBP*
  - Affects females almost exclusively; 1 M:28 F
    - Presumed lethal in male fetuses
  - Clinical features: Unilateral ichthyosiform skin lesions and ipsilateral limb defects range from shortening of the metacarpals and phalanges to absence of the entire limb. Nail changes are common.
    - Heart, lung, and kidneys can be involved.
    - Later: Intellect is usually normal.
  - Topical treatment with lovastatin/cholesterol clears skin over a few months.

- **Congenital X-linked dominant chondrodysplasia punctata** (Conradi–Hünermann syndrome, MIM 302960)
  - X-linked disorder, caused by variants in *EBP* in mosaic distribution
  - Primarily in females

○ Clinical features: congenital ichthyosiform erythroderma, transient swirls follow the lines of Blaschko. Short stature, rhizomelic shortening of extremities, cataracts
  ▪ Later: linear hyperkeratosis, pigmentary abnormalities, patchy alopecia, atrophoderma: "orange peel"-like skin with prominent pores
    • ID
○ Radiographic: asymmetry, epiphyseal stippling, severe scoliosis

# Evaluation and Management

*Pearl*: Advances in neonatal intensive care have improved the outlook for severe congenital ichthyosis, and genetic testing panels offer an earlier diagnosis and more accurate prognosis.

- Take a three-generation family history: common ethnicity, consanguinity, previous affected children, early deaths.
- Review prenatal history: polyhydramnios, fetal edema, IUGR, lack of spontaneous labor.
- Examine parents for subtle skin changes.
- Identify extradermal findings: CNS, eye, limbs.
- Examine and document cutaneous findings: nails, hair abnormalities.
  ○ Time of onset and clinical course
  ○ Scale pattern, quality, and color; presence of a collodion membrane, erythroderma, erosions, or blistering
  ○ Histology and dermatopathology: Examine hair microscopically for bamboo hair, trichorrhexis nodosa; skin biopsy sometimes needed for expert opinion
- Chronologic follow-up may allow tighter differential with time.
- Involve both dermatology and genetics consultants early.
- Genetic testing
  ○ Single gene testing is appropriate when phenotype is consistent with a distinctive, monogenic syndrome (**Netherton syndrome**).
  ○ Gene panels are appropriate when a well-defined phenotype does not have a single unique genetic cause (**lamellar ichthyosis**; **chondrodysplasia punctata**).
  ○ Exome sequencing may be appropriate for atypical or complex phenotypes after negative panel testing (erythroderma, blisters, and scales).
    ▪ Consider when there is clinical and genetic heterogeneity and a large number of candidate genes not covered in a panel
- Assemble a multidisciplinary team to optimize care.

- Utilize resources, support groups.
  ○ The Foundation for Ichthyosis and Related Skin Types (FIRST; http://www.firstskinfoundation.org) organizes medical consultations via a teledermatology program, facilitates contact between families with similar disorders, and provides patient information.
- Monitor for hypernatremic dehydration and hypothermia.
  ○ Infants should be in isolettes with increased humidity at 50–70%.
- Anticipate increased caloric needs.
  ○ Supplement calories, may need nasogastric feeds or gastrostomy.
- Appreciate high risk of infection.
  ○ Prophylactic antibiotics are *not* generally indicated.
  ○ Use sterile technique with dressing changes.
- Apply bland emollients (Vaseline or Aquaphor) regularly to aid shedding of scales and healing of fissures.
- Use treatments specific for the diagnosis.
  ○ Oral retinoids are helpful in some but harmful in other ichthyoses.
  ○ Pathogenesis-based therapies are useful in some ichthyoses (**CHILD syndrome**) and are likely to become increasingly utilized.
  ○ See https://www.clinicaltrials.gov for open research and therapeutic trials.

# Further Reading

Dinulos MB. (2014) Skin malformations. In: Hudgins L, Toriello HV, Enns GM, Hoyme HE, editors. *Signs and Symptoms of Genetic Conditions.* New York: Oxford University Press; pp. 475–96.

Glick JB, Craiglow BG, Choate KA, et al. (2017) Improved management of Harlequin ichthyosis with advances in neonatal intensive care. Pediatrics. 139:e20161003. PMID 27999114

Mazereeuw-Hautier J, Vahlquist A, Traupe Hi V, et al. (2018) Management of congenital ichthyososes. European guidelines of care: Part One. Br J Dermatol. [Epub ahead of print] PMID 30216406

Mazereeuw-Hautier J, Hernandez-Martin A, O'Toole EA, et al. (2018) Management of congenital ichthyoses: European guidelines of care: Part Two. Br J Dermatol. 2018 [Epub ahead of print] PMID 29897631

Richard G. (2017) Autosomal recessive congenital ichthyosis. In: Pagon RA, Adam MP, Ardinger HH, et al. editors. GeneReviews [Internet]. Seattle, WA: University of Washington, Seattle; 1993–2017. PMID 20301593

Sybert VP. (2017) *Genetic Skin Disorders.* 3rd ed. New York: Oxford University Press.

Yoneda K. (2016) Inherited ichthyosis: Syndromic forms. J Dermatol. 43:252–63. PMID 26945533

# 41

## Skin

## Vascular Malformations

## Clinical Consult

A term macrocephalic female was referred for a suspected diagnosis of Klippel–Trenaunay syndrome because of multiple capillary hemangiomas and a prominent vascular pattern over her back and flanks (Figure 41.1). She had macrocephaly, hemihypertrophy of the right leg, and 2–3 toe syndactyly. Her brain MRI showed hemimegalencephaly and perisylvian polymicrogyria. In view of her physical findings and MRI abnormalities, the diagnosis was revised to **megalencephaly–capillary malformation-polymicrogyria syndrome (MCAP)**. Genetic analysis revealed a mosaic variant in *PIK3CA* in 22% of the DNA sample obtained from skin. As expected, this variant was not present in peripheral blood. The nomenclature for this complex condition has evolved along with knowledge of its mosaic etiology and multisystem involvement.

## Definition

- Vascular birthmarks occur in 40–60% of infants; most are of no clinical significance.
- Categorized as capillary, venous, arterial, lymphatic, or combination types and as high-flow (arterial) or low-flow (venous)
- In isolation, the common nevus flammeus is a benign lesion.
  - Called nevus simplex, salmon patch or macular staining, "stork bites" or "angel kisses"
  - Commonly at the base of the neck, glabella, eyelids, and philtrum
  - Lesions become more obvious with crying, and they fade with age.
  - Those at the base of the neck may never totally disappear.
- Facial nevus flammeus can be striking in **Beckwith–Wiedemann** (MIM 130650), **Rubinstein–Taybi** (MIM 180849; Figure 41.2), and **Bohring–Opitz** (MIM 605039) syndromes (Figure 11.4).

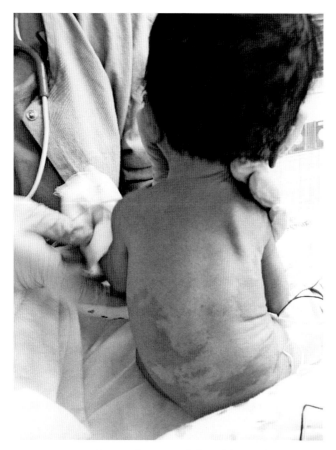

FIGURE 41.1  Newborn with macrocephaly and flat capillary hemangiomas of the back and flanks. Additional findings allowed the diagnosis of megalencephaly–capillary malformation–polymicrogyria syndrome (MCAP).

## Differential Diagnosis

### Macular Stains over the Back Midline

- Benign vascular birthmark that, when midline in the lower spine, can mark an occult spinal dysraphism, especially with an overlying hairy patch, underlying lipoma, or abnormal gluteal cleft.
- Spine imaging identifies lipoma, tethering, thickening of the filum.

### Port Wine Stains

- Isolated port wine stains are usually unilateral, asymptomatic. May occur anywhere on body. Can be subtle in infancy; more evident with age
- **Sturge–Weber syndrome** (MIM 185300)
  - ○ Sporadic disorder, due to a somatic, mosaic, activating variants in *GNAQ* in affected tissues
  - ○ Clinical features: facial port wine stain in V1/V2 dermatome distribution, leptomeningeal involvement (evident by age 1 year), glaucoma ~60%, seizures 80%
    - Later: ID or behavioral issues 70–85%, hemiparesis

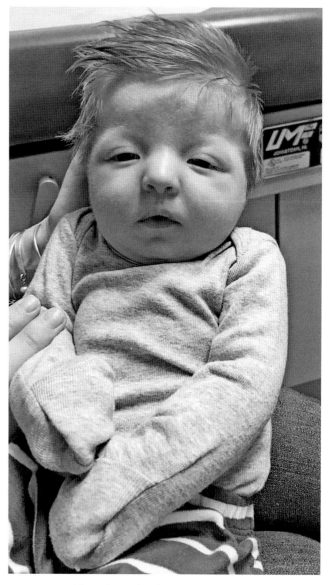

FIGURE 41.2  This infant with Rubinstein-Taybi syndrome has a prominent nevus flammeus.

### Segmental Overgrowth with Vascular Components

- *PIK3CA* related overgrowth spectrum (PROS)
  - ○ Overlapping, often severe, group of conditions with phenotypes that vary with the tissues that are affected by a mosaic *PIK3CA* somatic mutation.

*Pearl*: When PROS is suspected, gene testing should include a tissue other than blood: skin, saliva; preferably from an affected region.

- **CLOVES syndrome** (MIM 612918)
  - ○ Congenital *l*ipomatous asymmetric *o*vergrowth of the trunk, lymphatic, and capillary *v*enous and combination *v*ascular malformations, *e*pidermal nevi, *s*pine syndrome

- ○ Sporadic disorder, caused by mosaic somatic variants in *PIK3CA*
- ○ Clinical features: striking overgrowth, usually truncal lipomatous masses, combined lymphatic and vascular malformations. Connective tissue and epidermal nevi (see Figure 3.4)
  - ■ Skeletal: progressive overgrowth, scoliosis, macrodactyly
- **Klippel–Trenaunay syndrome** (KT, MIM 149000)
  - ○ Sporadic disorder, caused, in a few patients, by a somatic, mosaic variant in *PIK3CA*
    - ■ A second gene, *AGGF1*, that encodes an angiogenic factor, acts as a susceptibility factor for KT.
  - ○ Clinical features: vascular and lymphatic abnormalities, varicosities, capillary malformations, lymphangiomas (Figure 41.3). Segmental asymmetric overgrowth, usually in one lower extremity. May overlap with MCAP

- **Megalencephaly–capillary malformation–polymicrogyria syndrome** (MCAP, MIM 602501; see Clinical Consult)
  - ○ Sporadic disorder due to somatic mosaic variants in *PIK3CA*, or germline mutation in *PIK3R2* or *AKT3*, all of which are in the *P13K/AKT/mTOR* pathway
  - ○ Clinical features: midline facial capillary birthmarks, extensive capillary changes resemble cutis marmorata, may fade with age. Epidermal nevi, streaks follow lines of Blaschko, indicating mosaicism. Hyperelastic skin and "doughy" subcutaneous tissues
    - ■ Skeletal: variable growth dysregulation. macrosomia, segmental overgrowth of a limb or digit, toe syndactyly (especially 2–3). Lax joints
    - ■ CNS: hypotonia, megalencephaly, seizures ~33%, hemimegalencephaly, ventriculomegaly, hydrocephalus, Chiari malformation
      - • Polymicrogyria >50%, usually perisylvian
    - ■ Cardiac: Arrhythmias may cause unexpected death.

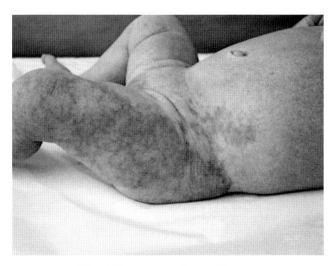

FIGURE 41.3 Klippel–Trenaunay syndrome with asymmetric capillary malformations and mild enlargement of one leg

- ■ Later: mild to severe DD, ID, autism ~33%
- **Proteus syndrome** (MIM 176929)
  - ○ Sporadic severe asymmetric overgrowth syndrome, caused by mosaic, somatic activating variants in *AKT1*
  - ○ Clinical features: capillary, venous, hemangiolipomatous and lymphatic malformations. Epidermal nevi and linear macular lesions, depigmented and hyperpigmented areas
    - ■ Skeletal: Segmental overgrowth is progressive; hemihyperplasia, macrodactyly, and exostoses may not be present in the newborn.
    - ■ CNS manifestations: hemimegalencephaly, abnormal corpus callosum
    - ■ Later: cerebriform hyperplasia of soles (a cardinal sign), increased risk for DVT, ID

## Other Syndromes with Hemangiomas

- **PHACE(S) syndrome** (MIM 606519)
  - ○ *P*osterior fossa abnormalities, *h*emangioma, *a*rterial, *c*ardiac, *e*yes, *s*ternum
  - ○ Underdiagnosed sporadic neurocutaneous syndrome, with no known responsible gene
  - ○ Clinical features: segmental hemangiomas of face and neck. Rarely, other components occur without a hemangioma.
    - ■ CNS: Dandy–Walker and posterior fossa anomalies, polymicrogyria, heterotopias, Moyamoya, anomalous vasculature
    - ■ Eye: coloboma, microphthalmia, abnormal retinal vessels, "morning glory" disc, optic nerve hypoplasia, cataracts
    - ■ Sternum: sternal agenesis, cleft or pit, raphe from umbilicus to sternum (Figure 41.4)
    - ■ Cardiac: aortic coarctation or dilatation, right aortic arch, tetralogy of Fallot

*Pearl*: Up to 20% of children with extensive segmental craniofacial hemangiomas may have PHACE(S) syndrome, even those with few non-hemangiomatous findings.

- SACRAL (LUMBAR) syndrome: *s*pinal dysraphism, *a*nogenital, *c*utaneous, *r*enal, and urologic *a*nomalies with *l*umbosacral hemangiomas
  - ○ Analogous to PHACE(S) syndrome, causing a similar phenotype affecting lower spine, renal, and genitourinary structures
  - ○ Rare, sporadic disorder, with no causative gene
  - ○ Clinical features: extensive perianal hemangiomas, tethered cord, occasionally lipoma, GU anomalies, hydronephrosis (Figure 41.5)
    - ■ Complications: urinary tract infection, skin breakdown, secondary infection

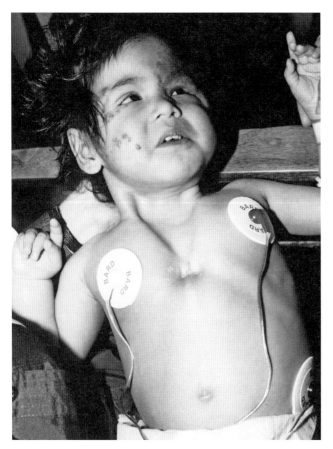

FIGURE 41.4 Hemangiomas of face and sternal cleft seen in PHACES syndrome.

## Evaluation and Management

- Imaging: can define the diagnosis
  - Brain MRI for macrocephaly or facial hemangioma

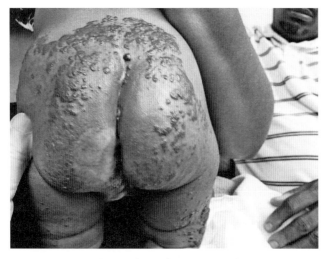

FIGURE 41.5 SACRAL syndrome shows severe and progressive hemangiomatous malformation involving the buttocks and perineum along with genitourinary malformations.

- Brain magnetic resonance angiography for arterial abnormalities in PHACE(S) syndrome
  - US or MRI of the spine for low sacral or perianal hemangioma or nevus flammeus
  - Echocardiogram
- Management is based on clinical phenotype.
  - Nevus flammeus in normal newborns: No intervention is needed for glabellar and posterior neck lesions.
  - Severe hemangiomatous disorders: Evaluate for CNS and other anomalies.
  - PROS: Treat conservatively, if possible. Surgery is complicated by non-healing incisions, chronic lymphatic drainage, and rapid tissue regrowth after debulking.
  - PHACE(S), PROS, Proteus: Manage risk of thrombosis due to venous stasis.
  - A recent clinical trial of a chemotherapeutic agent in PROS resulted in significant improvement and stabilization of symptoms (Venot et al. 2018).
- Genetic testing
  - For genes in *PIK3CA/AKT3/MTOR* pathway, include *a tissue other than blood*, preferably from an affected area
- Multidisciplinary approach: when many organ systems are involved
- Consider research trials for potential therapies, including mTOR inhibitors: https://clinicaltrials.gov.

## Further Reading

Garzon MC, Epstein LG, Heyer GL, et al. (2016) PHACE syndrome: Consensus-derived diagnosis and care recommendations. J Pediatr. 178:24–33. PMID 27659028

Greene AK, Goss JA. (2018) Vascular anomalies: From a clinicohistologic to a genetic framework. Plast Reconstr Surg. 141(5):709e–717e. PMID 29697621

Keppler-Noreuil KM, Rios JJ, Parker VE. (2015) PIK3CA-related overgrowth spectrum (PROS): Diagnostic and testing eligibility criteria, differential diagnosis, and evaluation. Am J Med Genet A. 167A:287–95. PMID 25557259

Luu M, Frieden IJ. (2016) Infantile hemangiomas and structural anomalies: PHACE and LUMBAR syndrome. Semin Cutan Med Surg. 35:117–23. PMID 27607319

Martinez-Lopez A, Blasco-Morente G, Perez-Lopez I, et al. (2017) CLOVES syndrome: Review of a PIK3CA-related overgrowth spectrum (PROS). Clin Genet. 91:14–21. PMID 27426476

Nathan N, Keppler-Noreuil KM, Biesecker LG. (2017) Mosaic disorders of the PI3K/PTEN/AKT/TSC/mTORC1 signaling pathway. Dermatol Clin. 35:51–60. PMID 27890237

Venot Q, Blanc T, Rabia SH, et al. (2018) Targeted therapy in patients with PIK3CA-related overgrowth syndrome. Nature. 558(7711):540–6. PMID AA29899452

# 42

## Skin

## Other Disorders

## Clinical Consult

A term baby girl, who was born to non-consanguineous East Indian parents, had white hair, pale irides, and roving eye movements. Red reflexes were apparent without an ophthalmoscope (Figure 42.1). She was otherwise nondysmorphic with a normal neurologic exam. Clinically, the most likely diagnosis was **oculocutaneous albinism type I.** This is the most common form of albinism that is recognizable in newborns. Other forms are more subtle in their clinical presentation and/or present later in life. She was referred for pediatric ophthalmology, dermatology, and genetics follow-up for possible molecular testing for albinism. While still in the nursery, the family was cautioned to use sun screen, sun-protective clothing, hats, and dark glasses to protect her eyes when outside. Referral for a low vision infant program was suggested.

## Pigmentary Abnormalities

- Disorders of melanin production are not uncommon in the newborn.
- Almost all systemic pigmentary disorders, such as albinism, piebaldism, and Waardenburg syndrome, are inherited.
- Oculocutaneous albinism (OCA) is the most common cause of decreased pigmentation in the newborn.
  - **OCA I** (MIM 203100)
    - Also called tyrosinase negative OCA
    - Autosomal recessive disorder, due primarily to variants in *TYR*
    - Clinical features: snow white hair, pink skin, blue eyes with iris transillumination defects, nystagmus, strabismus, head bobbing
    - Visual acuity 20/200-20/400
  - **OCA II** (MIM 203200)
    - Also called tyrosinase-positive albinism
    - Autosomal recessive disorder, caused by variants in *OCA2* (formerly called the P gene)
      - Most common form of albinism, especially in equatorial Africa

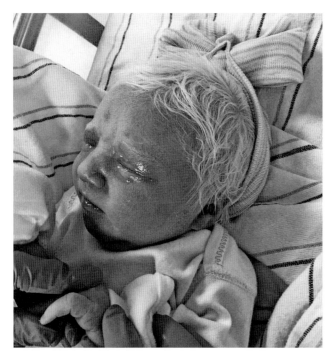

FIGURE 42.1 East Indian infant with oculocutaneous albinism. He has snow white hair and nystagmus.

- Clinical features: yellow brown hair, creamy pink skin, blue to yellow brown irides, nystagmus variably present. Generally less severe with some improvement with time

*Pearl*: Many infants with **Prader–Willi syndrome***  and Angelman syndrome are hypopigmented, and some may have mild albinism (Figure 42.2). This is seen in some but not all patients with a deletion of 15q11.2, especially when the mother transmits a concomitant recessive variant for *OCA2*.

- **Ocular albinism without skin and hair changes**
  - **Ocular albinism type I** (Nettleship–Falls type, MIM 300500)
    - X-linked disorder, due to variants in *GPR143*
    - Clinical features: hair color slightly lighter than sibs, nystagmus, impaired visual acuity, iris hypopigmentation
  - **Aland Island eye disease** (Forsius–Ericksson type, MIM 300600)
    - X-linked disorder, due to variants in *CACNA1F*
    - Clinical features: markedly impaired vision, nystagmus, astigmatism, foveal hypoplasia
- **Syndromic albinism**
  - **Chediak–Higashi syndrome** (MIM 214500)
    - Autosomal recessive disorder, due to variants in *LYST*
    - Clinical features: partial albinism, silvery hair, recurrent infections, later onset lymphoproliferative disorder
  - **Griscelli syndrome** (MIM 214450 type I; MIM 607624 type II)

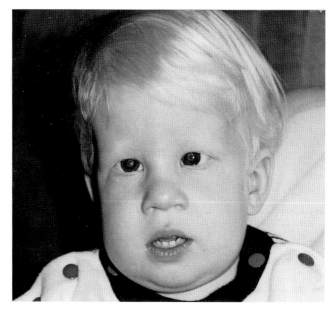

FIGURE 42.2 Prader–Willi syndrome in a two-year-old who presented as a neonate with white blond hair and hypotonia

- Autosomal recessive disorders, due to variants in *MYO5A* (type I) or *RAB27A* (type II)
- Clinical features: immunodeficiency, silvery hair
  - Similar to Chediak–Higashi syndrome (MIM 214500)
  - Later: hemophagocytic syndrome
  - **Hermansky–Pudlak syndrome** (MIM 614074)
    - Autosomal recessive disorder, genetically heterogeneous
    - Clinical features: mild OCA, easy bruising, bleeding diathesis; later onset presentation
  - **Piebaldism** (MIM 172800)
    - Autosomal dominant trait, due to variant in *KIT*
      - Rare disorder due to defective migration of neural crest cell derivatives
    - Clinical features: white forelock; stable, sometimes widespread patches of hypopigmented skin. Hands and feet spared
      - Normal health and life span
  - **Waardenburg syndrome**
    - Group of disorders (four main types), characterized by abnormal neural crest migration
    - Clinical features: white forelock (Figure 42.3) and hypopigmented skin in some, premature graying of hair, heterochromia, displacement of inner canthi, short palpebral fissures, medial eyebrow flare, distinctive nose with hypoplastic nares
      - Type 1 (MIM 193500)
        - Autosomal dominant disorder, due to mutation in *PAX3*
        - Clinical features: as listed previously and sensorineural hearing loss (25%), usually severe, occasionally unilateral

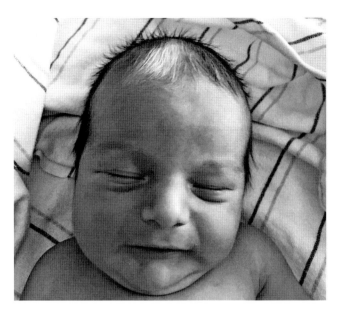

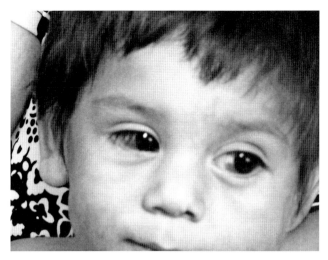

FIGURE 42.4  Ocular melanosis in an infant with phacomatosis pigmentovascularis: increased risks for glaucoma and melanoma.

FIGURE 42.3  White forelock in an infant with Waardenburg syndrome.

- Type 2 (MIM 193510)
  - A group of autosomal dominant disorders, due to variants in *PAX3, MITF, SNAI2,* or *SOX10*
    - 20X as common as type 1
  - Clinical features: as listed previously and sensori-neural hearing loss (50%). No displaced inner canthi
- Type 3 (Klein–Waardenburg syndrome, MIM 148820)
  - Autosomal dominant disorder due to variants in *PAX3*
  - Clinical features: as listed previously for type 1 and upper limb anomalies
- Type 4 (Shah–Waardenburg syndrome, MIM 277580)
  - Autosomal recessive disorder due to variants in *EDN3* or *EDNRB*. Also an autosomal dominant type, due to mutation in *SOX10*
  - Clinical features: as listed previously plus Hirschsprung disease
- **Other pigmentary abnormalities**
  - Extensive Mongolian spots with neurologic phenotype
    - Also called phacomatosis pigmentovascularis
    - Molecular mechanism unclear; mosaic somatic variants in *GNA11* and *GNAQ* reported
    - Clinical features: coexistence of a widespread vascular (usually capillary) nevus (nevus flammeus) and extensive Mongolian spots, or blue/slate/gray oculocutaneous melanosis (Figure 42.4)
      - Associated with other cutaneous nevi (e.g., anemicus, epidermal nevus, telangiectatic nevus) and/or neurologic problems
      - CNS: vascular abnormalities of circle of Willis; cerebral atrophy, cerebellar changes
  - Pigmentary mosaicism (previously hypomelanosis of Ito or incontinentia pigmenti achromians)

- A group of linear and swirled pigmentary disorders, caused by mosaicism for various chromosomal anomalies or somatic single gene mutations. Swirling pigmentation follows the lines of Blaschko (Figure 42.5A). These changes are usually not detectable in blood and require sampling of other tissues. No longer considered a specific entity. The following are examples:
  - **Pallister–Killian syndrome** (MIM 601803) due to mosaic 12p tetrasomy ( Figure 3.2)
  - Mosaic trisomy 7 (Figure 42.5B)
  - Mosaic triploidy
  - **Megalencephaly–capillary malformation–polymicrogyria syndrome** (MCAP, MIM 602501) due to mosaic variants in *PIK3CA*
  - **Curry–Jones syndrome** (MIM 601707; Figure 42.5C) due to mosaic variants in *SMO*
- Cutaneous features may not become apparent for a few weeks to months after birth.
  - Re-examine the baby unclothed.

## Cutis Aplasia

- A relatively common congenital skin defect consisting of hairless, full-thickness, "punched-out" lesions
  - Usually at the scalp vertex. Occasionally extensive. At birth, may resemble a fresh cigarette burn or appear as a healed scar.
  - Gradual healing, over several months, leaves a hairless atrophic scar (Figure 42.6A). If a large area, may need grafting
- Several genes have been identified in isolated or familial cutis aplasia and in syndromes featuring cutis aplasia.
- Chromosome disorders
  - **Trisomy 13\*** may have extensive or localized cutis aplasia at the vertex of the scalp (Figure 42.6B).

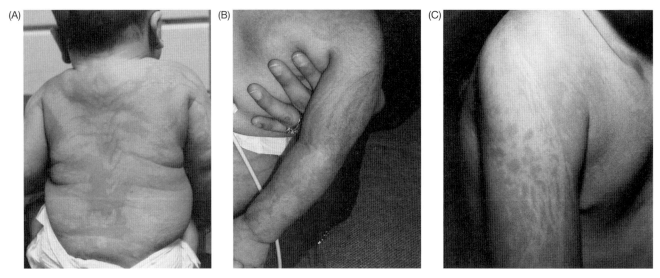

FIGURE 42.5  (A) Swirling mosaic pigmentation following the lines of Blaschko. (B) Abnormal pigmentary pattern seen in mosaic trisomy 7. (C) Streaky silvery pigmentary changes seen in Curry–Jones syndrome due to mosaic mutation in *SMO*.

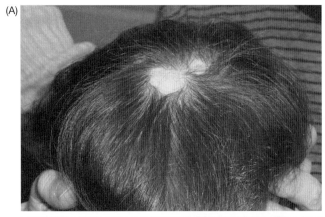

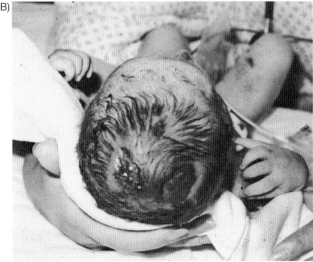

FIGURE 42.6  (A) Healed, hairless punched-out scalp defects at the vertex. (B) Extensive scalp defects in trisomy 13.

- ○ Deletions of 4p\*, 18q, and 19p13.3; maternal uniparental disomy for chromosome 14 and others
- Teratogens
  - ○ Methimazole
  - ○ Valproic acid
  - ○ Congenital rubella, varicella infections
- Syndromic cutis aplasia
  - ○ **Adams–Oliver syndrome** (MIM 100300, 614219)
    - ■ Autosomal dominant forms are due to variants in four genes: *ARHGAP3*, *RBPJ*, *EOGT*, and *NOTCH1*.
    - ■ Autosomal recessive form is due to variants in *DOCK6*.
    - ■ Clinical features: cutis aplasia (sometimes a tiny defect or may cover much of scalp), terminal transverse defects of toes or fingers or parts of limbs. Marked variability in expression within families (Figure 30.3)
      - • Rarely, scalp defects include absence of underlying skull and dura, exposing brain contents.
  - ○ **Scalp–ear–nipple syndrome** (Finlay–Marks syndrome, MIM 181270)
    - ■ Autosomal dominant disorder, due to variants in *KCTD1*
    - ■ Clinical features: extensive scalp cutis aplasia, minor ear abnormalities, underdeveloped nipples, toe syndactyly, scant body and pubic hair in adults
      - • Facial features: broad prominent forehead and displaced inner canthi
      - • Cutis aplasia heals slowly in childhood.
  - ○ **Johanson–Blizzard syndrome** (MIM 243800)
    - ■ Autosomal recessive disorder, due to homozygous or compound heterozygous variants in *UBR1*
    - ■ Clinical features: scalp defects, poor growth, dysmorphic features, hypoplasia of the alar wings of the nose
      - • Hypothyroidism, sensorineural hearing loss, imperforate anus, pancreatic exocrine insufficiency
      - • Later: oligodontia, ID

- ○ **Familial cutis aplasia** (MIM 107600)
  - ■ Autosomal dominant disorder, due to a variant in *BMS1*, a gene involved in ribosome biogenesis, recently identified in one family
  - ■ Clinical features: aplasia cutis at the vertex
- ○ Cutis aplasia caused by the death of an MZ co-twin
  - ■ The area of denuded skin can be extensive, covering large areas of the trunk; may be slow to heal (see Figure 4.3).
  - ■ Severe brain abnormalities, due to embolization of necrotic material from the deceased twin, are serious sequelae of this condition.

## Evaluation and Management

- Document family history: consanguinity, other affected individuals.
- Examine parents for heterochromia, deafness, hypopigmented areas, and cutis aplasia at the vertex.
- **Albinism**
  - ○ In **Waardenburg syndrome**, screen for hearing loss early and repeat several times in infancy and early childhood.
  - ○ Ophthalmologic exam and follow-up; refer to low vision specialists
  - ○ Use gene panels to evaluate large numbers of genes for isolated and syndromic albinism. Some genes for albinism await discovery.
  - ○ Advocate daily use of sunscreen, hats, long sleeves, to reduce risk of skin cancer and dark glasses to reduce photophobia.
- **Pigmentary dysplasias**
  - ○ Evaluate for chromosomal mosaicism and somatic single gene mosaicism: microarray in newborns may reveal the abnormality but later, skin biopsy for microarray will often be needed. Molecular analysis based on clinical features
  - ○ MRI of brain
- **Cutis aplasia**
  - ○ Examine the placenta for evidence of a fetus papyraceous and/or review US reports for history of twin gestation.
  - ○ Brain MRI if there is a deceased co-twin

- ○ Chromosome microarray
- ○ Gene testing based on clinical phenotype
  - ■ If isolated cutis aplasia is familial, no testing may be indicated.
  - ■ Single gene analysis for Johanson–Blizzard syndrome
  - ■ Gene panel for Adams–Oliver syndrome
- ○ Treat denuded areas as indicated by size: Small defects heal without treatment; others may require prolonged treatment and grafts.

## Further Reading

Bertsch M, Floyd M, Kehoe T, et al. (2017) The clinical evaluation of infantile nystagmus: What to do first and why. Ophthalmic Genet. 38:22–33. PMID 28177849

Federico JR, Krishnamurthy K. (2018) Albinism StatPearls [Internet]. Treasure Island (FL): StatPearls Publishing. PMID 30085560

Grob A, Grekin S. (2016) Piebaldism in children. Cutis. 97:90–2. PMID 26919497

Lewis RA. (2015) Ocular albinism, X-linked. In: Pagon RA, Adam MP, Ardinger HH, et al. editors. GeneReviews [Internet]. Seattle, WA: University of Washington, Seattle; 1993–2017. PMID 20301517

Mirzaa GM, Campbell CD, Solovieff N, et al. (2016) Association of MTOR mutations with developmental brain disorders, including megalencephaly, focal cortical dysplasia, and pigmentary mosaicism. JAMA Neurol. 73:836–45. PMID 27159400

Patel DP, Castelo-Soccio L, Yan AC. (2018) Aplasia cutis congenital: Evaluation of signs suggesting extracutaneous involvement. Pediatr Dermatol. 35(1):e59–e61. PMID 29178194

Que SK, Weston G, Suchecki J, Ricketts J. (2015) Pigmentary disorders of the eyes and skin. Clin Dermatol. 33:147–58. PMID 25704935

Ruggieri M, Praticò AD. (2015) Mosaic neurocutaneous disorders and their causes. Semin Pediatr Neurol. 22:207–33. PMID 26706010

Silberstein E, Pagkalos VA, Landau D, et al. (2014) Aplasia cutis congenita: clinical management and a new classification system. Plast Reconstr Surg. 134(5):766e–74e. PMID 25347652

Song J, Feng Y, Acke FR, et al. (2016) Hearing loss in Waardenburg syndrome: A systematic review. Clin Genet. 89:416–25. PMID 26100139

Thomas AC, Zeng Z, Rivière JB, et al. (2016) Mosaic activating mutations in *GNA11* and *GNAQ* are associated with phakomatosis pigmentovascularis and extensive dermal melanocytosis. J Invest Dermatol. 136(4):770–8. PMID 26778290

# Appendix

## Syndromes That Commonly Present in the Newborn

# 18

## Trisomy 21   Definition

- Down syndrome (DS) is caused by an extra copy of chromosome 21.
- Most common autosomal trisomy
- Incidence 1/629 live births
- Risk increases with advancing maternal age, but more are born to young mothers because of high birth rate.
- Chromosome anomaly
  - Trisomy 21: 47,XX,+21, 95%
  - Unbalanced translocation, often Robertsonian translocation (fusion of the long arms of two acrocentric chromosomes): 46,XX,der(14;21) (q10;q10),+21, 2–3%
    - Most translocations are de novo, but approximately 3–4% are familial.
  - Mosaicism: 47,XX,+21/46,XX, 1–2%
- Recurrence risk ~1% greater than for other women of the same age
  - Higher risk when a parent carries a translocation

## Diagnosis

- Prenatal screening
  - First trimester screening includes maternal serum screening for PAPP-A (low) and hCG (high) plus US measurement of nuchal translucency ( NT) between 10–14 weeks. Abnormal if ≥3mm
  - Maternal serum screening for DS in the second trimester includes evaluation of AFP (low), unconjugated estriol (low), hCG levels (high) and Inhibin A (high). Detection rate ~80% with 5% false positive rare.
  - cfDNA >10 weeks' gestation has 99.5% detection rate for DS.
    - False-positive rate is ~0.06%
    - Positive predictive value decreases with lower maternal ages.
    - Adequate fetal fraction of DNA (fetal DNA/total DNA) in maternal serum is necessary for interpretation.
      - Maternal obesity is associated with low fetal fraction and lower detection rate of DS.

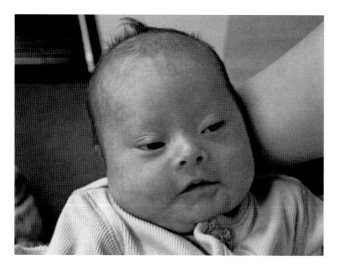

FIGURE 1S.1  Typical craniofacial findings in Down syndrome, including up-slanting palpebral fissures, midface underdevelopment, and downturned mouth corners.

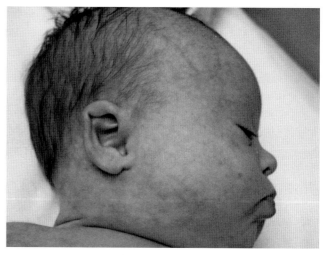

FIGURE 1S.2  Note overfolded ear helix and midface underdevelopment.

- Fetal US findings in DS
  - Abnormal >3mm nuchal translucency at 10–14 weeks
    - Absent nasal bone best measured at 13 or 14 weeks.
      - Noted in ~60% DS versus <1% of unaffected fetuses
      - Technically difficult; useful in high risk cases
    - "Soft signs" in the second trimester are present in ~50%: short long bones, echogenic bowel, nuchal thickening, pleural effusion, ventriculomegaly, pyelectasis, echogenic intracardiac focus.
      - 10–17% of unaffected fetuses have an isolated soft sign.
      - Risk for DS increases when several signs are present.
    - Other defects
      - Cardiac defects, particularly AVSD
      - "Double-bubble" or duodenal atresia, in 2.5%
      - Hydrops; common cause of late fetal demise
- Clinical features
  - Challenging diagnosis in the premature baby with DS
  - Hypotonia is almost universal.
  - Mild microcephaly, brachycephaly, central hair whorl, large fontanels, accessory (third) fontanel, redundant skin at the nape of the neck
  - Face: round, up-slanting palpebral fissures (Figure 1S.1), epicanthal folds, flat midface, small ears <3rd % ( 3% =3 cm in a term baby) with overfolded superior aspect of the helices (Figure 1S.2), open mouth, downturned corners of the mouth, protruding tongue, "theatrical" grimace

*Pearl*: To elicit a "theatrical grimace," gently scratch the bottom of the foot until the infant cries. The upslant of the palpebral fissures is accentuated, the tongue often protrudes, and the corners of the mouth turn down.

  - Hands: fifth finger clinodactyly, single flexion crease and short middle phalanx, broad hand with transverse palmar crease 45%

  - Feet: sandal gap, deep plantar crease
  - Cardiac defect 40–50%
    - Complete AVSD 37%
    - VSD 31%
    - ASD 15%
    - Partial AVSD 6%
    - TOF 5%
    - PDA 4%
  - GI anomalies
    - Duodenal atresia or stenosis (± annular pancreas) ~3.0%
      - Among all patients with duodenal atresia, ~28% have DS.
    - Hirschsprung disease <1%
    - Imperforate anus
  - Eye: strabismus, lacrimal duct obstruction, congenital cataracts 5%
  - Congenital anomalies in general are more common: hydrocephalus, cleft palate, tracheoesophageal fistula, hydronephrosis, hypospadias, small male genitalia
- Common complications
  - Feeding difficulties due to hypotonia, oral/pharyngeal dysfunction, GE reflux
  - Hearing loss 15%
    - Middle ear effusion contributes to conductive loss.
  - Transient myeloproliferative disorder (TMD) 10–30%
    - Asymptomatic DS infant: >5% blasts on routine peripheral smear
    - Symptomatic DS infant: hepatosplenomegaly, rash, hydrops, or life-threatening illness
    - Somatic mutation in *GATA-1* is necessary for occurrence of TMD.
    - Most resolve spontaneously.
      - ~20% of TMD progresses to acute megakaryocytic leukemia or myelodysplastic syndrome.

- Neurodevelopment
  - Average IQ 50–70
  - Developmental scales for DS are published: sit, 11 months; crawl, 17 months; walk, 26 months; first word, 18 months.
  - Cardiac anomalies do not predict a worse developmental outcome.
  - Neurobehavioral problems may arise with age: ADHD, anxiety, seizures, autism.

## Differential Diagnosis

o Hypotonic disorders
  - Hypothyroidism
  - Syndromes: **Beckwith–Wiedemann syndrome*** (MIM 130650), **Zellweger syndrome** (MIM 214100), **Prader–Willi syndrome*** (MIM 176270)
  - Chromosomal syndromes **Kleefstra syndrome** (9q34 deletion, MIM 610253), **Pallister–Killian syndrome** (12p tetrasomy mosaicism, MIM 601803), **Smith–Magenis syndrome** (17p11.2 deletion, MIM 182290)

*Pearl*: Rarely, an infant with DS lacks the expected facial features. Suspect a second diagnosis obscuring classic DS phenotype.

## Evaluation and Management

- Evaluations
  - Echocardiogram *before* discharge; necessary even without cardiac murmur
  - Follow American Academy of Pediatrics' health supervision guidelines for DS; use syndrome-specific growth and developmental charts: http://pediatrics.aappublications.org
  - Monitor for hypothyroidism, sleep apnea, respiratory and middle ear infections,
    - Later onset: diabetes mellitus, autoimmune disorders, obesity, asthma, short stature, GI issues, celiac disease, skin problems, cervical instability.
- Genetic testing
  - Chromosome analysis, *not* microarray, is the preferred test when DS is suspected.

- When a translocation is detected, test the parents.
- Positive cfDNA test for trisomy 21: Confirm with conventional chromosome analysis in cord or peripheral blood if not done by amniocentesis
- Microarray *does not rule out a translocation*.
  - Add FISH for chromosome 21 when urgent.
- Counsel the family.
  - Giving the diagnosis
    - As soon as possible, tell both parents that DS is suspected and testing has been ordered.
      - This avoids "rumors" or staff avoiding family.
    - Meet with parents together if possible.
    - Explain the diagnosis in a straightforward manner, stressing the positive.
      - Discuss strengths and abilities, not just anomalies and disabilities. Emphasize advances in medical care and improved quality of life and health.
    - Acknowledge grief. Limit the amount of information delivered during the first session.
    - Offer anticipatory guidance and appropriate referrals to local and national support organizations: https://www.ndss.org.
  - Enroll in early infant development program.
  - Offer genetic counseling especially if infant has a translocation

## Further Reading

Bull MJ; AAP Committee on Genetics. (2011) Health supervision for children with Down syndrome. Pediatrics. 128:393–406. PMID 21788214

Gray KJ, Wilkins-Haug LE. (2018) Have we done our last amniocentesis? Updates on cell-free DNA for Down syndrome screening. Pediatr Radiol. ;48(4):461–470. PMID 29550862

Tunstall O, Bhatnagar N, James B et al. (2018) Guidelines for the investigation and management of transient leukaemia of Down syndrome. Br J Haematol. 182(2):200–211. PMID 29916557

Versacci P, Di Carlo D, Digilio MC, Marino B. (2018) Cardiovascular disease in Down syndrome. Curr Opin Pediatr. 30(5)616-22. PMID 30015688

Zemel BS, Pipan M, Stallings VA, et al. (2015) Growth charts for children with Down syndrome in the United States. Pediatrics. 136:e1204–11. PMID 26504127

# 2S

## Trisomy 18

## Definition

- Second most common autosomal trisomy in live-born babies
- Due to extra copy of chromosome 18 in >90% of affected infants. Mosaicism and translocations account for the remainder.
- Incidence ~1/5,000 live-borns
- Associated with advanced maternal age
- 3:1 female predominance

## Diagnosis

- Prenatal findings
  o US findings: polyhydramnios, IUGR, choroid plexus cysts, clenched hands. Structural CNS abnormalities and CHD are common.
  o Abnormal maternal serum screening test (estriol, uE3, and AFP all low) may identify at-risk pregnancies.
  o Noninvasive prenatal diagnosis (cfDNA) has a sensitivity of ~97% and a false positive rate of <0.041%. Amniocentesis remains the gold standard for diagnosis because cfDNA can rarely have false-negative or false-positive results.

*Pearl*: A normal fetal US performed in a high-risk center almost always rules out trisomy 18. This can be reassuring when screening tests suggest an increased risk. The decision to terminate a pregnancy should never be made on the basis of a screening test alone.

- Clinical features
  o IUGR, clenched fists with overlapping fingers (2 over 3 and 5 over 4); hypoplastic nails (Figure 2S.1), reduced to absent finger flexion creases. Petite, triangular face with high nasal bridge, small mouth, high forehead; "fawn-shaped," "wind swept" ears. short sternum, underdeveloped pubic area (Figure 2S.2). The hands are frequently held up near the ears with elbows flexed.
  o Cardiac abnormalities >50%

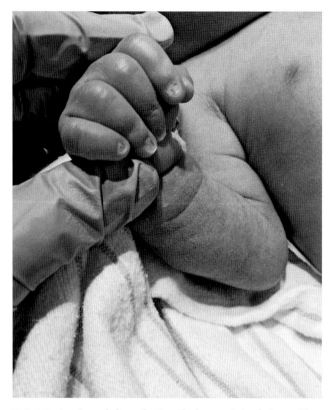

FIGURE 2S.1 Severely hypoplastic nails characteristic of trisomy 18.

○ Diaphragmatic hernia, radial hypoplasia, cleft lip/palate, omphalocele, tracheoesophageal fistula, postaxial polydactyly; brain abnormalities, particularly Dandy–Walker and variants
• Prognosis
○ This is a life-limiting disorder. 50% die in utero.
○ Of the live-born group, 50% die in first 2 weeks.
○ ~10% survive to 1 year.
○ Long-term survivors have severe ID and multiple medical problems.

*Pearl*: Intubation is characteristically very difficult in these infants due to the small mouth and oral cavity. In infants delivered without prenatal diagnosis, this can be a valuable clue to the diagnosis.

## Differential Diagnosis

• **Trisomy 13*** is often considered because of overlapping features, such as postaxial polydactyly and cardiac disease.
○ The facial features in these two disorders are quite distinct, and the bulbous nose in trisomy 13 is characteristic.
○ The classic clenched hand, nail hypoplasia, and absent finger flexion creases in trisomy18 are helpful in differentiating the two disorders.

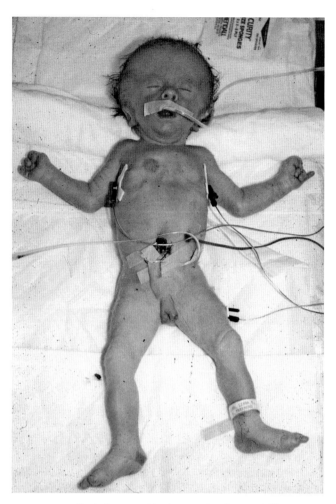

FIGURE 2S.2 Typical arm positioning seen in trisomy 18. Note triangular face, small mouth, short sternum, and overlapping fingers and underdeveloped pubic area.

• **Bowen–Conradi syndrome** (MIM 211180), or pseudo-trisomy 18, is an autosomal recessive "look-alike" syndrome with an almost equally poor prognosis.
○ Primarily occurs in the Hutterites, in whom homozygous mutations in *EMG* cause the condition
• **Marden–Walker syndrome** (MIM 248700) and **Pena–Shokeir syndrome** (Fetal Akinesia Deformation Sequence, MIM 208150) may present confusion, but the overall pattern and the prevalence of major structural abnormalities in trisomy 18 will help eliminate these diagnoses.
• **Distal arthrogryposis** syndromes may have similar hands without nail hypoplasia. The face, sternum, and presence of other anomalies should allow distinction.

## Evaluation and Management

• Prenatal diagnosis is increasingly common; careful parental counseling and a multidisciplinary team approach before delivery can best serve the infant and family.

- Recommend vaginal delivery, even in the presence of fetal indications for cesarean section, because operative delivery does not affect survival.
- Confirm all prenatal diagnosis (especially when made by cfDNA) with standard chromosome analysis to detect mosaicism, rare translocations, or other chromosome aberrations.
  ○ Collect cord blood or peripheral blood in a green-top, Na heparin tube.
  ○ If stillborn, biopsy the fetal side of placenta (rinse placenta in sterile saline, use sterile technique for biopsy, transport in sterile solution at room temperature) for chromosome analysis.
  ○ Significant controversy has arisen over optimal treatment for what had been considered a uniformly lethal disorder. Life may be extended with intensive support and invasive procedures, but the certainty of severe to profound intellectual disability remains.
  ○ We emphasize the benefits of family-centered comfort care and the option of perinatal hospice, including avoidance of intubation, multiple consults, and invasive procedures. Normal newborn care protocols and provision of nutrition are reasonable.
  ○ All options should be discussed with the family and, preferably, a plan agreed upon prior to delivery. The family's concerns and wishes should be carefully considered with the goal of quality of life being primary.
  ○ Bereavement support and infant photographs and footprints are important for the families of infants who die in the neonatal period.
- Major causes of death are central apnea, cardiac failure due to cardiac malformations, respiratory insufficiency due to hypoventilation, aspiration, upper airway obstruction, or a combination of these factors.
- Approximately 25% of infants may survive to be discharged home.

  ○ In infants surviving beyond several weeks, multidisciplinary cardiac, GI, and pulmonary management is indicated. Genetic consultation and support may be helpful in guiding management
  ○ G-tube feedings may ease feeding problems.
  ○ Cardiac surgery/palliation may be considered on an individual basis in infants surviving beyond a few months.
- The online support group SOFT (Support Organization for Trisomy 18, 13 and Related Disorders; https://trisomy.org), based in the United States, Europe, and Australia, provides information for families, especially those with longer-term surviving infants and children.

## Further Reading

Carey JC, Kosho T. (2016) Perspectives on the care and advances in the management of children with trisomy 13 and 18. Am J Med Genet C Semin Med Genet. 172:249–50. PMID 27643592

Dereddy NR, Pivnick EK, Upadhyay K, et al. (2016) Neonatal hospital course and outcomes of live-born infants with trisomy 18 at two tertiary care centers in the United States. Am J Perinatol. 34:270–5. PMID 27490773

Haug S, Goldstein M, Cummins D, et al. (2017) Using patient-centered care after a prenatal diagnosis of trisomy 18 or trisomy 13: A review. JAMA Pediatr. 171:382–7. PMID 28192554

Jacobs AP, Subramaniam A, Tang Y, et al. (2016) Trisomy 18: A survey of opinions, attitudes, and practices of neonatologists. Am J Med Genet A. 170:2638–43. PMID 27312333

Nelson KE, Rosella LC, Mahant S, et al. (2016) Survival and surgical interventions for children with trisomy 13 and 18. JAMA. 316:420–8. PMID 27458947

Pyle AK, Fleischman AR, Hardart G, Mercurio MR. (2018) Management options and parental voice in the treatment of trisomy 13 and 18. J Perinatol. 38(9): 1135–43. PMID 29977011

# 3S

## Trisomy 13

## Definition

- Trisomy 13 (T13) is caused by an extra copy of chromosome 13.
  - Associated with advanced maternal age
- Incidence 1/5,000 live births
  - Third most common autosomal trisomy
- Chromosomal findings
  - Trisomy 13: 47,XX,+13, 75%
  - Robertsonian translocation (long arms of two acrocentric chromosomes are joined at the centromere): 46, XX,+13,der(13;14), 20%
  - Other chromosome 13 anomalies: 5%
    - Mosaicism for T13
    - Partial duplication of chromosome 13
    - Unbalanced reciprocal translocation
    - Mosaicism for T13 and rearrangements of chromosome 13 are associated with a milder phenotype and longer survival.
- Recurrence risk ~1% when the infant has true T13
  - Higher risk when there is a familial translocation
- Morbidity and mortality are high.
  - Long-term survival poor
    - In utero death occurs in >40–50%.
    - Median survival is 7–10 days.
    - 25% die during the first day.
    - ~11% are alive at age 1 year.

## Diagnosis

- Prenatal findings
  - One-third of patients with T13 are diagnosed prenatally.
  - Most have congenital anomalies detectable by detailed fetal US, as early as 10 weeks of gestation.
    - Increased nuchal translucency, cystic hygroma in ~5–10%
    - IUGR
    - Cardiac defects >90%
    - Holoprosencephaly or a variant 66%
    - Omphalocele ~15%

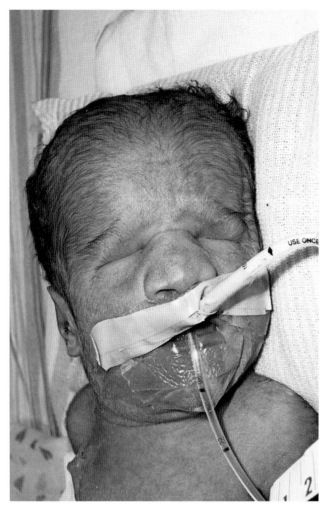

FIGURE 3S.1 Deep-set and small eyes and bulbous nose are characteristic of Trisomy 13 syndrome.

- ■ Genitourinary abnormalities ~35%
- ■ Polyhydramnios or severe oligohydramnios (from renal agenesis)
- • Prenatal testing
  - ○ cfDNA detection rate is ~96% sensitive for T13, with a false positive rate of 0.06%, slightly less accurate than for T21 or T18.
    - ■ In the presence of compatible fetal US abnormalities, a positive cfDNA screen is very helpful.
  - ○ Maternal serum screening in the first or second trimester does *not* provide a risk assessment for T13.
  - ○ Amniocentesis remains the gold standard for prenatal diagnosis.
- • Clinical features in the newborn
  - ○ Birth weight <2,500 g 33%
  - ○ Face: bulbous nasal tip, coarse facies (Figure 3S.1)
  - ○ Eyes: deep-set small eyes with short palpebral fissures, microphthalmia >75%, significantly increased frequency of holoprosencephaly with or without cyclopia
  - ○ Oral: Absence of the premaxilla causes a midline oral cleft and may alter the facial gestalt; it is commonly associated

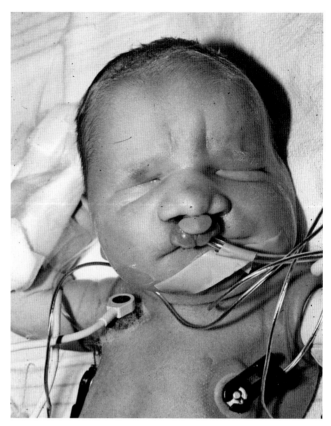

FIGURE 3S.2 Bilateral cleft and deep-set eyes. Typical nasal configuration apparent even with clefting.

with holoprosencephaly. bilateral cleft lip and palate also common (Figure 3S.2).
- ○ Scalp defects (cutis aplasia), usually at the vertex, 50%
- ○ Skeletal
  - ■ Postaxial polydactyly in ~50%
  - ■ Talipes/rocker bottom feet ~8%
- ○ Cardiac defects 80%
  - ■ Dextrocardia, atrial or septal defects, PDA
- ○ GI and GU: omphalocele, enlarged or polycystic kidneys
- ○ CNS anomalies
  - ■ Holoprosencephaly, microcephaly, ventriculomegaly
  - ■ Spina bifida, agenesis of corpus callosum
- ○ Surviving infants have profound ID, a high incidence of epilepsy, severe sensory impairments, self-abusive behavior, and feeding issues.

# Differential Diagnosis

- ○ **Trisomy 18***
  - ■ The face in T18 is distinct from that in T13. Facial features in T18 are small and delicate, whereas they are coarse in T13. The hands in T18 are clenched with overlapping fingers, and the nails are hypoplastic.

In T13, postaxial polydactyly is frequent and the nails are narrow and hyperconvex.

- o **Meckel syndrome** (MIM 249000)
    - ▪ Renal cysts and postaxial polydactyly can be seen in both Meckel syndrome and T13, but the frequent presence of encephalocele and hepatic fibrosis in Meckel syndrome is helpful in distinquishing the two diagnoses.
- o **Holoprosencephaly–polydactyly syndrome** (pseudo-trisomy 13 syndrome, MIM 264480)
    - ▪ Autosomal recessive lethal syndrome likely due to path-ogenic variants in ciliopathy genes in the Meckel/Joubert spectrum
    - ▪ Holoprosencephaly, oral clefts, cardiac anomaly, and pol-ydactyly are features in common with T13.
- o **Smith–Lemli–Opitz syndrome*** (SLOS, MIM 270400)
    - ▪ There is significant overlap between T13 and the severe presentation of SLOS, but the genital abnormalities in males and the Y-shaped 2–3 toe syndactyly in SLOS are distinctive.

# Evaluation and Management

- Evaluate all major organ systems to identify the range of anomalies.
- Genetic testing
    - o Chromosome analysis is preferred because it distinguishes between trisomy, translocations, and mosaicism. Use cord blood or peripheral blood sample.
    - o FISH provides a rapid preliminary diagnosis in 24–48 hours.
    - o Microarray only if chromosome analysis is normal.
        - ▪ Microarray does not detect translocations.
    - o Test parents when a translocation is detected in the infant.
- Prognosis: a severely life-limiting disorder that is usually lethal
    - o Each patient warrants a careful, individualized evaluation.
    - o Establish a treatment plan with the family, physicians and nurses (prenatally, if possible).
        - ▪ Balance the severity of the infant's problems with the wishes of the family and their ability to care for a mul-tiply handicapped child.

- ▪ Most families desire comfort care with bereavement counseling and home-based hospice/palliative care nursing support.
- ▪ When family and/or medical providers differ about management, a multidisciplinary care team, including an ethicist, may help reach consensus on major health care decisions.
    - o If the infant survives for 2 or 3 months, G-tube placement may make feeding easier for caretakers. Palliative cardiac surgery may be considered on an individual basis.
- Communicate with the family regularly and openly.
    - o Tell them about the suspected diagnosis as soon as possible.
    - o Establish rapport, listen and respond to their concerns, and respect their wishes to the extent possible.
    - o Communicate in a clear, consistent manner, avoiding med-ical jargon.
    - o Offer the family bereavement counseling and general sup-port from social services, home health, and palliative care providers.
    - o In longer term survivors a multidisciplinary approach is helpful to the family. Prolongation of life is possible in some of these children, although severe intellectual disability is certain. Emphasis on the quality of life is important.
    - o Provide information to families, especially useful for longer term survivors, available from SOFT (Support Organization for Trisomy 18, 13 and Related Disorders) at https://trisomy.org.

# Further Reading

Barry SC, Walsh CA, Burke AL, et al. (2015) Natural history of fetal trisomy 13 after prenatal diagnosis. Am J Med Genet. 167A:147–50. PMID 25339456

Carey JC. (2012) Perspectives on the care and management of infants with trisomy 18 and trisomy 13: Striving for balance. Curr Opin Pediatr. 24:672–8. PMID 23044555

Janvier A, Farlow B, Barrington K. (2016) Cardiac surgery for chil-dren with trisomies 13 and 18: Where are we now? Semin Perinatol. 40:254–60. PMID 26847083

Kroes I, Janssens S, Defoort P. (2014) Ultrasound features in trisomy 13 (Patau syndrome) and trisomy 18 (Edwards syndrome) in a consecutive series of 47 cases. Facts Views Vis Obgyn. 6:245–9. PMID 25593701

# 4S

## Turner Syndrome

## Definition

Turner syndrome (TS) causes gonadal dysgenesis because of partial or complete monosomy X.

- Incidence 1/2,500 live-born females
- Sporadic, low recurrence risk
  - Not associated with advanced maternal age
  - Rarely, a mother transmits a structurally abnormal X chromosome to her daughter or a father transmits a dicentric Y chromosome that is lost during cell division.
  - Monozygotic twins can be discordant for TS.

## Diagnosis

*Pearl.* Only one-third of babies with TS, usually those with lymphedema, is diagnosed as newborns. Consider TS in female infants *without* lymphedema who have IUGR, left-sided cardiac lesions (HLHS; CoA), or renal anomalies.

- Clinical features
  - Hydrops fetalis (Figure 5.2A) is often associated with fetal demise
  - Prenatal growth failure: mean BW deficit: 600 g
    - In 10%, BW deficit: >1,000 g
  - Craniofacial
    - Ptosis, epicanthal folds, lower canthal folds, down-slanting palpebral fissures, prominent ears
    - High arched palate, micrognathia
    - Low-set posterior hairline, excess posterior nuchal skin (Figure 5.2B), webbed neck
  - Cardiovascular 40–50%
    - Bicuspid aortic valve (BAV) 34%
    - CoA 19.1%
      - BAV and CoA are associated with loss of Xp.
    - Systemic venous abnormalities 8.1%
    - VSD 5.2%
    - Pulmonary venous abnormalities 4%
    - HLHS, single ventricle 3.5%

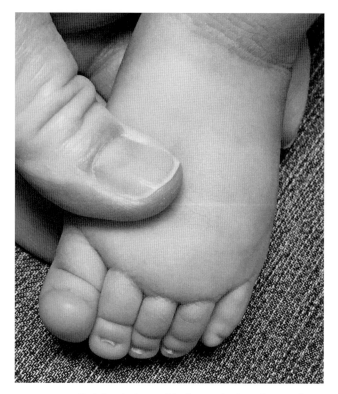

FIGURE 4S.1 Peripheral edema of the feet can be the only sign of Turner syndrome. The vertically oriented toenails can be brought down with gentle tension from Steri-Strips.

- ASD 1.7%
- Coronary artery abnormalities 1.6%
  o Extremities
    - Lymphedema ~1/3: neck, hands, feet (Figure 4S.1)
    - Spoon-shaped nails
  o Other: widely spaced nipples, shield-shaped chest
  o Renal anomalies 30–40%
    - Collecting system anomalies 20%, horseshoe kidney 10%, other 5%
  o Later onset
    - Cardiovascular: hypertension 50%, aortic dilation 3–8%
      • Aortic dissection occurs in adolescents and adults, even without preceding aortic root dilatation.
        • In ~10% of aortic dissections in TS, there is no preexisting cardiac anomaly or hypertension.
    - Skeletal: cubitus valgus, Madelung deformity
    - Short stature: caused by loss of *SHOX* on Xp or Yp
      • Height usually below normal by 3 years
        • 90% are short by 5 years
      • Mean untreated adult height 143 cm
        • Growth hormone treatment adds 11.9 cm.
    - Endocrine
      • Spontaneous puberty in one-third, more common with mosaicism
        • Spontaneous menses are uncommon.
      • Hypothyroidism
    - Infertility

- Pregnancy has been achieved with donor eggs.
  o Intelligence usually normal
    - Attention deficit, executive functioning problems, and learning disabilities are common.

*Pearl*: Females with TS can manifest X-linked recessive disorders such as hemophilia, muscular dystrophy, and fragile X syndrome.

- Chromosome findings
  o Monosomy X ~45%: 45,X
    - 70% of live-born patients with 45,X have lost a *paternal* sex chromosome.
    - Chromosome analysis cannot distinguish the parental origin of the X chromosome.
  o Mosaicism ~50%: 45,X/46,XX; 45,X/47,XXX
    - FISH: best for detecting mosaicism
    - 45,X/46,XX ~15%
      • Generally, milder phenotype, especially when prenatally diagnosed: taller stature, less renal dysfunction
      • Higher chance of spontaneous menarche, fertility
  o Structurally abnormal X chromosome
    - Deletion: 46,X,del(Xp)
    - Isochromosome: i(Xq) or i(Xp) is caused by two copies of the long (q) or short (p) arm connected by a centromere.
    - Ring: r(X)
      • When the X-inactivation center, *XIST*, is deleted, in 30% of r(X), there is ID.
    - Balanced or unbalanced X/autosome translocation
    - Marker chromosome ~3%: 46,X,+mar; 45,X/46,X,+mar
      • ID 66%
  o Y chromosome 5–10%: 45,X/46,XY, 45,X/46,XY/47,XYY; 45,X/46,X,idic(Y)
    - Increased risk of gonadoblastoma
    - 45,X/46,XY: When prenatally diagnosed with normal fetal US exam, most are phenotypically normal males.
    - 46,X,del(Y) males: Loss of *SRY* causes TS phenotype even without a 45,X cell line.

*Pearl*: A false-positive cfDNA maternal screening test for a fetal sex chromosome abnormality may be associated with a *maternal* X chromosome abnormality: ~10% of these mothers have 45,X/46,XX. Deletion of *STS* on Xp, which causes X-linked ichthyosis, may also produce a false-positive cfDNA test.

## Differential Diagnosis

- Cystic hygroma
  o Septated cystic hygroma in the first trimester: 1 in 285 pregnancies
    - Higher morbidity and mortality than increased nuchal translucency

- Cystic hygroma has high mortality even when chromosome analysis is normal.
  o Etiology
    - Chromosome aneuploidy 50%
      - After TS, **Down syndrome**\* is the most common cause.
    - Cardiac defects,\* **Noonan syndrome and other RASopathies**\*
- Hydrops fetalis\*
  o Congenital lymphedema syndromes
    - **Milroy disease** (MIM 153100)
    - **Distichiasis lymphedema syndrome** (MIM 153400)
    - **Microcephaly lymphedema syndrome** (MIM 152950)
  o **Noonan syndrome and other RASopathies**\*

## Evaluation and Management

- Evaluate for associated malformations.
  o Pediatric cardiology evaluation, echocardiogram is recommended even if fetal echocardiogram was normal
    - Plan to repeat a normal echocardiogram because aortic dilation can develop later.
  o Abdominal US
  o Hearing screen
- Chromosome analysis is the preferred diagnostic test.
  o A standard analysis of 30 metaphase cells can detect 10% mosaicism with 95% confidence. Note: Microarray can miss 45,X/47,XXX mosaicism.
  o Confirm positive prenatal tests with chromosome analysis on blood.
    - When normal, consider testing a second tissue type.
  o Add FISH or microarray under these circumstances.
    - For pure 45,X, suspected mosaicism, suspected TS with 46,XY: Add FISH with X and Y centromere probes.
    - For ring X, marker chromosome or X/autosome translocation: Add FISH for *XIST* and microarray.
    - When a female with 45,X has clitoromegaly or mixed gonadal dysgenesis, add FISH for *SRY* and microarray.
- Follow published clinical practice guidelines and consensus statements.

  o The Pediatric Endocrine Society: http://www.eje-online.org/content/177/3/G1.full.pdf+html
  o American Academy of Pediatrics: http://pediatrics.aappublications.org/content/111/3/692
- Counsel parents to anticipate otitis media, hearing loss, short stature, hypothyroidism, hypertension, hormonal replacement therapy.
- Refer to family support group.
  o Turner Syndrome Society: http://www.turnersyndrome.org
- Refer to Endocrinology before the onset of short stature to plan for growth hormone treatment.

*Pearl*: Straighten vertically oriented toenails by applying topical liquid adhesive (e.g., benzoin) to the toenail, letting it dry to a tacky consistency, and attaching one end of a Steri-Strip skin closure to the nail. Pull the Steri-Strip snugly to apply gentle tension to the nail. Keeping the Steri-Strip taut, attach the other end to the ventral surface of the toe. Reapply Steri-Strips daily until toenails are horizontal.

## Further Reading

Frías JL, Davenport ML; Committee on Genetics and Section on Endocrinology. (2003) Health supervision for children with Turner syndrome. Pediatrics. 111:692–702. PMID 12612263

Gravholt CH, Andersen NH, Conway GS, et al., (2017) Clinical practice guidelines for the care of girls and women with Turner syndrome: proceedings from the 2016 Cincinnati International Turner Syndrome Meeting. Eur J Endocrinol. 177:G1–G70. PMID 28705803

Kriksciuniene R, Zilaitiene B, Verkauskiene R. (2016) The current management of Turner Syndrome. Minerva Endocrinol. 41:105–21. PMID 26878561

Ranke MB. (2015) Why treat girls with Turner syndrome with growth hormone? Growth and beyond. Pediatr Endocrinol Rev. 12:356–65. PMID 26182480

Shankar RK, Backeljauw PF. (2018) Current best practice in the management of Turner syndrome. Ther Adv Endocrinol Metab. 9(1):33–40. PMID 29344338

Tokita MJ, Sybert VP. (2016) Postnatal outcomes of prenatally diagnosed 45,X/46,XX. Am J Med Genet A. 170A:1196–201. PMID 26789280

# 5S

# Wolf–Hirschhorn Syndrome

## Definition

- Wolf–Hirschhorn syndrome or 4p minus syndrome (WHS, MIM 194190) is caused by a contiguous, usually terminal, deletion on distal chromosome 4p.
  - Deletion of terminal 4p is "pure" in 55%.
  - An unbalanced translocation involves distal 4p in 45%.
  - Rare: ring chromosome 4, mosaicism for the deletion or other chromosome 4 rearrangement

*Pearl*: Unbalanced familial translocations are a common cause of WHS. Recommend chromosome analysis with FISH for the terminal end of 4p for the parents of a child with WHS.

  - Deletion size ranges from 2 to >20 Mb.
    - Severity and risk of death increase with the size of the deletion.
  - The classic deletion includes a 200-kb region at 4p16.3, 1.4–1.9 Mb from the terminal end of 4p. Some are interstitial deletions.
    - Two critical regions: proximal WHSCR1 (two genes are responsible for the phenotype: *WHSC1* and *WHSC2*) and the more distal WHSCR2
      - A de novo novel probably pathogenic nonsense variant in *WHSC1* has been reported in a patient with syndromic intellectual disability who has a phenotype that overlaps WHS.
      - Note: More distal deletions that encompass only *WHSCR2* do not produce the WHS phenotype.
- Incidence 1/20,000 to 1/50,000 live births
- Females predominate: 2 F:1 M
- Mortality
  - Infant mortality ~17%
  - Mortality by 2 years ~21%
  - Median survival 34+ years for de novo deletions; 18+ years for unbalanced translocations

## Diagnosis

- Prenatal findings
  - Microcephaly, congenital heart disease 50%, IUGR, oral clefting, other structural anomalies
  - Perinatal distress 30%

- Clinical features
  - Poor growth; low birth weight 81%
  - Craniofacial
    - Hypertelorism, prominent eyes, arched eyebrows, broad nose (Figure 5S.1)
    - Broad high nasal bridge and long nose flow into a prominent glabella, creating a straight line in profile—similar to a Greek warrior helmet (Figure 5S.2)
    - Exotropia, ptosis, optic nerve defects, coloboma
    - Conductive hearing loss 40%
    - Short philtrum
    - Oral clefts 30% (Figure 5S.3)
    - Thin upper lip, tented mouth, downturned corners

*Pearl*: Microcephaly and other key features may not be present when there is an unbalanced translocation or larger deletion due to the dosage effect of genes from the reciprocal chromosome.

  - GU malformations 30–50%
  - Skeletal: vertebral defects, fused ribs, clubfeet, split hand
  - GI: feeding problems, GERD, failure to thrive. G tube may be required.
  - CNS
    - Microcephaly 90%
    - Structural brain anomalies ~80%

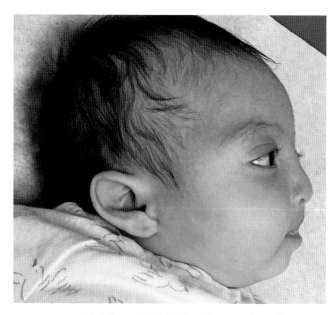

FIGURE 5S.2  This infant with Wolf–Hirschhorn syndrome has a broad and prominent nose that resembles an ancient Greek warrior's helmet.

- Thin corpus callosum, enlarged lateral ventricles, decreased white matter, cortical atrophy, cerebellar hypoplasia (posterior lobe)

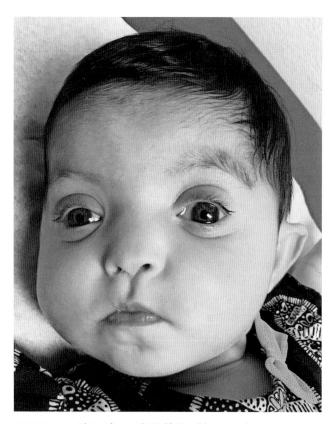

FIGURE 5S.1  This infant with Wolf-Hirschhorn syndrome has a terminal deletion of chromosome 4p and the typical facial features of hypertelorism, arched eyebrows, prominent eyes, and a broad nose.

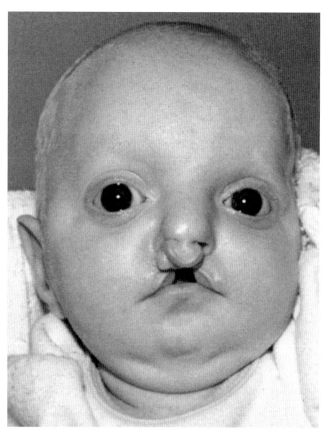

FIGURE 5S.3  Bilateral cleft lip is relatively common in Wolf–Hirschhorn syndrome.

- Hypotonia, developmental delay
  - Later onset
    - Seizures >90%
      - The critical region for seizures contains the candidate gene *PIGG*.
      - Various seizure types
      - Peak incidence 6–12 months
      - Often triggered by fever
      - Distinctive electroencephalogram (EEG) pattern 90%
      - With treatment, seizures resolve in up to 55%.
    - Intellectual disability: mild 10%, moderate 25%, severe 65%
    - Poor expressive language; gestural vocabulary increases with time
    - Many milestones are achieved in late childhood or young adulthood: walking independently 20%, with support 25%, self-feeding 10%, daytime sphincter control 10%.
- Microarray is the preferred first diagnostic test.
  - Microarray identifies all deletions and most translocations.
    - Approximately half of the translocations are not visible with conventional chromosome analysis but are evident with FISH or microarray.
    - FISH may miss 5% of deletions detectable on microarray.
    - However, 20% of WHS translocations cannot be identified as such by microarray because the partner chromosome is an acrocentric short arm. The microarray will identify these rearrangements as deletions.
      - Follow up with chromosome analysis to detect these translocations.
  - Unbalanced translocations can be familial, inherited from a carrier parent, or de novo.
    - Follow up all unbalanced translocations with parental FISH and chromosome analysis.

## Evaluation and Management

- Evaluate for other anomalies.
  - Echocardiogram, ECG
  - Abdominal US
  - Dilated eye exam
  - Swallow study for suspected GERD
  - Evaluate renal function with BUN, Cr, urinalysis
- Chromosomal microarray is preferred first test; follow with chromosome analysis for the following indications:
  - When microarray reveals a "pure" 4p terminal deletion, order chromosome analysis to detect "silent" acrocentric translocations missed on microarray.

- Test parents with FISH and conventional chromosome analysis to rule out a balanced translocation, when the baby has an unbalanced translocation.
- Multidisciplinary conference with parents to discuss prognosis and plan for care
- Anticipate and plan for common problems and counsel parents about:
  - Feeding problems, failure to thrive, poor growth
    - Monitor growth parameters using WHS-specific growth charts (Antonius, 2008).
    - Caloric requirements are less than expected and should *not* be based on expectations for typical infants.
    - Treat GERD, and consider early G tube placement.
      - Do not overfeed after a G tube has been placed.
  - Sleep apnea is common; consider a sleep study.
  - Seizures begin at 6 months–3 years.
    - Treat with valproate and/or phenobarbital.
    - EEG, follow up with a neurologist
    - Optimal management of seizures can improve outcome.
  - Frequent hospitalizations in early years
    - With chronic infections, evaluate for immunodeficiency: specific antibody responses, mitogen studies, B cell counts, T cell subsets; quantitative IgA, IgG, IgM
- Refer for genetic counseling, early intervention/infant development program, and parent support group.
  - http://4p-supportgroup.org

## Further Reading

Antonius T, Draaisma J, Levtchenko E, et al. (2008) Growth charts for Wolf–Hirschhorn syndrome (0–4 years of age). Eur J Pediatr. 167:807–10. PMID 17874131

Battaglia A, Carey JC, South ST. (2015) Wolf–Hirschhorn syndrome: A review and update. Am J Med Genet C Semin Med Genet. 169:216–23. PMID 26239400

Battaglia A, Filippi T, Carey JC. (2008) Update on the clinical features and natural history of Wolf–Hirschhorn (4p-) syndrome: Experience with 87 patients and recommendations for routine health supervision. Am J Med Genetics C Semin Med Genet. 148C:246–251. PMID 18932224

Ho KS, South ST, Lortz A, et al. (2016) Chromosomal microarray testing identifies a 4p terminal region associated with seizures in Wolf–Hirschhorn syndrome. J Med Genet. 53:256–63. PMID 26747863

Lozier ER, Konovalov FA, Kanivets IV, et al. (2018) De novo nonsense mutation in WHSC1 (NSD2) in patient with intellectual disability and dysmorphic features. J Hum Genet. 63(8):919–922. PMID 29760529

South ST, Whitby H, Battaglia A, et al. (2008) Comprehensive analysis of Wolf–Hirschhorn syndrome using array CGH indicates a high prevalence of translocations. Eur J Human Genet. 16:45–52. PMID 17726485

# 6S

## Chromosome 5p Deletion Syndrome

## Definition

- Chromosome 5p deletion syndrome (5p-, cat cry syndrome, cri du chat, MIM 123450) is caused by a deletion of the distal short arm of chr 5, which includes 5p12.
  - The phenotype is determined by the size and position of the deletion and whether other microarray abnormalities are present.
  - Deletions range in size from 560 kb to 40 Mb; there is no common recurring breakpoint.
  - Genes that encode Semaphorin F (*SEMAF*) and δ-catenin (*CTNND2*) map to the critical region for facial dysmorphism and ID at 5p15.2.
  - The high-pitched, cat-like cry has been mapped to proximal 5p15.32, a distal band on chr 5p.
    - Rarely, when a small deletion is limited to 5p15.3, the cat-like cry occurs alone, without other features of the syndrome.
    - Similarly, interstitial deletions that do not include the distal band, 5p15.3, may lack the typical cry.
- Incidence 1/15,000 to 1/50,000 live births
- This deletion is usually de novo with a low recurrence risk. However, it is important to identify the familial cases because they have a high recurrence risk.
  - Deletion—recurrence risk low; paternal origin in 80–90%
    - De novo terminal deletion 80–90%
      - Autosomal dominant multigenerational inheritance of small terminal 5p deletions is rare but reported.
    - De novo interstitial deletion 3–5%
  - Translocation
    - De novo translocation
    - Familial translocation 10–15%—recurrence risk is high.

*Pearl*: Parental chromosomal analysis/FISH should be performed routinely to rule out a familial translocation.

# Diagnosis

Most features of 5p- are nonspecific and common, but the pattern of anomalies, especially the cry, makes this syndrome recognizable.

- Prenatal findings
  - IUGR; other findings uncommon
  - Cell free DNA panels available to evaluate for microdeletions in appropriate situations

- Clinical features
  - Unexplained IUGR and postnatal growth delay
  - Face: mild microcephaly, round face, mild hypertelorism, down-slanting palpebral fissures and epicanthal folds, strabismus, optic nerve abnormalities, preauricular tags, micrognathia, broad nasal bridge (Figure 6S.1A)
  - Other anomalies: hypospadias, cryptorchidism, syndactyly, renal anomalies 6–18%, cardiac defects 18–30%

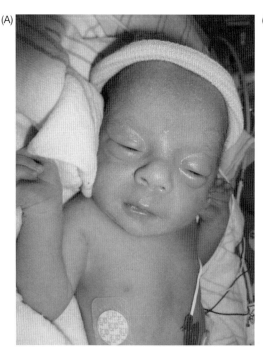
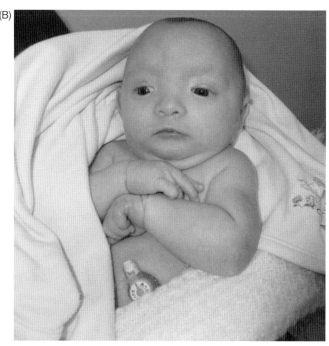
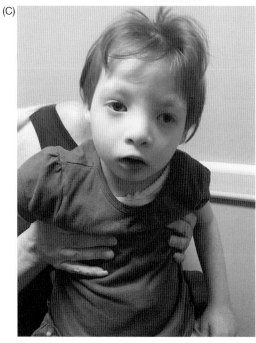

FIGURE 6S.1  Child with 5p- at birth (A), at several months of age (B), and at 5 years of age (C). G tube still in use at age 5.

- o Clinical features are more severe in patients with other microarray abnormalities.
- o CNS anomalies 30%; mega cisterna magna, cerebellar hypoplasia, underdevelopment of brain stem
  - ▪ Seizures are rare.
  - ▪ Abnormal high-pitched, mewing cry is pathognomonic, but it is not present in all affected individuals.
    - • The unusual cry is the single best diagnostic sign.
    - • When present in infancy, it persists through approximately age 1 year.
  - ▪ Hypotonia
  - ▪ Hearing loss ~8%
- o Late diagnosis is not uncommon, especially when symptoms are mild.
  - o In one study, 42% of patients were diagnosed in the newborn period, 81% in the first year, and 18% between 13 months and 47 years. Figures 6S.1B and 6S.1C show the same infant as shown in Figure 6S.1A at ages 9 months and 5 years.
- • Medical complications/development/behavior
  - o Mean IQ 48 (range, <40–75)
  - o GE reflux, poor feeding, hypotonia, cyanotic episodes
  - o Neurodevelopmental effects
    - ▪ Most children are affectionate and gentle; up to 50% are hyperactive (squirmy as infants), distractable; some are aggressive. Autism has been reported.
    - ▪ Hyperacusis 70–80%
    - ▪ Development progresses without regression.
      - • Many skills can be achieved despite severe ID.
      - • 50% walk by age 3 years; all walk eventually.
      - • Language acquisition is slow: 25% use short sentences by age 4½ years, and almost all do so by age 10 years.
    - ▪ Children reared at home do significantly better than those who have been institutionalized.
- • Life expectancy
  - o Childhood mortality is higher when the 5p deletion is part of an unbalanced translocation (~18.5%) compared to a terminal 5p deletion (~4.8%).
    - ▪ Common causes of death: pneumonia, respiratory distress, cardiac defects
  - o Life expectancy is near normal when there is no major organ involvement.
    - ▪ Patients >60 years old have been reported.
- • Differential diagnosis
  - o Other disorders that cause IUGR
    - ▪ Chromosome microdeletions or duplications
    - ▪ Fetal alcohol spectrum disorder
  - o Deletions of chromosome 5p may unmask autosomal recessive disorders localized within the deleted segment such as:
    - ▪ **Primary ciliary dyskinesia** (PCD, MIM 608644)

- • Autosomal recessive disorder, caused by biallelic pathogenic variants in *DNAH5*, at 5p15.2. Individuals with a 5p deletion and PCD have recurrent sinopulmonary infections.

# Evaluation and Management

- • Evaluate for other anomalies.
  - o Echocardiogram
  - o Abdominal US
  - o Ophthalmology examination
- • Genetic testing
  - o Chromosome microarray is the preferred first-tier test.
    - ▪ FISH for the 5p telomere is also diagnostic, but microarray is preferred because other gains or losses will also be detected.
  - o When a *terminal* 5p deletion is detected on microarray
    - ▪ Order chromosome analysis to rule out an unbalanced translocation with an acrocentric chromosome.
    - ▪ Perform chromosome analysis or FISH for 5p (depending on size of deletion) on both parents to detect a familial translocation or inversion.
- • Refer for early infant intervention, occupational therapy, physical therapy, and speech therapy.
- • If feeding problems do not resolve, a G tube should be considered.
- • Monitor for associated long-term problems: chronic otitis media, sensorineural hearing loss, scoliosis.
  - o Utilize syndrome-specific growth charts for 5p.
- • Genetic counseling for recurrence risks
- • Refer families to 5p- online support groups.
  - o https://www.criduchat.org
  - o https://fivepminus.org

# Further Reading

Cerruti Mainardi P. (2006) Cri du chat syndrome. Orphanet J Rare Dis. 1:33. PMID 16953888

Guala A, Spunton M, Tognon F, et al. (2016) Psychomotor development in cri du chat syndrome: Comparison in two Italian cohorts with different rehabilitation methods. Sci World J. 2016:3125283. PMID 28004033

Marinescu RC, Mainardi PC, Collins MR, et al. (2000) Growth charts for cri-du-chat syndrome: An international collaborative study. Am J Med Genet. 94:153–62. PMID 10982972

Nguyen JM, Qualmann KJ, Okashah R, et al. (2015) 5p deletions: Current knowledge and future directions. Am J Med Genet C Semin Med Genet. 169:224–38. PMID 26235846

# 7S

# Chromosome 22q11.2 Deletion Syndrome

## Definition

- Deletion of a critical region of 1.5 Mb on chromosome 22q
- Originally called DiGeorge syndrome and velocardofacial syndrome (VCF) based on different phenotypes in early reports
  - In 1965, Dr. Angelo DiGeorge, an endocrinologist, reported a patient with severe cardiac disease, immune deficiency, and hypoparathyroidism.
  - In 1978, Dr. Robert Shprintzen, a speech pathologist, reported patients with cleft palate, cardiac defects, and a characteristic face.

*Pearl*: The 22q11.2 deletion syndrome is the preferred name for this condition. Avoid using other terms that create false distinctions and diagnostic confusion: DiGeorge, partial DiGeorge syndrome, Shprintzen syndrome, velocardiofacial syndrome, CATCH 22, conotruncal anomaly face syndrome, and so on.

- The 22q11.2 deletion syndrome disrupts the formation of structures derived from the third and fourth branchial pouches, thymus, aortic arch, palate, face, and parathyroid glands.
- Repetitive elements at 22q11.2 predispose this region to recurrent rearrangements. Typical and atypical 22q11.2 deletions and duplications cause a varied phenotype.
- Incidence 1:4,000. Most common microdeletion syndrome
  - Mild cases without cardiac or palate defects are underascertained.
    - ~70% diagnosed as newborns, usually those with cleft palate, cardiac defect, or hypocalcemia
- 90% de novo; 10% familial
  - Mothers are affected more often than fathers (Figure 7S.1).
- *TBX1*, within the deleted segment, is a candidate for major findings of 22q deletion.

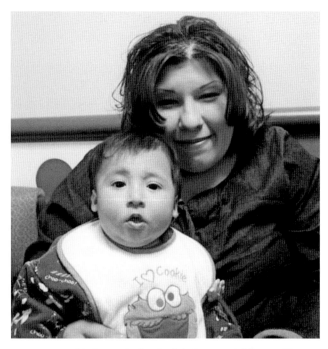

FIGURE 7S.1  Mother and infant both with 22q11.2 deletions. Note that the typical features are less apparent in the mother.

## Diagnosis

- Craniofacial dysmorphic features: variable. Face is characteristic but often subtle in newborns and non-Caucasians.
  - Long, myopathic face; small tented mouth
  - Lateral margins of the nose are parallel; nose lacks normal modeling.
  - Periorbital fullness, hooded eyelids (Figure 7S.2)
  - Asymmetric crying face
    - An excellent clue that can be missed when intubated or if the baby does not cry during the exam
  - Ears small, posteriorly rotated, minor helical anomalies
- Growth
  - Poor postnatal growth, < 3rd percentile, ~40%
- Cardiac >75%
  - Most defects are conotruncal: septal defects, TOF 20%, interrupted aortic arch type B, right aortic arch, truncus arteriosus, vascular rings 5%
- Palatal defects >70%
  - Cleft palate, submucous cleft palate, bifid uvula
  - Velopharyngeal incompetence ~90%
- Limbs
  - Long, slender fingers
  - Clubfeet and camptodactyly not uncommon
  - Postaxial polydactyly-occasional
- Immune deficiency
  - Hypoplastic, absent thymus
    - Low T cell subset; may resolve with age

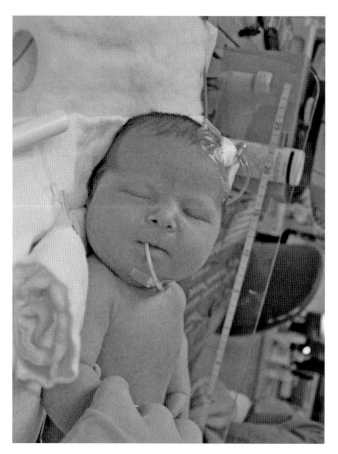

FIGURE 7S.2  Newborn with 22q11.2 deletion.  Subtle facial findings include small mouth, lateral build up to nasal bridge, mild micrognathia and periorbital fullness.

*Pearl:* Low lymphocyte count may be a useful sign in newborns. Be suspicious for this diagnosis when chromosome analysis fails, because abnormal T cells may not respond to phytohemagglutinin.

- Humoral B cell immune deficiency
- Abnormal immunoglobulins
- Hypocalcemia ~50%
  - Usually transient; may recur
  - May cause neonatal seizures
- Skeletal
  - Scoliosis; vertebral anomalies
- Gastrointestinal
  - Abnormal swallowing, dysmotility
  - Nasopharyngeal regurgitation, a feature in many patients
  - Constipation
  - Hirschsprung disease
  - Imperforate anus, malrotation, diaphragmatic hernia, tracheoesophageal fistula
- Renal ~30%
  - Agenesis, multicystic dysplastic kidney
  - *CRKL* haploinsufficiency drives renal abnormalities.
- Hearing loss: conductive, sensorineural

- Ophthalmic
  - Strabismus
  - Sclerocornea
  - Tortuous retinal vessels
  - Posterior embryotoxon
- Psychiatric issues
  - ADHD, obsessive–compulsive disorder (OCD), anxiety
  - Autistic spectrum ~20%
  - Adults: schizophrenia, depression ~25%
- Developmental delays
  - Walking: mean 18 months
  - Language delay
  - Average IQ 70–90
    - Verbal IQ > performance IQ
- Prenatal diagnosis
  - Allows optimal clinical management after delivery.
    - Use of irradiated blood products
    - Monitoring calcium
  - Conotruncal heart defects are the most common finding in the fetus.

# Differential Diagnosis

- Teratogens
  - **Isotretinoin embryopathy** (Accutane)
  - **Maternal diabetes** may act through disruption of similar pathway.
  - **Fetal alcohol spectrum disorder**
- Atypical 22q11.2 chromosome abnormalities
  - Small, atypical, or distal deletions (MIM 611867) or duplications (MIM 608363) of 22q11.2
    - May not be detected by FISH
- Single gene disorders
  - **Alagille syndrome** (MIM 118450)
    - Autosomal dominant trait, due to mutation in *JAG1* or, less commonly, ~7%, chr 20p12 deletion
    - Clinical features: primarily right-sided cardiac defects, posterior embryotoxon, vertebral anomalies
  - **CHARGE syndrome** (MIM 214800)
  - **Oculo-auricular-vertebral syndrome** (OAVS, MIM 164210)
    - Craniofacial and ear abnormalities more prominent in OAVS, not subtle
  - **VACTERL association** (MIM 192350)
  - Other causes of severe combined immunodeficiency
  - *TBX1* mutation, without deletion, can cause typical findings of 22q deletion.

# Evaluation and Management

- Prenatal diagnosis
  - For fetal conotruncal or other major cardiac defect, offer amniocentesis with microarray or cfDNA with microdeletion panel. Recommend confirming cfDNA diagnosis with amniocentesis.
  - When diagnosis is established, counsel family and plan delivery.
    - Refer to pediatric cardiologist and cardiac surgeon.
    - Deliver at a tertiary level facility with appropriate on-site services: NICU, pediatric cardiology.
    - Make arrangements for pediatric cardiothoracic surgery if needed.
- Diagnostic testing
  - Microarray is preferred test: It detects typical and atypical deletions and duplications.
  - FISH detects typical 22q11.2 deletions.
  - Test parents to identify inherited deletion.
- Evaluate for other anomalies.
  - Echocardiogram
  - Renal US
  - Hearing screening at birth and as clinically indicated—at least yearly for first few years of life. Audiology and ENT as needed
- Laboratory studies
  - Monitor serial ionized serum calcium.
  - Quantify T cell subsets.
    - Avoid live vaccines until T cell numbers have normalized.
    - Consider immunology referral.
    - Use irradiated blood products at surgery until immune status is known.
- Anticipate feeding problems, especially postoperatively. Utilize occupational therapy.
- Emphasize the critical need for intensive speech therapy and possible surgery for velopharyngeal insufficiency
- Refer to infant development program.
- Utilize growth charts specific for 22q deletion syndrome.
- Refer to support group.
  - International 22q11.2 Foundation: 22q.org
  - 22q and You Center at the Children's Hospital of Philadelphia– links to support groups

# Further Reading

Bassett AS, McDonald-McGinn DM, et al.; International 22q11.2 Deletion Syndrome Consortium. (2011) Practical guidelines for managing patients with 22q11.2 deletion syndrome. J Pediatr. 159:332–9. PMID 21570089

Levy-Shraga Y, Gothelf D, Goichberg Z, et al. (2017) Growth characteristics and endocrine abnormalities in 22q11.2 deletion syndrome. Am J Med Genet A. 173:1301–8. PMID 28421700

McDonald-McGinn DM, Sullivan KE, Marino B, et al. (2015) 22q11.2 deletion syndrome. Nat Rev Dis Primers. 1:15071. PMID 27189754

Tang KL, Antshel KM, Fremont WP, Kates WR. (2015) Behavioral and psychiatric phenotypes in 22q11.2 deletion syndrome. J Dev Behav Pediatr. 36:639–50. PMID 26372046

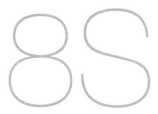

# Achondroplasia

## Definition

- Achondroplasia (MIM 100800) is the most common short-limbed skeletal dysplasia.
- Autosomal dominant disorder, caused by a heterozygous gain-of-function mutation in *FGFR3*, at chromosome 4p16.3
  - Recurrent pathogenic variant >99%: p.Gly380Arg (G380R)
  - De novo change >85%
    - Advanced paternal age is common.
- Incidence ~1/15,000 to 1/25,000
- Infant mortality is increased related to stenosis of the foramen magnum and central sleep apnea.
- Recurrence risk
  - When both parents are unaffected, the recurrence risk is <<1% due to rare germline mosaicism in the father.
  - When one parent is affected, the recurrence risk is 50% (Figure 8S.1).
  - When both parents are affected, the risk is 25% for homozygous lethal achondroplasia, 50% for heterozygous achondroplasia, and 25% for average stature.

## Diagnosis

*Pearl*: A fetal skeletal dysplasia that is diagnosed by fetal US early in pregnancy is *not* achondroplasia, which is diagnosed no earlier than the late second trimester, if at all.

- **Clinical features are distinctive**
  - Diagnosis is usually clinical. Radiographs are confirmatory.
  - Craniofacial: macrocephaly, prominent forehead, depressed nasal bridge, underdeveloped midface as seen in this newborn and at age 1 (Figures 8S.2)
  - **Skeletal findings**
    - Increased upper-to-lower segment ratio: average newborn upper segment:lower segment ratio =1.7
      - Upper segment: top of the head to top of pubic ramus
      - Lower segment: top of pubic ramus to bottom of heel
    - Rhizomelia: short proximal long bones

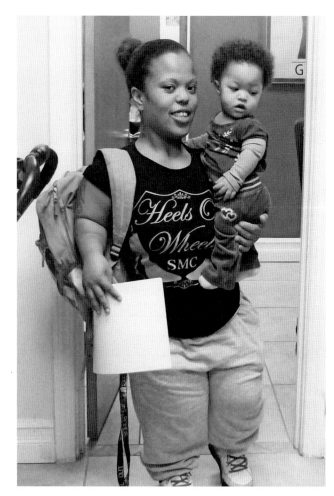

FIGURE 8S.1 Autosomal dominant achondroplasia in a mother and infant.

- ■ Trident-shaped hand: subtle gap between the distal middle and ring fingers. Fingers are of similar length.
- ■ Thoracolumbar gibbus
- ■ Hyperextensible knee joints, reduced elbow extension, extra skin in deep folds
- o Hypotonia, mild to moderate
- o Normal cognitive development; gross motor delayed
- • **Radiographic features**
  - o Small, cuboid vertebral bodies, short pedicles
    - ■ Interpedicular distance does not increase as it should, from cervical to sacral vertebrae.
  - o Small iliac wings, narrow sciatic notches
  - o Short tubular bones, metaphyseal flaring
  - o Short proximal and middle phalanges
- • **Common problems**
  - o Respiratory insufficiency, small chest, airway collapse
  - o GE reflux
  - o Sleep apnea, usually obstructive due to relatively large adenoids and tonsils and midface hypoplasia. Central sleep apnea most often due to compression at the foramen magnum

- o CNS
  - ■ Hypotonia with an otherwise normal neurologic exam resolves over time.
  - ■ Narrow foramen magnum can compress the spinal cord, causing long tract signs, hypotonia, asymmetric reflexes, prolonged ankle clonus, and central apnea.
  - ■ Hydrocephalus ~6% <2 years
    - • Lateral ventricles are normally larger and extra-axial fluid is often present.
    - • Plot head circumference on achondroplasia growth curves for males and females.
    - • Hydrocephalus can be overdiagnosed.

*Pearl*: SIDS is increased (~7%) in achondroplasia due to craniocervical cord compression.

- • **Later complications**
  - o Otitis media, middle ear dysfunction, conductive hearing loss
  - o Exaggerated lumbar lordosis, lumbar stenosis, genu varum, tibial overgrowth

## Differential Diagnosis

- • Achondroplasia can be overdiagnosed as it is better known and more common than other skeletal dysplasias.
- • **Hypochondroplasia** (MIM 146000)
  - o Autosomal dominant skeletal dysplasia, caused by a different heterozygous pathogenic variant in the same gene, *FGFR3*
  - o Clinical features: uncommonly diagnosed in the newborn but macrocephaly can occur in infancy. Milder than achondroplasia: prominent forehead, flat midface. Proportions are usually normal at <2 or 3 years.
    - ■ Diminished IQ 9–25%, ADHD, learning difficulties
- • **Thanatophoric dysplasia** (MIM 187600)
  - o Lethal autosomal dominant skeletal dysplasia, caused by a heterozygous pathogenic variant in *FGFR3*, usually p.Lys650Glu
  - o Clinical features: more severe than achondroplasia: macrocephaly, small facial features. Severe rhizomelia of all limbs, redundant rolls of skin, sausage-like fingers, narrow thorax, short ribs
    - ■ Pulmonary hypoplasia causes lethality in pregnancy or perinatal period; rare survival past infancy with extraordinary medical support

*Pearl*: Despite their names, **achondroplasia** and **pseudoachondroplasia** (MIM 177170) have little in common. Pseudoachondroplasia is a distinct and unrelated skeletal dysplasia with a normal appearance at birth. Short stature and a

(A)

(B)

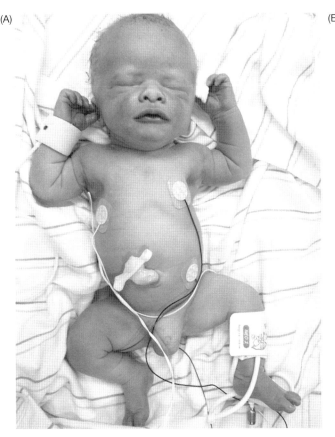
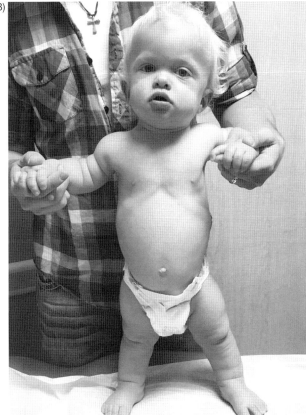

FIGURE 8S.2 (A) Newborn shows typical clinical findings of achondroplasia with macrocephaly, mild rhizomelic shortening, and a slightly small chest. (B) Same child at age 1 year.

waddling gate present in the first 2 years of life due to a pathogenic variant in the *COMP* gene.

- **Homozygous achondroplasia**
  - Lethal skeletal dysplasia
  - 25% risk with each pregnancy when both parents have achondroplasia
  - Clinical features: respiratory insufficiency due to severely restricted chest size

## Evaluation and Management

- Genetic testing: targeted mutation analysis for known *FGFR3* mutation. May not be necessary if clinical/radiologic diagnosis is clear
- Counsel parents *prior* to hospital discharge.
  - Offer a positive prognosis.
  - Head support: Avoid excessive motion of head or hyperflexion of the head onto the chest.
    - Avoid infant swings, sling-back baby seats, soft front-loading baby carriers, umbrella-style strollers, walkers and jumpers.
    - Support head in car seat.

- Avoid aggravating lumbar gibbus.
  - Keep baby relatively horizontal.
  - Discourage early sitting and weight bearing.
- Increase truncal tone with "tummy time."
- Prompt medical evaluation for apnea/snoring/respiratory distress.
- **CNS imaging**: Neuro signs and symptoms should guide imaging for possible cord compression.
  - Weakness, decreased or asymmetric movement, apnea, weak suck, poor feeding, sweating, sustained clonus, asymmetric reflexes, delayed developmental milestones per AAP guidelines for achondroplasia
  - Increasing head circumference on achondroplasia-specific growth curves, clonus and worsening or persistent hypotonia
  - Abnormal sleep study: central sleep apnea
  - MRI is the most useful modality in assessing the foramen magnum. CT can also be helpful.
- **Anticipate common complications**
  - Respiratory
    - Respiratory insufficiency
      - Small thorax and decreased compliance limit respiration
    - Obstructive and central apnea
      - Order sleep study on emergent basis

- Refer to neurosurgery if imaging measurements of foramen magnum suggest cord compression.
- Treat with CPAP
  ○ Neurologic status, hydrocephalus
- Measure head circumference closely through the first 1 or 2 years of life.
- Monitor for cervicomedullary junction cord compression and foramen magnum narrowing based on clinical symptoms.
- Utilize an experienced pediatric radiologist.
  - Compare with achondroplasia-specific norms for head circumference, lateral ventricle size, and foramen magnum measurements
- Clinical follow-up
  ○ Use AAP guidelines for health supervision: http://pediatrics.aappublications.org/content/116/3/771.full?sid=7c6d8c08-341f-498e-a968-9cec515d032e.
  ○ Use achondroplasia-specific growth and developmental charts.
  ○ Monitor hearing annually, and treat otitis media to prevent conductive hearing loss.
  ○ Later: monitor for genu varum, obesity, and spinal stenosis. Instruct to avoid gymnastics and high-impact sports. Leg lengthening surgery available to older individuals; important to pursue with experienced surgeon after psychosocial evaluation of patient and family.
  ○ Counsel regarding developmental milestones.
- Low muscle tone <2 years
- Speech delay indicates probable middle ear disease.
- Normal intelligence overall; may be slightly lower than that of siblings, although this has not been widely studied

○ Novel treatment protocols are under active investigation and trials are currently enrolling patients.
- C-type natriuretic peptide antagonizes *FGFR3* downstream signaling by inhibiting *MAPK* pathway: https://www.clinicaltrials.gov.
- Refer to support groups such as Little People of America: http://www.lpaonline.org.

# Further Reading

Hoover-Fong JE, McGready J, Schulze KJ, et al. (2007) Weight for age charts for children with achondroplasia. Am J Med Genet A. 143A:2227–35. PMID 17764078

Horton WA, Rotter JI, Rimoin DL, et al. (1978) Standard growth curves for achondroplasia. J Pediatr. 93:435–8. PMID 690757

Ireland PJ, Pacey V, Zankl A, et al. (2014) Optimal management of complications associated with achondroplasia. Appl Clin Genet. 7:117–25. PMID 25053890

Pauli RM, Legare JM. Achondroplasia. (2018) In: Adam MP, Ardinger HH, Pagon RA, Wallace SE, Bean LJH, Stephens K, Amemiya A, editors. GeneReviews®[Internet]. Seattle (WA): University of Washington, Seattle; 1993–2018. PMID 20301331

Trotter TL, Hall JG; American Academy of Pediatrics Committee on Genetics. (2005) Health supervision for children with achondroplasia. Pediatrics. 116:771–83. PMID 16140722

Tunkel D, Alade Y, Kerbavaz R, et al. (2012). Hearing loss in skeletal dysplasia patients. Am J Med Genet A. 158A:1551–5. PMID 22628261

White KK, Bompadre V, Goldberg MJ, et al. (2016) Best practices in the evaluation and treatment of foramen magnum stenosis in achondroplasia during infancy. Am J Med Genet A. 170:42–51. PMID 26394886

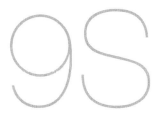

# Beckwith–Wiedemann Syndrome

## Definition

- Beckwith–Wiedemann syndrome (BWS, MIM 130650) is an autosomal dominant overgrowth syndrome caused by disruption of imprinted genes on chromosome 11p15.5.
- Incidence 1/11,000; mild cases may not be ascertained.

*Pearl*: BWS occurs more often with ART: 1/4,000, primarily from hypomethylated maternal alleles on chromosome 11p15.5.

- Usually sporadic
  - Positive family history 15%
  - 1 M:1 F
  - MZ twins are usually concordant but may be discordant, as in Figure 9S.1.

- Molecular etiology: epigenetic aberrations, abnormal methylation patterns, paternal uniparental disomy, mutations, deletions, duplications in two imprinted gene clusters on chromosome 11p15.5. Rarely, BWS is caused by mosaic genome-wide paternal uniparental isodisomy involving all chromosomes.
  - Detection rate for molecular testing is 75–80%; normal results in blood can be due to mosaicism and do not rule out BWS
- Prenatal findings: macrosomia, macroglossia, visceromegaly, polyhydramnios
  - Large placenta with mesenchymal dysplasia; long, thick umbilical cord
- Clinical features: prematurity, LGA, hypoglycemia 50%, hyperinsulinemia 5%, visceromegaly, limb asymmetry, hemihyperplasia (hemihypertrophy), omphalocele, diastasis recti, umbilical hernia. Cardiomegaly usually resolves spontaneously.
- Nevus flammeus, macroglossia, malar flattening, infraorbital creases, prominent eyes, posterior ear creases, helical or lobular pits or indentations (Figure 9S.2).
  - Rare: cleft palate, polydactyly, diaphragmatic hernia, extra nipples, genital anomalies
- Embryonal tumors (Wilms tumor and hepatoblastoma) 7.5%
  - Tumor surveillance is advised every three months until age 8 years

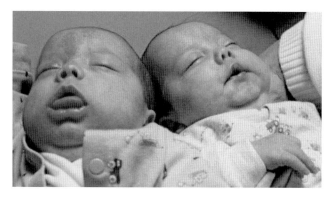

FIGURE 9S.1 These monozygotic twins are discordant for Beckwith–Wiedemann syndrome. This syndrome is more common after conception using ART.

## Differential Diagnosis

- These disorders cause large birth weight, hemihyperplasia, macroglossia, neonatal hypoglycemia or hyperinsulinism.
  - Chromosome anomalies
    - **Down syndrome**\*
    - **Deletion 9q, dup 11p15.5**

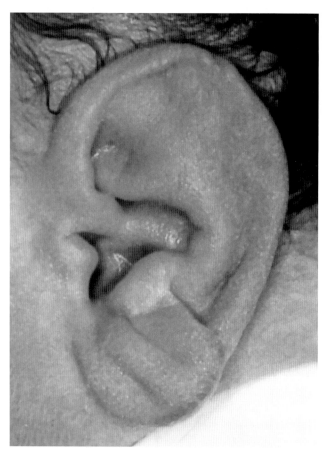

FIGURE 9S.2 Creases, pits, and indentations in the lobule are useful diagnostic signs in Beckwith–Wiedemann syndrome. They can also occur on the posterior surface of the helix and lobule.

- **Cantu syndrome** (MIM 239850)
- **CLOVES** or **Proteus syndromes** (MIM 176920)
- **Costello syndrome** (MIM 218040) or other **RASopathy**\*
- Congenital disorders of glycosylation
- **Congenital hypothyroidism, hypopituitarism**
- **Infant of a diabetic mother**\*
- **Kabuki syndrome** (MIM 147920, 300867)
- **KATP channel-related hyperinsulinism** (MIM 601820)
- **Klippel–Trenaunay syndrome** (MIM 149000)
- Metabolic defects: fatty acid oxidation, glycogen storage, lysosomal storage, mitochondrial
- **Neurofibromatosis type 1** (MIM 162200)
- **Perlman syndrome** (MIM 267000)
- **Simpson–Golabi–Behmel syndrome** (MIM 312870)
- **Sotos syndrome** (MIM 117550)
- **Transient neonatal diabetes mellitus type 1** (MIM 601410)
- Vascular lymphatic tongue malformation with cystic hygroma

## Evaluation and Management

- Document pregnancy history: subfertility, ART, polyhydramnios, large fetal size.
- Record family history: parental birth weights, asymmetry, macroglossia, omphalocele.
- Examine parents: posterior ear creases and pits.

*Pearl:* Examine parents' baby pictures, even when family history is negative.

- Evaluate for associated anomalies.
  - Placental size, histology, and length of umbilical cord
    - Helpful in mild BWS or in preterm babies
  - Abdominal US to establish baseline. Evaluate any renal anomalies for possible tumor.
  - Echocardiogram
- Monitor for complications.
  - Consult endocrinology for severe persistent hypoglycemia, which may require prolonged diazoxide and partial pancreatic excision.
  - Macroglossia can affect breathing, sleep, and feeding.
    - Feeding may be easier when prone.
    - Sleep study
    - Jaw usually grows to accommodate the large tongue
    - Reduction glossectomy may be indicated for persistent sleep apnea and/or feeding problems. The surgically altered tongue can have a good appearance and normal function. An experienced surgical team is needed for this complex procedure to reduce complications.

- Implement tumor surveillance ASAP using established protocols.
  - Include infants with hemihyperplasia and others without all features of BWS.
    - When MZ twins are discordant, monitor *both* twins for tumors.
  - Abdominal US every 3 months until age 8 years
  - Serum AFP level every 3 months until age 4 years
    - Follow downward trend as the normally elevated newborn AFP decreases over first year.
    - Rising AFP supports hepatoblastoma.
- Molecular genetic testing
  - Test individuals with two or more signs: LGA, hemihyperplasia, macroglossia, omphalocele, hyperinsulinism, placentomegaly, visceromegaly.
  - Sporadic BWS
    - Order chromosome 11p15.5 methylation panel (methylation-sensitive PCR or MLPA).
    - If negative, order *CDKN1C* gene analysis and microarray.
  - Familial BWS
    - Order *CDKN1C* gene analysis, and follow with 11p15.5 methylation panel.
    - When negative, order microarray.
  - To detect mosaicism, test a tissue other than blood.
  - Chromosome analysis identifies chromosome 11p15.5 rearrangements; ~1% of all BWS.

*Pearl*: BWS, an overgrowth disorder, and Russell–Silver syndrome (MIM 180860), an IUGR disorder, are "mirror image" syndromes. A loss-of-function pathogenic variant in the growth-regulation gene *CDKN1C* causes BWS, whereas a gain-of-function pathogenic variant in the same gene causes Russell–Silver or IMAGe syndromes (MIM 614732), another IUGR syndrome.

- Long-term outcome generally good
  - Intelligence usually normal
    - ID more common with prematurity, untreated hypoglycemia, duplication of paternal chromosome 11q15.5
  - Reassure parents that size and facial appearance typically normalize, often by 9–11 years.
    - Expect final height in upper normal range.
- Recommend outpatient genetic follow-up.

## Further Reading

Baskin B, Choufani S, Chen YA, et al. (2014) High frequency of copy number variations (CNVs) in the chromosome 11p15 region in patients with Beckwith–Wiedemann syndrome. Hum Genet. 133:321–30. PMID 24154661

Eggermann T, Binder G, Brioude F, et al. (2014) *CDKN1C* mutations: Two sides of the same coin. Trends Mol Med. 20:614–22. PMID 25262539

Mussa A, Russo S, De Crescenzo A, et al. (2016) (Epi)genotype–phenotype correlations in Beckwith–Wiedemann syndrome. Eur J Hum Genet. 24:183–90. PMID 25898929

Õunap K. (2016) Silver–Russell syndrome and Beckwith–Wiedemann syndrome: Opposite phenotypes with heterogeneous molecular etiology. Mol Syndromol. 7:110–21. PMID 27587987

Prada CE, Zarate YA, Hopkin RJ. (2012) Genetic causes of macroglossia: Diagnostic approach. Pediatrics. 129:e431–7. PMID 22250026

Weksberg R, Shuman C, Beckwith JB. (2010) Beckwith–Wiedemann syndrome. Eur J Hum Genet. 18:8–14. PMID 19550435

Wilkins-Haug L, Porter A, Hawley P, Benson CB. (2009) Isolated fetal omphalocele, Beckwith–Wiedemann syndrome, and assisted reproductive technologies. Birth Defects Res A Clin Mol Teratol. 85:58–62. PMID 19107956

# 10S

## CHARGE Syndrome

## Definition

- CHARGE syndrome (MIM 214800) is an autosomal dominant disorder caused by heterozygous mutation or deletion in *CHD7* on chromosome 8q12.1.
    o Usually sporadic; mild cases can be familial.
    o Increased mean paternal age
- CHARGE is an acronym:
    o *C*oloboma
    o *H*eart defect
    o *A*tresia choanae
    o *R*etardation of growth or development
    o *G*enitourinary anomalies
    o *E*ar and hearing anomalies
    o Some authors suggest adding *C*left lip or palate and *H*istory in the family to the acronym
- Prevalence 1/8,500 to 1/12,500 (North America)
- Recurrence risk
    o 1–3%, when mutation is de novo, due to germ line mosaicism in a parent
    o 50%, when parent is affected
- Mortality
    o Survival to 5 years: 70%
    o Highest mortality in the first year, especially with choanal atresia and cardiac defects or tracheoesophageal (TE) fistula

## Diagnosis

- Diagnosis is clinical; criteria are evolving.
    o Cardinal features: coloboma, choanal atresia/stenosis, typical external ear anomaly, dysfunction of various cranial nerves, facial palsy (Figure 10S.1), semicircular canal hypoplasia (most distinctive sign) or vestibular dysfunction
    o Supportive features: cleft lip/palate, cardiac or esophageal malformation, deafness, hypogonadotropic hypogonadism, growth retardation, ID, family member with a cardinal or two supportive features

*Pearl*: Assume that a newborn with a facial palsy and microphallus has CHARGE syndrome until proven otherwise.

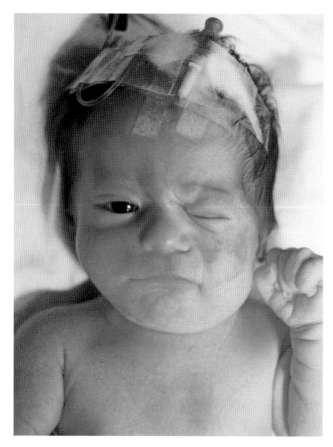

FIGURE 10S.1 This infant with a right facial palsy has CHARGE syndrome. Note the square forehead.

- Minimal diagnostic criteria have not been established.
  - CHARGE has a variable phenotype.
    - Affected identical twins have been strikingly discordant.
  - Consider CHARGE in infants without some cardinal features.
    - More severely affected individuals are overrepresented in the medical literature.
- Clinical features
  - Normal to low normal birth weight and length
  - Face: square forehead, bitemporal narrowing, facial asymmetry, small tented mouth
    - Unilateral or bilateral facial paralysis ~50%
  - Eyes: colobomas (iris, retina, optic nerve), bilateral colobomas 70–80%
    - Approximately half of colobomas are iridal. Others are detected with retinal exam.
    - Hypoplastic optic nerves, nystagmus, microphthalmia, anophthalmia

*Pearl*: Among patients with iris coloboma, almost 20% have CHARGE syndrome.

- Nose: choanal atresia or stenosis 65%
  - Laryngeal cleft, subglottic stenosis, tracheomalacia, vocal cord paralysis
- Ears: characteristic dysplastic pinnae 95–100%: deficient lobule and inferior helix, discontinuous antihelix and antitragus, triangular concha (Figure 10S.2). The ear anomaly can be mild or subtle.
  - Hypoplastic auditory canal
  - Inner ear anomalies >90%
    - Absent or hypoplastic semicircular canals predict *CHD7* mutation.
    - Visualize semicircular canals in the newborn on a plain profile skull X-ray or CT scan of the temporal bones.
    - Mondini dysplasia is a helpful sign but it is not pathognomonic for CHARGE syndrome.
- Cleft lip and/or palate 15–25%
- TE fistula 20–30%; diaphragmatic hernia infrequent
- Cardiac 50–85%
  - Conotruncal defects (e.g., TOF) 33%
  - AV canal, VSD, ASD, coarctation, PDA
  - Right aortic arch, aberrant subclavian artery
- Renal 10–40%: agenesis, horseshoe, cystic kidneys
- Genital: micropenis, cryptorchidism
  - Labial hypoplasia in females

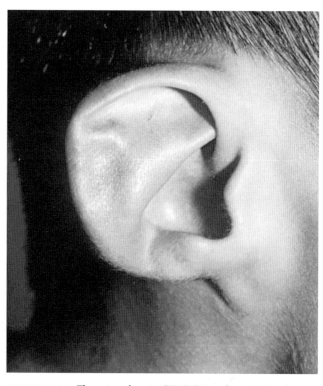

FIGURE 10S.2 The external ear in CHARGE syndrome is simple, with a triangular-shaped concha, a diagonally oriented antihelix, and a deficient lobule.
SOURCE: Courtesy of Kenneth L. Jones, MD, University of California, San Diego, CA.

- Extremities: polydactyly, split hand/foot, thumb hypoplasia, clubfoot
- CNS: arhinencephaly, hypoplastic olfactory bulbs
  - Microcephaly, usually postnatal
  - Cerebellar hypoplasia, cerebellar vermis hypoplasia, Chiari I malformation
- Functional problems in newborns
  - GI: swallowing and feeding problems 80%, GE reflux >50%, tube feeding ~90%
  - Postnatal growth failure
  - Mixed deafness 60–90%
  - Facial palsy causes dry eyes; treat with artificial tears
- Later findings
  - Hypothalamopituitary dysfunction: growth hormone deficiency, delayed puberty
  - Cardiac arrhythmia
  - Thermal dysregulation
  - Severe combined immunodeficiency, thymic dysfunction, recurrent infection
  - ID 70%, autism

## Differential Diagnosis

- Teratogens*
  - **Diabetic embryopathy***
  - **Alcohol,*** hydantoin, isotretinoin, methimazole, thalidomide
- Chromosome disorders
  - **Cat eye syndrome** (inv dup 22q11, MIM 115470)
  - **Trisomies 13*, 18***
  - 11qter deletion, 13qter deletion, **22q11.2 deletion***
- Syndromes
  - **Burn–McKeown syndrome** (MIM 608572)
    - Autosomal recessive disorder, caused by biallelic pathogenic variants in *TXNL4A*
    - Clinical features: choanal atresia, coloboma of lower eyelids, deafness, cleft lip/palate, cardiac defects, normal intellect
  - **Kabuki syndrome** (MIM 147920)
    - Autosomal dominant multiple congenital anomaly disorder caused by a pathogenic variant in *KMT2D*
    - Clinical features: long palpebral fissures, everted lower lid, arched eyebrows hypoplastic laterally, large ears, cleft palate, fetal pads, cardiac and other anomalies (Figure 12.4)
  - **Kallmann syndrome** (hypogonadotropic hypogonadism 1 with or without anosmia, MIM 308700)
  - Holoprosencephaly from various causes often includes choanal atresia
  - **VATER/VACTERL* association** (MIM 192350) (Figure 18S.1)

## Evaluation and Management

- Pregnancy history: ART, maternal diabetes, teratogenic exposures, thyroid disorders, Graves disease,
- Examine parents for anosmia, coloboma, facial palsy, hearing loss.
  - Affected parents have been unaware of their own retinal coloboma until examined by an ophthalmologist.
- Evaluate for associated anomalies.
  - Choanal atresia: pass a No. 6 French NG tube in each nostril.
  - Ophthalmology evaluation
  - Cardiology consult
  - Hearing screening
  - Random cortisol, glucose
    - Endocrinology consult and follow-up for hypopituitarism, micropenis
  - Complete blood count for severe combined immunodeficiency
- Imaging
  - Echocardiogram
  - Renal US
  - Imaging for inner ear anomalies: temporal bone CT (Mondini malformation), plain skull film in profile (semicircular canals)
- Genetic testing
  - Chromosome microarray
  - *CHD7* sequencing and deletion/duplication analysis (https://www.ncbi.nlm.nih.gov/gtr)
    - Test infants with classic and atypical phenotypes.
      - Pathogenic variant detected in 70% of tested patients; >90% when most diagnostic criteria are met
      - A negative test does not rule out CHARGE: 10–30% have no detectable mutation.
    - *CHD7* mutation database: https://www.chd7.org
    - After identifying a pathogenic variant in *CHD7*, test parents for that specific mutation.
- Follow in a multidisciplinary team (e.g., craniofacial clinic) with audiology, occupational, and speech therapy.
- Follow in outpatient endocrinology and genetics clinics.
  - Some have benefited from growth hormone therapy.
  - Treat hypogonadotrophic hypogonadism to avoid osteoporosis.
- Refer for early infant intervention services, programs for low vision and hearing impaired.
- Refer parents to support groups: https://www.chargesyndrome.org.

## Further Reading

Bergman JEH, Janssen N, Hoefsloot LH, et al. (2011) *CHD7* mutations and CHARGE syndrome: The clinical implications of an expanding phenotype. J Med Genet. 48:334–42. PMID 21378379

Hale CL, Niederriter AN, Green GE, Martin DM. (2016) Atypical phenotypes associated with pathogenic *CHD7* variants and a proposal for broadening CHARGE syndrome clinical diagnostic criteria. Am J Med Genet A. 170A:344–54. PMID 26590800

Hsu P, Ma A, Wilson M, et al. (2014) CHARGE syndrome: A review. J Paediatr Child Health. 50:504–11. PMID 24548020

van Ravenswaaij-Arts C, Martin DM. (2017) New insights and advances in CHARGE syndrome: Diagnosis, etiologies, treatments, and research discoveries. Am J Med Genet C Semin Med Genet. 175(4):397–406. PMID 29171162

Verloes A. (2005) Updated diagnostic criteria for CHARGE syndrome: A proposal. Am J Med Genet. 133A:306–8. PMID 15666308

Wong MT, Schölvinck EH, Lambeck AJ, van Ravenswaaij-Arts CM. (2015) CHARGE syndrome: A review of the immunological aspects. Eur J Hum Genet. 23:1451–9. PMID 25689927

# 11S

# Cornelia de Lange Syndrome

## Definition

- Cornelia de Lange syndrome (CdLS, MIM 122470) is a cohesinopathy that is caused by pathogenic variants in genes associated with cohesin molecules that hold sister chromatids together during mitosis.
- Incidence 1/10,000 live births; mild cases may not be ascertained.
- Usually sporadic but familial cases have been reported
- Recurrence risk 1.5%; germ line mosaicism occurs in apparently unaffected parents.
- Prenatal findings: IUGR, microcephaly, micrognathia, diaphragmatic hernia, cardiac and limb anomalies
  - Low pregnancy-associated plasma protein A in first and second trimesters
- Variable phenotypes
  - Severe, classic CdLS has dominated clinical reports.
  - Milder phenotypes can be difficult to recognize and may be responsible for the greater number of affected patients.
- Clinical features
  - In classic CdLS, IUGR, with growth parameters <10th percentile
  - Craniofacial features: long eyelashes; thick arched eyebrows appear full but neatly "penciled," not bushy; synophrys; ptosis 50%; short nose with concave nasal bridge and upturned nasal tip; broad nose; long and/or, smooth, flat, prominent philtrum; thin upper lip vermillion; downturned mouth; cleft palate 20% (Figure 11S.1)
  - Congenital anomalies
    - Skeletal: small hands and feet, brachydactyly, hand oligodactyly, ulnar ray deficiency (Figure 11S.2), absent forearm, radioulnar synostosis in one-third, toe syndactyly, hip dysplasia 10%
    - Skin: hypertrichosis, cutis marmorata
    - GI: gastroesophageal reflux >90% is often severe, malrotation 10%, volvulus, intestinal obstruction, diaphragmatic hernia 1% (Figure 21.2), pyloric stenosis 4%

*Pearl*: When an upper extremity defect occurs with diaphragmatic hernia, consider Cornelia de Lange syndrome.

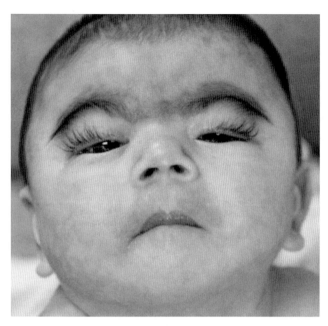

FIGURE 11S.1  This is the classic appearance of an infant with Cornelia de Lange syndrome. Note the long eyelashes, arched penciled eyebrows, synophrys, and long prominent philtrum.

- ■ Cardiac 25%, GU anomalies, vesicoureteral reflux 40%, cryptorchidism
- ■ CNS: enlarged ventricles and cisterna magna, thin white matter, brainstem and cerebellar vermis aplasia
  - • Seizures ~25%, hypertonia, low-pitched growling cry
  - • Sensorineural and conductive hearing loss 60%
  - • Later: speech delay, IQ 30–60, autism
    - • Rarely, normal IQ
- o Transient thrombocytopenia 10%
- o Immunodeficiency, humoral and cellular
  - ■ Chronic infections >50% in classic CdLS: sinopulmonary, sepsis, oral candidiasis, herpes, varicella, meningitis

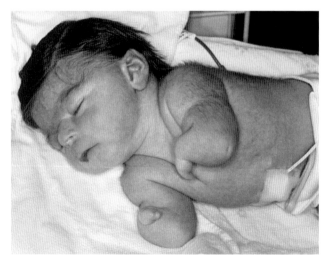

FIGURE 11S.2  This infant with Cornelia de Lange syndrome has bilateral ulnar hypoplasia and monodactyly.

- ■ Reduced T cell subsets
- • Molecular etiology: seven known cohesion genes
  - o Autosomal dominant
    - ■ *NIPBL* (5p13.1, MIM 608667) 60%, may be mosaic
      - • Classic CdLS is usually caused by pathogenic variant in *NIPBL*.
    - ■ *SMC3* (10q25, MIM 606062) 1–2%
    - ■ *RAD21* (8q24.1, MIM 606462) <1%
    - ■ *BRD4* (19p13.12) rare
    - ■ *ANKRD11* (16q24.3) rare
  - o X-linked
    - ■ *HDAC8* (Xq13.1, MIM 300269) 4% (Figure 11S.3)
    - ■ *SMC1A* (Xp11.22, MIM 300040) 1–2%
  - o Somatic mosaicism, especially *NIPBL* variants—23%

## Differential Diagnosis

- • Deletion chromosome 2q31 syndrome
- • Partial duplication of chromosome 3q
- • **Fetal alcohol spectrum disorder***
- • **Fryns syndrome** (MIM 229850)

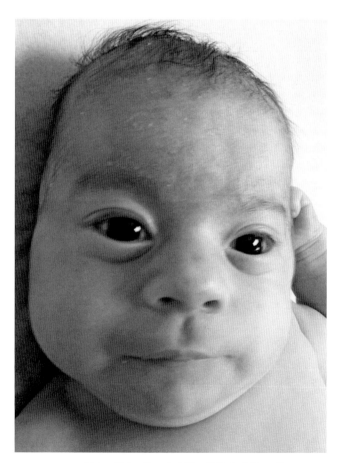

FIGURE 11S.3  This mildly affected girl has X-linked Cornelia de Lange syndrome caused by a copy number variant that disrupted *HDAC8*.

- **KBG syndrome** (MIM 148050) is caused by a heterozygous pathogenic variant in *ANKRD11*. Clinical features include hypertelorism, synophrys and bushy eyebrows, long philtrum and thin vermillion border of the upper lip, brachydactyly.
- **Rubinstein-Taybi syndrome** (MIM 1808049, 613684) is caused by a heterozygous pathogenic variant in *CREBBP* or *EP300*. Clinical features include microcephaly, arched eyebrows, long eyelashes, broad nasal bridge, beaked nose, broad thumbs and halluces.

## Evaluation and Management

- Document family history: affected relatives, intellectual disability, microcephaly, congenital anomalies, infant deaths.
- Examine relatives for mild CdLS features.
- Evaluate for associated anomalies.
  - Cleft palate, bifid uvula
  - Echocardiogram, abdominal US, imaging for malrotation, EEG
  - Audiology evalaution, Brainstem Auditory Evoked Response (BAER)
  - Monitor CBC for platelet count
- Evaluate immunoglobulins and T cell subsets, especially with recurrent infections.
- Manage poor feeding, treat GE reflux aggressively and proactively.
  - Gastrostomy for severe feeding dysfunction, aspiration risk
  - Treat reflux long term in conjunction with gastroenterology.
- Genetic testing
  - SNP microarray
  - CdLS gene panel: sequencing and deletion/duplication testing
  - To detect mosaicism, test buccal cheek sample at same time as blood.
  - Test parents pathogenic variant detected in their baby.
    - Parents without CdLS features are rarely carriers, ~1%.
  - Consider exome sequencing when other tests are negative.

- Utilize expert consensus guidelines (Kline, 2018). Monitor with CdLS growth charts at http://www.cdlsusa.org.
- Early infant intervention program. Utilize assisted communication devices and interactive computer programs.
- Counsel regarding serious infection, aspiration, pneumonia, chronic GI problems especially reflux.
- Genetic counseling
- Support group: http://www.cdlsusa.org

## Further Reading

Boyle MI, Jespersgaard C, Brøndum-Nielsen K, et al. (2015) Cornelia de Lange syndrome. Clin Genet. 88:1–12. PMID 25209348

Cereda A, Mariani M, Rebora P, et al. (2016) A new prognostic index of severity of intellectual disabilities in Cornelia de Lange syndrome. Am J Med Genet C Semin Med Genet. 172:179–89. PMID 27148700

Huisman SA, Redeker EJ, Maas SM, et al. (2013) High rate of mosaicism in individuals with Cornelia de Lange syndrome. J Med Genet. 50:339–44. PMID 23505322

January K, J Conway L, Deardorff M, et al. (2016) Benefits and limitations of a multidisciplinary approach to individualized management of Cornelia de Lange syndrome and related diagnoses. Am J Med Genet C Semin Med Genet. 172:237–45. PMID 27145433

Jyonouchi S, Orange J, Sullivan KE, et al. (2013) Immunologic features of Cornelia de Lange syndrome. Pediatrics. 132:e484–9. PMID 23821697

Kline AD, Moss JF, Selicorni A, et al. (2018) Diagnosis and management of Cornelia de Lange syndrome: first international consensus statement. Nat Rev Genet. 19:649–666. PMID 29995837

Mehta D, Vergano SA, Deardorff M, et al. (2016) Characterization of limb differences in children with Cornelia de Lange syndrome. Am J Med Genet C Semin Med Genet. 172:155–62. PMID 27120260

Nizon M, Henry M, Michot C, et al. (2016) A series of 38 novel germline and somatic mutations of NIPBL in Cornelia de Lange syndrome. Clin Genet. 89:584–9. PMID 26701315

Schrier SA, Sherer I, Deardorff MA, et al. (2011) Causes of death and autopsy findings in a large study cohort of individuals with Cornelia de Lange syndrome and review of the literature. Am J Med Genet A. 155A:3007–24. PMID 22069164

# 12S

## Diabetic Embryopathy

## Definition

- Pregestational maternal diabetes, type 1 or 2 (DMII), is a human teratogen, increasing the risk for congenital malformations, miscarriage, prematurity, preeclampsia, asphyxia, and perinatal death.
  - Among infants of diabetic mothers (IDM), 5–12% have a congenital anomaly, compared to 2–3% in the general population.
    - Infants of gestational diabetics have weakly increased risks for anomalies; OR is seldom >2.
    - Infants of gestational diabetics with obesity have higher risks approaching risks of Type I diabetics
  - Glycemic control and HgbA1c levels correlate with congenital anomalies; risk of anomalies increases to 15–17% for HgbA1c >7.
  - The prevalence of DMII has doubled worldwide in the past 30 years and continues to rise.
  - Maternal obesity (BMI >30) without diabetes is associated with an intermediate risk for similar patterns of congenital anomalies.
  - The severity and timing of hyperglycemia may affect the type of anomaly.
  - Underlying genetic or epigenetic factors may lower the threshold for particular anomalies in a given patient.
- Common features in IDM
  - **Congenital anomalies**: Data abstracted from large registry reports suggest increased risks for the following isolated anomalies:
    - Cardiac: heterotaxy, atrioventricular septal defects, D-transposition, total anomalous pulmonary venous return, hypoplastic left heart syndrome
    - CNS: microcephaly, holoprosencephaly, anencephaly, encephalocele, spina bifida
    - Ear anomalies
    - Renal anomalies, agenesis
    - Omphalocele
    - Orofacial clefts
    - Anorectal anomalies

- **Specific phenotypes associated with diabetic embryopathy-** these also occur in infants who are not born to diabetic mothers:
  - **Caudal regression syndrome/sacral agenesis** (MIM 600145)
    - IDM causes an increased risk for caudal regression: aOR 22.06.
      - However, only 17% of infants with caudal regression have a diabetic mother.
    - Clinical features
      - Agenesis or dysgenesis of the caudal spine, may include both lumbar and sacral elements
      - High termination of a club-shaped spinal cord: most common presentation
      - Occult neural tube defect, spinal cord tethering, genital malformations
      - Sirenomelia: most severe manifestation of caudal regression
        - Maternal DM in 5%
    - Sequelae: bowel and bladder incontinence, orthopedic issues; similar to infants with spina bifida
  - **Oculoauriculovertebral spectrum** (OAVS, hemifacial microsomia, MIM 164210)
    - Clinical features: ear, ocular, vertebral, cardiac defects
      - In IDM, these are usually isolated anomalies. Full spectrum of OAVS is less common in IDM.
  - **Femoral-facial syndrome** (femoral hypoplasia unusual facies syndrome, MIM 134780)
    - ~35% are IDM.
    - Genetic factors unrelated to IDM likely play a role.
    - Clinical features: microretrognathia, long philtrum, short nose, round face, cleft palate ~20%, occasional cleft lip (Figure 12S.1),
      - Skeletal: symmetric or asymmetric short or absent femurs, preaxial polydactyly, radial–humeral synostosis, humeral absence, vertebral defects, tibial defects
  - **Holoprosencephaly** (HPE, MIM 236100)
    - IDM have a >20-fold increased risk for HPE.
    - Clinical features: Midline facial features can be subtle—hypotelorism, absent frenulum. Absent nasal septum, choanal atresia, premaxillary agenesis
      - CNS anomalies can be severe or mild: lobar, semilobar, and alobar HPE.
      - Septo-optic dysplasia, pituitary dysfunction: hypernatremia (from diabetes insipidus), micropenis
  - **Preaxial hallucal polydactyly** (MIM 601759)
    - Clinical features: bilateral or unilateral polydactyly of great toe; proximal implantation (Figure 12S.2)
  - **VATER/VACTERL association** (MIM 192350)
    - Clinical features: heart defects, vertebral anomalies, renal agenesis, anal atresia
  - Lumbocostovertebral syndrome
    - Vertebral and rib defects with lateral body wall hernia

*Pearl*: IDM with significant macrosomia may appear microcephalic because the baby's body is larger than expected for the normal head size.

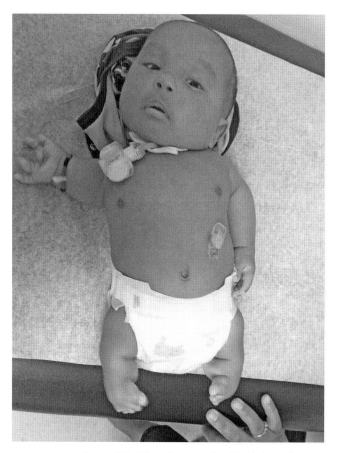

FIGURE 12S.1 Femoral-Facial syndrome in this IDM baby with Pierre Robin sequence, bilateral femur absence, unilateral humerus absence and caudal regression.

  - **Associated clinical problems**
    - Birth weight. IDM with congenital anomalies are generally heavier at birth and deliver earlier than infants with similar congenital anomalies in nondiabetics.

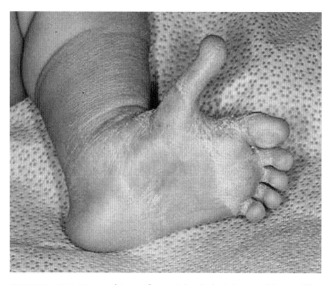

FIGURE 12S.2 Unusual type of preaxial polydactyly, possibly specific for diabetic embryopathy.
SOURCE: Courtesy of Margaret Adam, MD, University of Washington, Seattle, WA.

- IUGR: consequence of poorly controlled diabetes when severe hyperglycemia occurs around fertilization
  - Small size may be due to reduced inner cell mass.
- Feeding dysfunction
  - Prolonged poor feeding: common among term IDM without major congenital anomalies. Etiology is obscure.
    - Consider an undiagnosed encephalopathy.
    - Feeding usually slowly improves; occasionally requires short-term G tube.
- Hypertrophic cardiomyopathy (HCM)
  - Cardiac hypertrophy 38%; usually septal but may include myocardium
    - Asymmetric septal hypertrophy most common and least severe type
    - Dilated hypertrophic cardiomyopathy
      - In extreme cases, massive hypertrophy may lead to fetal or neonatal death.
    - Most resolve by 6 months.
    - Unclear role of HCM as risk factor for hypertension and insulin resistance in later life
- Small left colon syndrome
  - Mimics Hirschsprung disease but resolves with conservative therapy
  - Most common cause of intestinal obstruction in IDM
- Neurodevelopmental effects
  - Children of poorly controlled diabetics are more likely to have slightly reduced IQ and ADHD.

- Imaging
  - Echocardiogram to identify cardiac defects, monitor for HCM
  - Abdominal US, skeletal radiographs, spine US and/or radiographs
  - Head imaging for suspected HPE or unexplained poor feeding
- Genetic testing
  - Microarray, especially when pattern of multiple anomalies is not typical
  - In IDM with VATER/VACTERL spectrum anomalies: Consider chromosome breakage studies (DEB) for Fanconi anemia.
  - In IDM with holoprosencephaly:
    - Chromosomal testing to rule out T13 and T18 and/or SNP microarray
    - Holoprosencephaly gene sequencing panel for common mutations
- Refer babies with caudal regression/sacral agenesis to a spina bifida multidisciplinary team.
- Monitor developmental status.
- Continue diabetic care for mother post-delivery to achieve optimal glycemic control in the interpregnancy period. *Plan* all future pregnancies. Recommend:
  - Daily multivitamin supplement for mother with supplemental periconceptional folic acid, to achieve 2–5 mg/day
  - Early diagnosis and management of pregnancy allows timely insulin treatment if indicated
  - First trimester fetal US for abnormalities

## Differential Diagnosis

- Chromosome anomalies
- Teratogens: Valproic acid has some similar effects.
- Single gene disorders
  - **Fanconi anemia** (MIM 227650) especially with VACTERL anomalies
  - **Congenital hyperinsulinism** (nesidioblastosis, MIM 256450)
  - Overgrowth syndromes

## Evaluation and Management

- Pregnancy history: Document when DM was diagnosed, level of glycemic control, HgbA1c, treatment, maternal BMI, hypertension, smoking, teratogenic exposure.
- Examine for anomalies in other organs: uvula, palate, femurs, gluteal crease, anal wink.

## Further Reading

Adam MP, Hudgins L, Carey JC, et al. (2009) Preaxial hallucal polydactyly as a marker for diabetic embryopathy. Birth Defects Res A Clin Mol Teratol. 85:13–9. PMID 18798547

Correa A, Gilboa SM, Besser LM, et al. (2008) Diabetes mellitus and birth defects. Am J Obstet Gynecol. 199:237.e1–9. PMID 18674752

Johnson JP, Carey JC, Gooch WM, et al. (1983) Femoral hypoplasia—Unusual facies syndrome in infants of diabetic mothers. J Pediatr. 102:866–72. PMID 6854450

Nasri HZ, Houde Ng K, Westgate MN, et al. (2018) Malformations among infants of mothers with insulin-dependent diabetes: Is there a recognizable pattern of abnormalities? Birth Defects Res. 110(2):108–113. PMID 29377640

Ornoy A, Reece EA, Pavlinkova G, et al. (2015) Effect of maternal diabetes on the embryo, fetus, and children: Congenital anomalies, genetic and epigenetic changes and developmental outcomes. Birth Defects Res C Embryo Today. 105:53–72. PMID 25783684

Parnell AS, Correa A, Reece EA. (2017) Pre-pregnancy obesity as a modifier of gestational diabetes and birth defects associations: A systematic review. Matern Child Health J. 21:1105–20. PMID 28120287

# 13S

# Fetal Alcohol Spectrum Disorder

## Definition

- Fetal alcohol spectrum disorder (FASD), a nondiagnostic term, includes all manifestations of prenatal alcohol exposure (PAE).
  - Fetal alcohol syndrome (FAS): this diagnosis can be made when all major criteria are met (growth impairment, facial features, brain and neurobehavioral involvement) with or without PAE. Most severe FASD phenotype
  - Partial FAS: this diagnosis is used when most, but not all, growth, facial, and neurobehavioral manifestations are present; criteria depend on documentation of PAE.
  - Alcohol-related neurodevelopmental disorder: this diagnosis requires neurologic sequelae and confirmed PAE without growth or facial features. Most common FASD phenotype
  - Alcohol-related birth defects: this term is used when there is ≥1 FASD-related congenital anomaly and documented PAE without facial, growth, or neurologic sequelae. Associated with first trimester binge drinking
  - Fetal alcohol effects: this term is out of favor; no established diagnostic criteria
  - Prenatal alcohol exposure: documented intoxication, ≥6 drinks/week for ≥2 weeks, ≥3 drinks on ≥2 occasions during pregnancy (Hoyme et al., 2016)
- Incidence: FASD 9/1,000 live births; FAS 0.5–2/1,000 (United States)
  - FASD is the leading cause of intellectual disability. It is more common than Down syndrome, spina bifida, and HIV combined
  - Underascertained in infancy
    - ADHD, executive functioning deficits cannot be ascertained until childhood.
    - Often missed, misdiagnosed later in childhood
- Maternal alcohol use is common in pregnancy.
  - 20% of all pregnant women in the United States consume alcohol at some point during pregnancy.
  - One in 30 consumes >2 ounces of absolute alcohol/day.
  - ~2% are binge drinkers: ≥3 drinks consumed in one sitting.

*Pearl*: Mothers may deny or underreport PAE. Ask about general health before tactfully asking about any history of alcohol use, especially in the months *before* the positive pregnancy test.

- High-risk groups
  ○ Maternal anxiety, depression, ID, drug abuse, social isolation, physical abuse, low socioeconomic or educational level
  ○ Children in orphanages, foster care, adoptees; prisoners, Aboriginal, Native American, Alaskan Native populations
- High prevalence areas for FASD
  ○ South Africa (13–20%), Russia (4–5%), Croatia, Lazio region, Italy; remote areas of Alaska, Canada, Australia
- Dose and timing
  ○ Alcohol can damage fetal CNS throughout gestation.
    ■ Most sensitive period: first trimester
  ○ The highest risk is associated with heavy episodic or "binge" drinking, as this results in the highest blood-alcohol levels.
  ○ Moderate consumption (1–2 ounces of absolute alcohol/day) affects growth and behavior *without* dysmorphic features in ~11%.
  ○ No safe level of alcohol use in pregnancy has been established; however, an occasional drink or a single binge episode should *not* cause FAS.
- Genes modify FASD phenotype.
  ○ FAS in <50% fetuses of chronically alcoholic women
  ○ Monozygotic twins are usually concordant; dizygotic twins are often discordant.
- Comorbidities
  ○ Inadequate prenatal care, malnutrition, iron-deficiency anemia, smoking, and use of other drugs increase preterm birth, miscarriage, stillbirth, fetal death.

*Pearl*: Maternal smoking and alcohol exposure are synergistic, increasing the odds ratios for preterm delivery and low birth weight by more than the sum of their individual risks.

- FAS diagnosis: *All* of the following clinical categories must be represented with a negative evaluation for other causes:
  ○ ≥2 Facial features
    ■ Short palpebral fissures <10th percentile, smooth philtrum, thin upper lip (Figure 13S.1)
  ○ Height and/or weight ≤10th percentile
  ○ CNS
    ■ Small brain, corpus callosum dysgenesis, cerebellar vermis hypoplasia, migration abnormalities, nonfebrile seizures
  ○ Neurobehavior
    ■ Hypotonia, poor suck, shrill cry
  ○ With or without PAE
    ■ See University of Washington four-digit diagnostic code: https://depts.washington.edu/fasdpn/htmls/4-digit-code.htm.

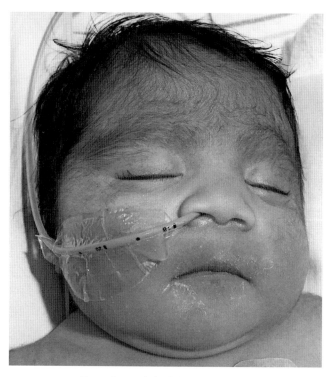

FIGURE 13S.1  This infant with fetal alcohol syndrome has a long, smooth philtrum and a thin upper lip that lacks a Cupid's bow appearance.

- Additional features
  ○ Head circumference (HC): usually modestly reduced
    ■ HC: −1 SD 24%; <−3 SD 10%
      • Cognitive impairment is not more severe in microcephalic group.
  ○ Craniofacial: ptosis, strabismus, microphthalmia, coloboma, optic nerve hypoplasia, microtia, prominent horizontal ear crus in the concha, hearing loss, maxillary hypoplasia, micrognathia, cleft palate* (Figure 13S.2)
  ○ Cardiac: septal defects, TGA, TOF
    ■ More cardiac anomalies with heavy drinking (OR 3.76) than with binge drinking (OR 2.49).
  ○ Musculoskeletal: nail hypoplasia, clinodactyly, camptodactyly, "hockey stick" palmar crease (extending into web between index and middle fingers), vertebral defects, scoliosis, radioulnar synostosis
  ○ Renal: kidney agenesis, hypoplasia, dysplasia, horseshoe kidney
  ○ Later findings
    ■ Receptive and expressive language disorders 76–81%
    ■ Visual impairment 62%
    ■ Chronic serous otitis media 77%
    ■ Conduct disorder 90%
- Early diagnosis and intervention before age 6 years improve outcome.
  ○ Consider FASD for the following:
    ■ Low BW, or confirmed PAE, with or without congenital anomalies

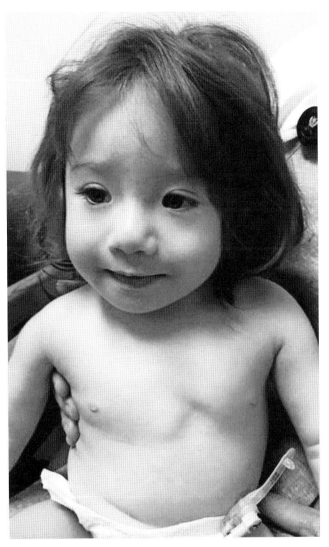

FIGURE 13S.2 This child with fetal alcohol syndrome has a cleft palate, short palpebral fissures, telecantus, and epicanthal folds. Note the nevus flammeus on the forehead, the chest wall asymmetry, and the gastric feeding tube.

- Jitteriness, shrill cry, irritability, poor feeding, hyperacusis, difficulty habituating to stimuli

## Differential Diagnosis

- o Chromosome anomalies
  - **Cri du chat syndrome\*** (5p-, MIM 123450)
  - **Williams syndrome\*** (MIM 194050)
  - **Duplication 15q syndrome** (MIM 608636)
  - **Down syndrome\***
  - **22q deletion syndrome\*** (MIM 192430)
- o Teratogens\*
  - **Anticonvulsant exposure**
  - Toluene (methylbenzene) embryopathy
  - **Maternal PKU** (MIM 261600)

- o Syndromes
  - **Coffin–Siris syndrome** (MIM 135900)
  - **Cornelia de Lange syndrome\*** (MIM 122470)
  - **Dubowitz syndrome** (MIM 223370)
  - **Noonan syndrome\*** (MIM 163950)
  - **Oculodentodigital syndrome** (MIM 164200)

*Pearl:* Women with ID may abuse alcohol. When FASD is suspected, order fragile X testing and microarray.

## Evaluation and Management

- Independently document /confirm family and social histories.
- Document prenatal care, nutrition, teratogen exposures during *and* prior to pregnancy, timing and amount: alcohol, tobacco, drugs, solvents, glues, spray paint, lacquer.
- Self-reporting does not identify all women with alcohol use disorders but routine use of T-ACE screening questions, which were developed for pregnant women, and other tools that reduce stigma, can help identify mothers of infants at increased risk for FASD. T-ACE scoring: 2 points for more than 2 drinks for T (**t**olerance); 1 point each for ACE. Positive total score is 2 points or more.
  - o **T**- How many drinks does it **t**ake to make you feel high?
  - o **A**- Has anybody every **a**nnoyed you by complaining about your drinking?
  - o **C**- Have you ever felt you ought to **c**ut-down on your drinking?
  - o **E**- Have you ever needed a drink (**e**ye-opener) first thing in the morning to get going?
- Examine parents for dysmorphic features, intellectual disability, psychiatric problems, mood disorders, microcephaly.
- Use FASD diagnostic algorithms (Cook 2016; Hoyme 2016).
- Evaluate for associated anomalies
  - o Brain MRI
  - o Echocardiogram
  - o Ophthalmology evaluation
  - o Abdominal US
  - o Hearing screening
- Genetic testing
  - o Chromosomal microarray
  - o Consider fragile X testing and other gene testing consistent with the phenotype.
- Notify social services.
  - o In the United States, the law mandates reporting FASD to child protective services, making appropriate referrals and a plan of safe care.
- Anticipate common problems:
  - o Feeding, growth, constipation
  - o Sleep
  - o SIDS
  - o Cognitive impairment, challenging behaviors
- Refer for early infant intervention.

*Pearl*: In FASD, stimulant medication does not improve, and may worsen, symptoms of ADHD.

- Recommend resources for caregivers:
  - http://www.nofas.org
  - https://www.fasworld.com

## Further Reading

Chiodo LM, Sokol RJ, Delaney-Black V, et al. (2010) Validity of the T-ACE in pregnancy in predicting child outcome and risk drinking. Alcohol. 44:595–603. PMID 20053522

Cook JL, Green CR, Lilley CM, et al.; Canada Fetal Alcohol Spectrum Disorder Research Network. (2016) Fetal alcohol spectrum disorder: A guideline for diagnosis across the lifespan. CMAJ. 188:191–7. PMID 26668194

Del Campo M, Jones KL. (2017) A review of the physical features of the fetal alcohol spectrum disorders. Eur J Med Genet. 60:55–64. PMID 27729236

Hoyme HE, Kalberg WO, Elliott AJ, et al. (2016) Updated clinical guidelines for diagnosing fetal alcohol spectrum disorders. Pediatrics. 138:e20154256. PMID 27464676

Montag AC. (2016) Fetal alcohol-spectrum disorders: identifying at-risk mothers. Int J Womens Health. 8:311–323. PMID 27499649

Popova S, Lange S, Shield K, et al. (2016) Comorbidity of fetal alcohol spectrum disorder: A systematic review and meta-analysis. Lancet. 387:978–87. PMID 26777270

Treit S, Zhou D, Chudley AE, et al. (2016) Relationships between head circumference, brain volume and cognition in children with prenatal alcohol exposure. PLoS One 11:e0150370. PMID 26928125

Williams JF, Smith VC; Committee on Substance Abuse. (2015) Fetal alcohol spectrum disorders. Pediatrics. 136:e1395–406. PMID 26482673

# 14S

## Incontinentia Pigmenti

### Definition

- Incontinentia pigmenti (IP, MIM 308300) is an X-linked dominant multisystem disorder that typically affects females.
  - It is prenatally lethal in almost all affected males.
  - Females survive because some of their cells express a normal gene product from their other X chromosome.
    - Most affected females show a markedly skewed X-chromosome inactivation pattern.
- A heterozygous pathogenic variant in, *IKBKG* (*NEMO*) is detected in ~85% of affected individuals.
  - *IKBKG* is important for many immune and inflammatory processes and protects against apoptotic processes.

### Diagnosis

- Skin abnormalities typically go through four phases: 50% have skin changes in infancy. Stages frequently overlap.
  - **Stage 1**: Erythematous, vesiculated blisters, pustules appear along the lines of Blaschko.
    - Crops appear every 1 or 2 weeks, often present at birth but may occur in utero. Most commonly, lesions involve the extremities, but they can occur elsewhere (Figure 14S.1A).
  - **Stage 2**: verrucous phase with warty papules, hyperkeratosis, or plaque-like lesions, follows or may occur simultaneously with blisters. Lesions follow the lines of Blaschko (Figure 14S.1B).
  - **Stage 3**: Hyperpigmentation remains after resolution of earlier phases. Linear and swirled hyperpigmentation is in a "marble cake" pattern, most often on the trunk but also on extremities (hyperpigmentation and evolving stages are shown in Figure 14S.1C)
  - **Stage 4**: pallor, atrophy, scarring, hypopigmented streaks, usually on the backs of the legs

*Pearl*: Use a Wood's light, which emits long wave ultraviolet light, to see hypochromic streaks on the backs of the legs of possible carrier mothers. Pigmentary changes often disappear by adulthood and may not be evident on routine examination.

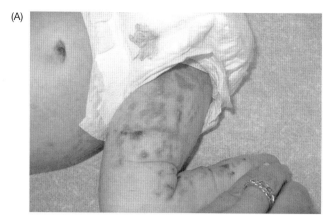

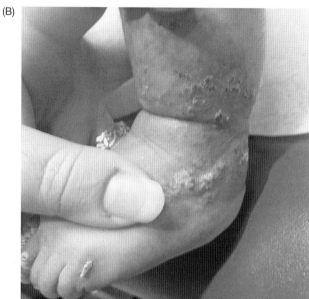

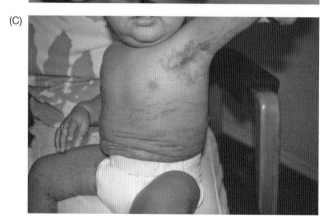

FIGURE 14S.1 Evolving stages of IP in infancy. (A) Blisters on extremities. (B) Evolving verrucous stage changes and (C) "marble cake" swirled hyperpigmentation.
SOURCE: Angela Scheuerle MD, University of Texas Southwestern.

- Other skin findings
  - Patchy alopecia, particularly at the vertex. Sparse hair common in childhood
  - Nail dystrophy, usually mild, 40%

- CNS
  - Microcephaly 4%
  - Seizures, ID in approximately one-third
  - Occasional neonatal encephalopathy with multiple infarcts and hemorrhage. Treatment with corticosteroids has been successful in at least one case.
- Ophthalmologic
  - Cataracts, microphthalmia, abnormal retinal vessels with a risk for retinal detachment
- Skeletal
  - Hemivertebrae 20%
- Later
  - Dental: hypodontia, conical teeth, 80%
  - Unilateral breast aplasia
  - Other CNS, skeletal, ocular, and dermatologic findings are common but variable and usually not evident in the newborn.
- Rare affected males may have normal gene function in some cells.
  - Klinefelter syndrome: 47,XXY karyotype
  - Postzygotic mosaicism for a mutation in *IKBKG*

## Differential Diagnosis

- Infection: Herpes zoster, varicella cause blisters
- Diffuse cutaneous mastocytosis
- **Hypomelanosis of Ito** (MIM 300337) mosaic conditions, both chromosomal and single gene. Mosaicism could be confused with a later phase of IP in which the blistering phase occurred in utero and resolved.
  - Consider skin biopsy for chromosome analysis or molecular testing depending on the clinical presentation.
- Erythema toxicum

## Evaluation and Management

- Document family history: other affected female relatives, multiple miscarriages, a lack of males in the mother's family.
- Examine the mother for features involving hair, nails, teeth, and skin. Ask about seizures or learning problems.
  - Use a Wood's light in a dark room to visualize hypochromic streaks on the back of the mother's legs.
- Evaluate for associated anomalies.
  - Consider CNS imaging and neurology consultation for seizures or other neurologic symptoms.
  - Pediatric ophthalmology assessment in the first months of life
  - Skin biopsy generally not necessary but, if done, can be expected to show multiple eosinophils and large dyskeratotic cells

- Gene testing
  - Chromosome analysis in affected males
  - Gene analysis identifies mutation in~85% of female patients.
    - Particularly useful when mother's carrier state cannot be ascertained clinically (e.g., no family history, no clinical findings of IP, and no hypochromic streaks on the mother's legs)
- Refer for infant developmental assessment and, if necessary, early infant program and neurodevelopmental monitoring.
- Genetic consultation for recurrence risk assessment and molecular testing

## Further Reading

Greene-Roethke C. (2017) Incontinentia Pigmenti: A Summary Review of This Rare Ectodermal Dysplasia With Neurologic Manifestations, Including Treatment Protocols. J Pediatr Health Care. (6):e45–e52. PMID 28870493

Happle R. (2016) The categories of cutaneous mosaicism: A proposed classification. Am J Med Genet A. 170A:452–9. PMID 26494396

Ruggieri M, Praticò AD. (2015) Mosaic neurocutaneous disorders and their causes. Semin Pediatr Neurol. 22:207–33. PMID 26706010

Scheuerle AE, Ursini MV. (2015) Incontinentia pigmenti. In: Pagon RA, Adam MP, Ardinger HH, et al, editors. GeneReviews [Internet]. Seattle, WA: University of Washington, Seattle; 1993–2017. PMID 20301645

Soltirovska Salamon A, Lichtenbelt K, Cowan FM, et al. (2016) Clinical presentation and spectrum of neuroimaging findings in newborn infants with incontinentia pigmenti. Dev Med Child Neurol. 58:1076–84. PMID 27121774

Swinney CC, Han DP, Karth PA. (2015) Incontinentia pigmenti: A comprehensive review and update. Ophthalmic Surg Lasers Imaging Retina. 46:650–7. PMID 26114846

# 15S

## Prader–Willi Syndrome

## Definition

- Prader–Willi syndrome (PWS, MIM 176270), a neurodevelopmental disorder characterized by hypotonia and poor feeding in infancy, is caused by loss or inactivation of a set of genes on the paternally-derived chr 15q11.2.
- Gene expression in the 15q11.2 critical region is determined by the methylation pattern and the parent of origin.
  - o In PWS, genes normally expressed only from the *paternally derived* chr 15q11.2 are lost or silenced.
  - o In **Angelman syndrome** (AS, MIM 105830), an acquired microcephaly syndrome, genes from the *maternally-derived* chr 15q11.2 are deleted or inactive.
- Incidence 1/10,000 to 1/30,000 live births

## Diagnosis

- Clinical features: bitemporal narrowing, almond-shaped eyes (Figure 15S.1), downturned corners of the mouth, thick saliva
  - o Hypotonia: is universal, contributes to hypoventilation, poor feeding, GERD, failure to thrive (Figure 1.2)
    - ▪ Reflexes are present; no tongue fasciculations
  - o Hypopigmentation with 15q deletion (Figures 42.2, 15S.2)
    - ▪ Locus for **oculocutaneous albinism, type II** (MIM 203200) is 15q12.
  - o Small hands, feet
  - o Hypogonadism
    - ▪ Cryptorchidism 80–90%
    - ▪ Clitoral and labial hypoplasia are underrecognized.

*Pearl*: Males with PWS are diagnosed earlier than females because their genital abnormalities are more obvious.

  - o Congenital anomalies: rare
  - o BW and length: 15–20% less than unaffected siblings.
    - ▪ Low birth weight occurs in 34%.
    - ▪ Prematurity occurs in 26%
- Later
  - o Hyperphagia, lack of satiety, obesity >1 year
    - ▪ Delayed gastric emptying; vomiting rare

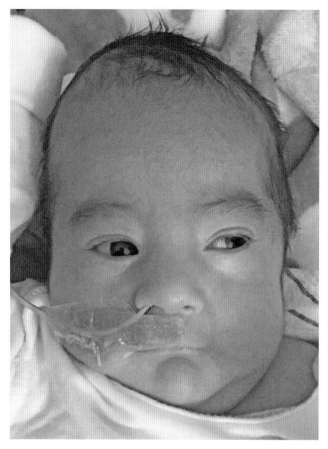

FIGURE 15S.1  This hypotonic infant with Prader–Willi syndrome has characteristic "almond-shaped" eyes and narrow bifrontal diameter. Note the NG tube for feeding.

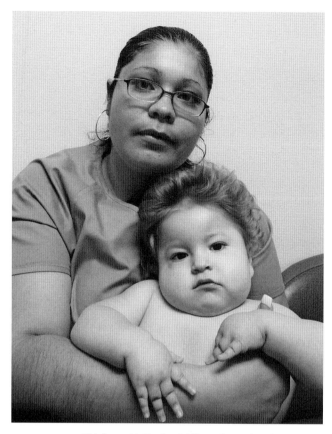

FIGURE 15S.2  This boy with Prader–Willi syndrome has decreased skin pigmentation and fairer hair compared to his normally pigmented mother. Note his bifrontal narrowing.

*Pearl*: Patients with PWS are not candidates for gastric bypass surgery because they continue to overeat. The chance of gastric rupture increases after surgery.

- ○ Strabismus
- ○ Hypothalamic, GH/IGF-1 defects
- ○ Neurobehavior
  - ■ Delayed milestones, ID: IQ 60–70
  - ■ OCD, ADHD, autism, psychosis 5–10%
  - ■ Skin picking, increased pain tolerance
- • Mortality 1.25–3% per year
  - ○ Children: SIDS, respiratory and GI infections, central adrenal insufficiency
    - ■ No increased mortality in growth hormone (GH)-treated group
  - ○ Adults: choking on food (especially hot dogs), gastric rupture, COPD, obesity
- • Molecular subtypes
  - ○ Chromosome 15q11.2 deletion ~65–75%
    - ■ Typical deletions: there are two common proximal breakpoints, BP1 and BP2; one distal breakpoint, BP3
      - • Type I deletion: BP1–BP3, includes more genes expressed in brain
        - • More obsessive–compulsive, self-injurious behaviors

- • Type II deletion: BP2–BP3
- • Usually de novo, low recurrence risk
- ■ Small atypical deletions (~8%): include *SNORD* (small nucleolar organizing RNAs) gene cluster
  - • Recurrence risk 50% for offspring of carrier fathers
- ○ Maternal uniparental disomy for chr 15 (matUPD15) ~20–30%
  - ■ Two maternally-derived copies of chr 15 remain after "rescue" of a trisomy 15 conception.
    - • Associated with advanced maternal age
    - • Rarely mosaic
    - • Recurrence risk <1%
  - ■ Rare familial chr 15 Robertsonian translocation or marker chromosome
- ○ Chr 15 imprinting center (IC) defect <5%
  - ■ Paternal chr 15 IC deletion, mutation (15%), or epimutation causes failure to reset to a paternal epigenetic pattern on chr 15 during spermatogenesis.
  - ■ Recurrence risk: 50% for offspring of carrier fathers

## Differential Diagnosis

- • Chromosome anomalies
  - ○ **Chromosome 1p36 deletion syndrome** (MIM 607872)

- ○ **Maternal UPD14** (Temple syndrome, MIM 616222)
  - ■ Also caused by **deletion of paternally-derived 14q32**
- ○ **Chromosome 15q11.2–q13 duplication syndrome** (MIM 608636)
- Hypotonia* syndromes
  - ○ HIE, CNS infection
  - ○ **Congenital myotonic dystrophy** (MIM 160900)
  - ○ **Spinal muscular atrophy** (MIM 253300)
  - ○ **Congenital muscular dystrophy** (MIM 607855)
  - ○ **Glycogen storage disorder II** (Pompe syndrome, MIM 232300)
  - ○ **Angelman syndrome** (AS, MIM 105830)

## Evaluation and Management

- Examine for congenital anomalies and other causes of hypotonia.*
- Evaluate for associated anomalies: cryptorchidism, hip dysplasia, central or obstructive sleep apnea.

*Pearl*: Unexplained hypotonia and poor suck in a term infant without congenital anomalies should prompt testing for PWS.

- Genetic testing
  - ○ Microarray and DNA methylation test for chr 15q11.2 (MLPA, methylation-specific PCR) diagnoses 99% of patients with PWS.
    - ■ Microarray detects deletion, mosaicism, and some UPD.
    - ■ Methylation detects deletion, UPD, and IC defects but does not distinguish between them.
    - ■ Methylation distinguishes between PWS and AS.
  - ○ Uniparental disomy test (microsatellite analysis) detects matUPD15; requires blood from both parents.
    - ■ If negative, sequence IC on chr 15q11.2. If that is negative, sequence *SNORD* gene cluster.
  - ○ Chromosome study: balanced translocation, inversion <1%.
    - ■ When a baby has a translocation, inversion, or marker chromosome, test parents.
- Manage feeding problems conservatively.
  - ○ Facilitate oral feeding: OT, special (cleft palate) nipples.
    - ■ Establish regular feeding schedule. PWS babies rarely wake for feedings.
    - ■ Treat GERD.
    - ■ Be patient. NG feeding can last several weeks.
  - ○ Early growth hormone therapy may reduce the need for gastrostomy tube placement. Gastrostomy should be a last resort as it increases the risk for later gastric rupture.
- Follow published health supervision guidelines.

- ○ http://pediatrics.aappublications.org/content/127/1/195
- Offer anticipatory guidance.
  - ○ Hyperphagia and obesity begin in late infancy.
    - ■ Avoid choking hazards: hot dogs.
  - ○ IUGR: Check for hypothyroidism.
  - ○ Scoliosis, temperature instability, unexplained fever, developmental delay
  - ○ SIDS (independent of GH therapy), respiratory insufficiency, infections
    - ■ During febrile illnesses, monitor cardiac status with telemetry and evaluate for central adrenal insufficiency.
- Growth hormone and other therapies
  - ○ GH treatment is standard of care in PWS. It improves stature, lean body mass, BMI, HC, fatigue, hypotonia, speech, and gross motor development.
    - ■ Begin GH in infancy before onset of hyperphagia, obesity
    - ■ Sleep study prior to and after onset of GH therapy
    - ■ Consult Endocrinology early
  - ○ *N*-acetylcysteine improves skin-picking behavior.
  - ○ Consider clinical trials for hyperphagia therapy.
    - ■ https://www.clinicaltrials.gov
- Refer to early infant intervention program.
- Coordinate outpatient care.
  - ○ Refer to PWS specialty clinic or multidisciplinary team of physical, occupational and behavioral therapists, nutritionist, and pediatric endocrinologist.
  - ○ Utilize PWS Medical Alert booklet.
    - ■ https://pwsausa.org/wp-content/uploads/2015/11/newMAbookfinal.pdf
  - ○ Use PWS growth charts, available with or without GH treatment.
- Refer parents for family support.
  - ○ Prader–Willi Syndrome Association: https://www.pwsausa.org
  - ○ Foundation for Prader–Willi Research: https://www.fpwr.org
  - ○ Offer smartphone app to families: https://www.prader-willi-world.com.

## Further Reading

Angulo MA, Butler MG, Cataletto ME. (2015) Prader–Willi syndrome: A review of clinical, genetic, and endocrine findings. J Endocrinol Invest. 38:1249–63. PMID 26062517

Butler MG, Lee J, Cox DM, et al. (2016) Growth charts for Prader–Willi syndrome during growth hormone treatment. Clin Pediatr (Phila). 55:957–74. PMID 26842920

Butler MG, Lee J, Manzardo AM, et al. (2015) Growth charts for non-growth hormone treated Prader–Willi syndrome. Pediatrics. 135:e126–35. Erratum in: Pediatrics. 135:946. PMID 25489013

Cassidy SB, Schwartz S, Miller JL, Driscoll DJ. (2012) Prader–Willi syndrome. Genetics Med. 14:10–26. PMID 22237428

Deal CL, Tony M, Höybye C, et al. (2013) Growth Hormone Research Society workshop summary: Consensus guidelines for recombinant human growth hormone therapy in Prader–Willi syndrome. J Clin Endocrinol Metab. 98:E1072–87. PMID 23543664

Kalsner L, Chamberlain SJ. (2015) Prader–Willi, Angelman, and 15q11–q13 duplication syndromes. Pediatr Clin North Am. 62:587–606. PMID 26022164

McCandless SE; Committee on Genetics. (2011) Clinical report— Health supervision for children with Prader-Willi syndrome. Pediatrics. 127:195–204. PMID 21187304

Miller JL, Angulo M. (2014) An open-label pilot study of *N*-acetylcysteine for skin-picking in Prader–Willi syndrome. Am J Med Genet A. 164A:421–4. PMID 24311388

Singh P. Mahmoud R, Gold GA, et al. (2018) Multicenter study of maternal and neonatal outcomes in individuals with Prader-Willi syndrome. J Med Genet. 55:594–598. PMID 29776967

# 16S

## Noonan Syndrome and Related Disorders

## Definition

- Noonan syndrome (NS) is the most common disorder in a group of conditions caused by pathogenic variants in genes in the RAS–mitogen-activated protein kinases (MAPK) signal transduction pathway, called RASopathies. Mutations interfere with normal morphogenesis and growth.
- Incidence of NS: 1/1,000 to 1/2,500; other RASopathies are rare.

## Diagnosis

- Prenatal diagnosis
  - The prenatal presentations of Noonan, cardiofaciocutaneous (CFC), and Costello syndromes overlap.
  - Shared features
    - Polyhydramnios, most common in CFC
    - Increased NT, cystic hygroma, hydronephrosis, fetal edema, pleural effusion, congenital heart disease, and fetal macrosomia
    - Cardiac defects such as hypertrophic cardiomyopathy (HCM), septal defects, arrhythmia, valve thickening/dysplasia are suggestive of Costello syndrome, though also seen in CFC syndrome
    - 9–17% of chromosomally normal fetuses with these prenatal findings have a pathogenic variant in a RAS–MAPK pathway gene.
  - Differential diagnosis includes other causes of congenital heart disease, hydrops, and peripheral lymphedema.
  - Gene sequencing panels may be useful prenatally, but turn-around time and frequent prematurity limit utility.
- **Noonan syndrome** (NS, MIM 163950)
  - Autosomal dominant trait, caused by heterozygous pathogenic variants in a growing number of genes: *PTPN11* 50%, *SOS1* 11%, *RAF1* 5%, *KRAS* ~1.5%, *NRAS* 0.2%, *RIT1* <1%, *RRAS* <1%
    - Rarely: *SOS2, RASA2, RRAS, SYNGAP1*
  - Clinical findings

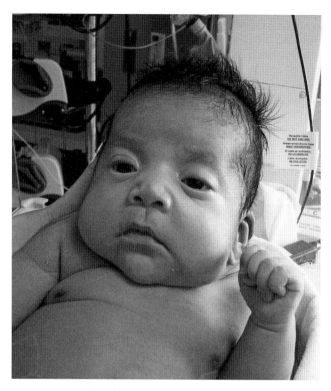

FIGURE 16S.1 This infant has mild ptosis, hypertelorism, retroverted ears, and redundant skin consistent with diagnosis of Noonan syndrome

- Face: down-slanting palpebral fissures, ptosis, posteriorly rotated ears, uplifted lobules, hypertelorism, redundant nuchal skin, webbing (Figure 16S.1). Intrafamilial variability is common.

*Pearl*: Edema often confounds the diagnosis of NS in neonates. It is also a clue to the diagnosis of a RASopathy because edema and hydrops are common presenting signs in these disorders.

- Growth: normal at birth with later fall off. Stature normal in 50% of NS adults (without growth hormone therapy)
- Cardiac: pulmonic stenosis 50–60%, HCM 20%, secundum ASD 6–10%
- Skeletal: pectus excavatum, carinatum; vertebral abnormalities and scoliosis
- Cryptorchidism
- Rarely lethal
○ Medical complications
- Feeding problems generally resolve by ~18 months.
  - Tube feedings required in ~25%.
  - G tube occasionally required.
- Hearing loss 10%
- Hematologic problems: thrombocytopenia, bleeding diathesis
  - Bleeding complications ~40%, serious in 18%

- Baseline screening coagulation tests are indicated prior to invasive procedures/surgery.
- Later: increased risk for cancers, including juvenile myelomonocytic leukemia (JMML) and rhabdomyosarcoma
- Severe variants in RAS–MAPK pathway genes that are usually present only as somatic mutations in isolated JMML have been reported with early lethality in NS.
■ Lymphatic problems
- Cystic hygroma and hydrops
- Later: Lymphatic dysplasia, especially symmetric or asymmetric swelling of the lower legs, is relatively common.
■ Developmental
- Developmental delay and learning problems; 30% have some autistic features
- Intelligence often within the normal range
  - IQ <70 in ~20%
• **Cardiofaciocutaneous syndrome** (CFC, MIM 115150)
- Autosomal dominant trait, caused, in 60–90% by heterozygous pathogenic variants in four genes: *KRAS, BRAF, MEK1, MEK2.*
- Early lethality due to hydrops is not rare.
○ Clinical findings
■ Face: more "coarse" than NS, relative macrocephaly, high forehead with bitemporal narrowing, absent to sparse eyebrows and lashes, deeply grooved philtrum (Figure 16S.2)

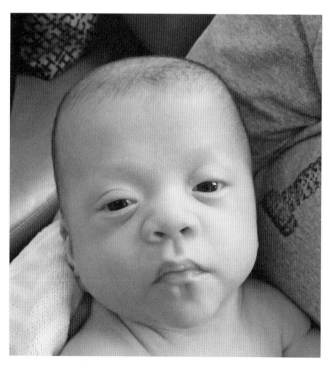

FIGURE 16S.2 This infant with cardiofaciocutaneous syndrome has nearly absent eyebrows and lashes, a deeply grooved philtrum, and mildly coarse features.

- Ectodermal features are prominent.
  - Dry, hyperkeratotic skin
  - Ichthyosis, eczema
  - Sparse, friable curly hair, sparse/absent eyebrows and lashes
- Cardiac defects in most patients
  - Pulmonic stenosis, HCM
- Neurologic problems
  - Seizures
  - Developmental delay, hypotonia, moderate to severe ID, behavior issues and autism
- **Costello syndrome** (MIM 218040)
  - Autosomal dominant disorder, caused by heterozygous missense mutation in *HRAS*
  - Clinical features: prenatal overgrowth followed by severe failure to thrive (see Figures 3.3A and 3.3B), poor feeding, vomiting, GERD
    - Distinctive face with coarse curly hair, loose skin.
    - Cardiac defects: HCM, septal defects, arrhythmia, and valve thickening/dysplasia
    - Hypoglycemia and arrhythmias are best discriminating features in the newborn
    - Intellectual disability is moderate and children are friendly and sociable.
    - Malignancies 15%: rhabdomyosarcoma most common
- **Noonan syndrome with lentigines** (previously called LEOPARD syndrome, MIM 151100)
  - Autosomal dominant disorder, caused by heterozygous mutation in *PTPN11* (most common), *RAF1, BRAF*
  - Clinical features: *l*entigines, *E*KG *c*onduction abnormalities, *o*cular hypertelorism, *p*ulmonic stenosis, *a*bnormal genitalia, and *d*eafness (defining the formerly used acronym)
    - Usually milder phenotype than NS
    - Café au lait spots in infancy; lentigines later. Inguinal and axillary freckling/lentigines
    - Cardiac defects, especially HCM
  - Difficult to distinguish from NS in infancy but later HCM, deafness, and café au lait spots are good discriminators
- **Noonan syndrome with loose anagen hair** (MIM 607721)
  - Autosomal dominant disorder, caused by recurrent heterozygous variant in *SHOC2*
  - Clinical features: similar to NS
    - Poor growth, growth hormone deficiency
    - Cardiac defects: dysplastic mitral valve and septal defects
    - Sparse thin hair. Diagnosis by hair microscopy
    - Hairless, darkly pigmented skin with eczema or ichthyosis
- **Neurofibromatosis type 1** (NF1, MIM 613113)
  - Autosomal dominant highly variable disorder, caused by heterozygous variant or deletion of *NF1*
  - Clinical features: Café au lait macules rarely present in the immediate neonatal period. Optic tract gliomas may present in the first year and rarely in the neonate. Plexiform neurofibromas are an uncommon finding in newborns and nearly all of the other features present in later infancy or childhood.
    - More often appreciated early when a parent is affected
    - When the diagnosis is apparent in the neonate, NF1 is often caused by a large deletion that includes the *NF1* gene.
    - Some patients with an *NF1* mutation have features of both Noonan syndrome and NF1 (MIM 601321).
- **Legius syndrome** (MIM 611431)
  - Autosomal recessive disorder, caused by heterozygous variants in *SPRED1*
  - Clinical features: usually not appreciated in newborns
    - Multiple café au lait spots without neurofibromas
    - Other later clinical problems are similar to NF1.

# Evaluation and Management

- Examine newborn for associated anomalies.
  - Newborn hearing screening and chronologic hearing screening
  - Order coagulation testing if surgical intervention is planned or there are any signs of excessive bruising or bleeding in NS.
    - Activated thromboplastin time, prothrombin time, and von Willebrand panel
    - For clinical symptoms of bleeding, obtain activity levels for factors VII, VIII, IX, XI, and XII, and consider referral to hematology.
- Echocardiogram is essential in NS, CFC and CS.
- Opthalmology evaluation in all these syndromes indicated.
- Dermatologic consultation and follow up needed for several of these conditions.
- Cranial imaging should be guided by symptoms and not done as baseline studies.
- Utilize published management guidelines for NS, CFC, CS and NF1.
- Monitor development and behavior for autistic symptoms frequent in Noonan syndrome and especially CFC syndrome.
- Refer to appropriate support group after diagnosis. Links to some include: CFCsyndrome.org; https://www.teamnoonan.org/; https://www.nfnetwork.org/community/nf-chat/; costellosyndromeusa.com

*Pearl*: A normal echocardiogram in an affected newborn *should be repeated before discharge* and as an outpatient because cardiomyopathy in the RASopathies can develop postnatally and progress rapidly.

- Genetic testing
  - A gene sequencing panel that includes the known genes in the RAS pathway is more cost-effective than serial single gene analysis.
  - If negative, add deletion/duplication tests for these genes.

# Further Reading

Allanson JE, Roberts AE. (2016) Noonan syndrome. In: Pagon RA, Adam MP, Ardinger HH, et al. editors. GeneReviews [Internet]. Seattle, WA: University of Washington, Seattle; 1993–2017. PMID 20301303

Conger B, Santa Cruz M, Rauen KA. (2014) Cardio-facio-cutaneous syndrome: Clinical features, diagnosis, and management guidelines. Pediatrics. 134:e1149–62. PMID 25180280

Digilio MC, Lepri F, Baban A, et al. (2011) RASopathies: Clinical diagnosis in the first year of life. Mol Syndromol. 1:282–289. PMID 22190897

Ferner RE, Huson SM, Thomas N, et al. (2008) Guidelines for the diagnosis and management of individuals with neurofibromatosis 1. J Med Genet. 44(2):81–8. PMID:17105749

Garg S, Brooks A, Burns A, et al. (2018) Autism spectrum disorder and other neurobehavioural comorbidities in rare disorders of the Ras/MAPK pathway. Dev Med Child Neurol. 59(5):544–549. PMID 28160302

Mason-Suares H, Toledo D, Gekas J, et al. (2017) Juvenile myelomonocytic leukemia-associated variants are associated with neo-natal lethal Noonan syndrome. Eur J Hum Genet. 25:509–511. PMID 28098151

Myers A, Bernstein JA, Brennan M, et al. (2014) Perinatal features of the RASopathies: Noonan syndrome, cardiofaciocutaneous syndrome and Costello syndrome. Am J Med Genet A. 164A:2814–21. PMID 25250515

Stevenson DA, Schill L, Schoyer L, et al. (2016) The Fourth International Symposium on Genetic Disorders of the Ras/MAPK Pathway. Am J Med Genet A. 170:1959–66. PMID 27155140

# 17S

## Smith–Lemli–Opitz Syndrome

## Definition

- Smith–Lemli–Opitz syndrome (SLOS, MIM 270400) is a cholesterol biosynthesis disorder, first described in 1964.
- SLOS is the prototypic metabolic disorder that causes multiple congenital anomalies. SLOS affects many organ systems because cholesterol is vital for steroid hormone synthesis, bile salts, cell membranes, and CNS function.
- Autosomal recessive disorder, caused by biallelic variants in *DHCR7*, the gene responsible for the last step in the cholesterol synthesis pathway
  - Pathogenic variants cause elevated 7-dehydrocholesterol (7-DHC).
  - Sequence analysis detects variants in 96%.
- Incidence 1/20,000 to 1/40,000
  - Females are underascertained because abnormal genitalia in males brings them to medical attention.
  - More common in Caucasians of European origin
  - Rare in Asians and Africans

## Diagnosis

- Phenotype is broad: from mild to severe to early embryonic lethality
- **Prenatal findings**
  - Maternal serum screening results can suggest the diagnosis.
    - Very low estriol (uE3) in the context of other normal serum markers (AFP, HCG) and fetal US abnormalities
  - Fetal US: oligohydramnios, anhydramnios, increased nuchal translucency 50%, IUGR 70%, hypospadias, congenital heart disease 90%, postaxial polydactyly

*Pearl*: A fetus affected with SLOS rarely has a normal fetal US.

  - Diagnostic testing
    - Amniotic fluid
      - 7-DHC elevated
      - Sequence analysis for *DHCR7*

- **Clinical features in newborns**
  - Distinctive dysmorphic features may be obscured by intubation, tape, and edema.
  - IUGR
  - Microcephaly 80%, ptosis, cataracts 20%, short nose with anteverted nares (Figure 17S.1), cleft palate, micrognathia, nuchal edema
  - CNS anomalies
    - Abnormal cerebellum and corpus callosum
    - Holoprosencephaly 5%
  - Cardiac anomalies >50%
    - Atrioventricular canal 25%, primum ASD 20%, PDA at term 18%, membranous VSD 10%, HLHS
  - Limb anomalies
    - Postaxial polydactyly hands/feet 25–50% (Figure 17S.2A)
    - Hypoplastic or proximally placed thumb
    - Y-shaped syndactyly of toes 2–3; a cardinal feature of SLOS that is rare in other disorders (Figure 17S.2B)
  - Genital anomalies
    - Undervirilized male genitalia: hypospadias, bifid scrotum, sex reversal in 46,XY males
  - **Common complications**
    - Gastrointestinal
      - Poor feeding, failure to thrive; these may be *only* signs in mild cases
      - Gastroesophageal reflux, dysmotility
      - Pyloric stenosis, Hirschsprung disease
      - Cholestatic liver disease; may improve with cholesterol and bile acid supplementation
    - Behavior
      - Hypotonia, irritability
      - Sleep cycle disturbance
      - Later: tantrums, moderate to severe ID, autism 75%

## Differential Diagnosis

- Other causes of low (<0.5 MoM) or undetectable (<25 ng/ml) maternal serum uE3
  - **X-linked ichthyosis** (steroid sulfatase deficiency, MIM 308100)
    - Incidence 1/3,000; most common cause of low uE3 in male fetuses
    - Deletion on the X chromosome detectable with FISH testing.
  - Anencephaly, hypopituitarism, midline brain defects, various causes of adrenal insufficiency, **Zellweger syndrome** (MIM 214100), **multiple sulfatase deficiency** (MIM 272200), **trisomy 18\***
- Syndromes with shared features
  - **Fanconi anemia** (MIM 227650)
    - IUGR, microcephaly, hypoplastic thumbs, genital anomalies in males

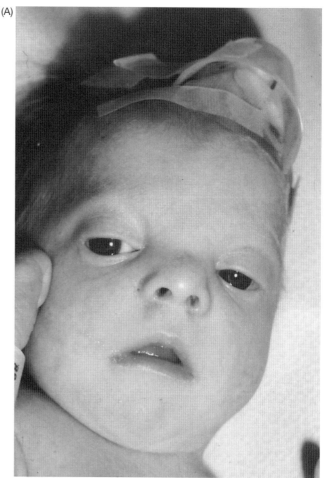

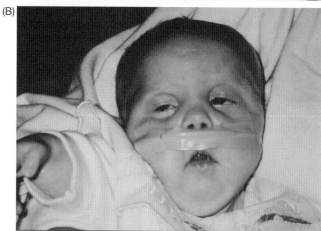

FIGURE 17S.1 A AND B  Facial features in SLOS. Note ptosis, anteverted nares, and facial hypotonia.

  - **Otopalatodigital syndrome, type II** (MIM 304120)
    - Cleft palate, micrognathia more severe than in SLOS, face dissimilar and hands distinctive
  - **Trisomy 13\***
    - Polydactyly and CHD overlap with SLOS, but face is dissimilar.

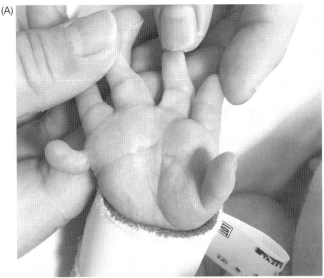

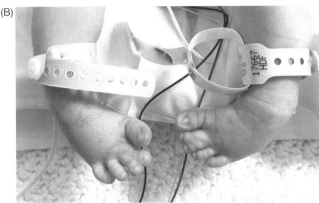

FIGURE 17S.2 Limb findings in SLOS include (A) postaxial polydactyly of hands or feet and (B) characteristic Y-shaped 2–3 toe syndactyly.

o **Talipes equinovarous–atrial septal defect–Robin sequence–persistence of left superior vena cava syndrome** (TARP, MIM 311900)
  ▪ X-linked recessive, due to variants in *RBM10*
  ▪ Hypotonia, cleft palate, micrognathia, CHD, occasional polydactyly
  ▪ Clubfeet are more common in TARP than in SLOS.

## Evaluation and Management

• Family history: consanguinity, reproductive loss, siblings with IUGR, microcephaly or congenital anomalies
• Note distinctive features: ptosis, ambiguous genitalia, Y-shaped 2–3 toe syndactyly. Examine palate carefully; visualize uvula.
• Evaluate for associated abnormalities.
  o Brain imaging: US, MRI
  o Echocardiogram

o Biochemical testing, serial LFTs
o Abdominal US; rectal biopsy if Hirschsprung disease is suspected
• Diagnostic testing
  o 7-DHC: consistently elevated; diagnostic
  o *DHCR7* gene analysis: sequencing and, if necessary, deletion/duplication testing
    ▪ Specific pathogenic variants may correlate with severity and prognosis.
  o Gene panel or exome sequencing may unexpectedly detect SLOS in mildly affected children with poor growth or hypotonia who lack recognizable dysmorphic or other cardinal features of SLOS.

*Pearl*: Serum cholesterol can be low, but it is an unreliable sign in SLOS. A low cholesterol value supports the diagnosis of SLOS, but a normal value does not exclude it.

• Confer with specialists as needed: ophthalmology, gastroenterology, neurology.
• Manage feeding problems.
  o G tube is often needed.
• Consider dietary therapy and nutritionist consult.
  o Fat-soluble vitamin supplements
  o Most patients are treated with cholesterol supplementation, which may improve cholestasis, behavior, motor skills, and growth, although data on benefits are conflicting.
    ▪ Cholesterol does not cross the blood–brain barrier. No pharmacologic treatment improves or prevents ID in SLOS.
    ▪ Start oral cholesterol supplementation at 100 mg/kg/day, divided TID.
    ▪ Hospital pharmacy can compound purified cholesterol powder or a crystalline or aqueous suspension
    ▪ Liquid pasteurized egg yolks are a food-based source of cholesterol.
• Avoid drugs that increase 7-DHC levels: haloperidol, trazadone, aripiprazole (Abilify).
• Refer to SLOS support group.
  o http://www.smithlemliopitz.com
• Refer to early infant developmental program.
• Consider participation in ongoing clinical trials using statins and antioxidants. www.clinicaltrials.gov
  o Research may offer improved therapeutic targets.

## Further Reading

Bianconi SE, Cross JL, Wassif CA, et al. (2015) Pathogenesis, epidemiology, diagnosis and clinical aspects of Smith–Lemli–Opitz syndrome. Expert Opin Orphan Drugs. 3:267–80. PMID 25734025

Diaz-Stransky A, Tierney E. (2012) Cognitive and behavioral aspects of Smith–Lemli–Opitz syndrome. Am J Med Genet C Semin Med Genet. 160C:295–300. PMID 23042585

Donoghue SE, Pitt JJ, Boneh A, White SM. (2018) Smith-Lemli-Opitz syndrome: clinical and biochemical correlates. J Pediatr Endocrinol Metab. 31(4):451–459. PMID 29455191

Haas D, Haege G, Hoffmann GF, Burgard P. (2013) Prenatal presentation and diagnostic evaluation of suspected Smith–Lemli–Opitz

(RSH) syndrome. Am J Med Genet A. 161A:1008–11. PMID 23532938

Nowaczyk MJ, Irons MB. (2012) Smith–Lemli–Opitz syndrome: Phenotype, natural history, and epidemiology. Am J Med Genet C Semin Med Genet. 160C:250–62. PMID 2305995

Witsch-Baumgartner M, Lanthaler B. (2015) Birthday of a syndrome: 50 years anniversary of Smith–Lemli–Opitz syndrome. Eur J Hum Genet. 23:277–8. PMID 24824134

# 18S

## VATER / VACTERL Association

## Definition

- VATER/VACTERL association (MIM 192350) defines a group of congenital anomalies that occur together, in various combinations, more often than expected by chance.
  - VATER or VACTERL, used interchangeably here, is not a "syndrome" because there is no evidence for a single etiology.
- Etiology: unknown but likely heterogeneous
  - Homozygous variants in *HAAO* and *KYNU* have been reported in 4 affected patients with cardiac, renal, limb and vertebral anomalies and low nicotinamide adenine dinucleotide (NAD) levels. These genes encode enzymes in the kynurenine pathway that produces NAD from tryptophan. Similar defects in the embryos of null mice were reversed with dietary niacin supplementation. (Shi et al, 2017)
    - Usually sporadic
    - Low recurrence risk when features are typical
    - Risk factors
  - ART
    - Esophageal atresia aOR 4.5
    - Anorectal atresia aOR 3.7

## Diagnosis

- VATER/VACTERL is an acronym.
  - *V*ertebral defects (or *V*SD)
  - *A*nal atresia (Figure 18S.1)
  - *T*racheo*e*sophageal (TE) fistula
  - *R*enal or *r*adial (Figure 18S.2) defects
  - VACTERL adds a "C" for *C*ardiac* and an "L" for *L*imb.*
  - Other features
    - Single umbilical artery
    - Normal BW
    - Lack of dysmorphic features or neurologic signs
- The diagnosis is clinical. Other causes must be excluded.
  - Requires three anomalies in the VATER spectrum
  - No anomalies outside the VATER spectrum

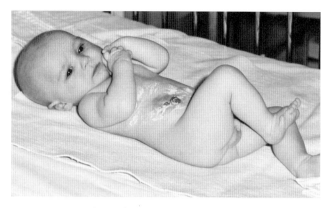

FIGURE 18S.1 Infant with VATERL association has an imperforate anus and an abnormal fifth metatarsal and little toe. Note his normal birth weight and nondysmophic face.

## Differential Diagnosis

- Chromosome anomalies
  - Aneuploidy: **Down syndrome,** * **trisomy 18** *
  - **22q11.2 deletion syndrome** * (MIM 192430)
  - Microdeletions of 7q, 13q, 16q24.1 (*FOXF1*), Xq26 (*ZIC3*)
  - **Maternal uniparental disomy for chr 16** (matUPD16)
    - Occurs when a trisomy 16 conceptus loses the paternal copy of chr 16 to restore disomy
    - Clinical features: TE fistula, anal anomalies,* hydronephrosis, renal* agenesis, absent gall bladder, single umbilical artery
      - Features atypical for VATER: respiratory failure
- Teratogens
  - **Maternal pregestational diabetes** *
    - VACTERL spectrum anomalies are more common in infants of poorly controlled pregestational diabetic mothers.
    - Features atypical for VATER: ear and brain anomalies, sacral agenesis, preaxial polydactyly
  - **Valproic acid embryopathy**
    - Present in ~10% of exposed infants

- Clinical features: radial ray defects; cardiac, renal anomalies
- Features atypical for VATER: low BW 10%, spina bifida 1–3%, tall forehead, flat nasal bridge, shallow philtral ridges, thin upper lip, cleft palate (Figures 6.2, 19.1)
- **Alveolar capillary dysplasia** (MIM 265380)
  - Heterozygous deletion or pathogenic variant in *FOXF1* at chr 16q24.1
  - Clinical features: anal and other GI atresias, cardiac, renal anomalies in 80%
    - Features atypical for VATER: lethal lung disorder
- **CHARGE syndrome** * (MIM 214800)
  - Autosomal dominant disorder, due to pathogenic variant in *CHD7*
  - Clinical features: cardiac anomalies, TE fistula
    - Features atypical for VATER: coloboma, choanal atresia, cranial nerve involvement, IUGR (Figures 10S.1, 10S.2)
- **Currarino syndrome** (MIM 175450)
  - Autosomal dominant trait, caused by pathogenic variant in *MNX1*
    - Or a **7q deletion, that includes 7q36.3**
  - Clinical features: anal anomalies, "sickle-shaped" sacrum, intraspinal or presacral mass (anterior meningomyelocele), sacral or pelvic teratoma, tethered cord, urogenital anomalies, bicornuate uterus
- **Fanconi anemia** (MIM 227650)
  - Autosomal recessive chromosome instability disorders that cause increased chromosome breakage with DEB
  - Clinical features: thumb anomalies, TE atresia, and other VATER anomalies affect 33% of children with Fanconi anemia (Figure 18S.3).

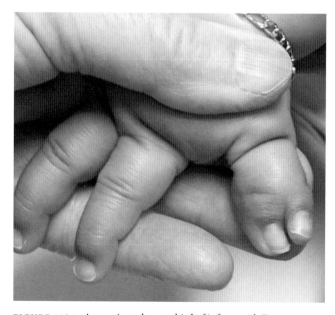

FIGURE 18S.3 Approximately one-third of infants with Fanconi anemia have congenital anomalies in the VATER/VACTERL spectrum. As a "rule of thumb," test any child with a thumb anomaly for Fanconi anemia with a chromosome breakage study.

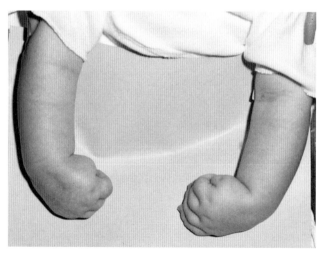

FIGURE 18S.2 The same infant has clubbed hands because of radial hypoplasia.

- Median age for aplastic anemia is 7 years.
- Features atypical for VATER: microcephaly,* ptosis, microphthalmia, café au lait macules
  - **VATER + hydrocephalus** (MIM 300514)
    - X-linked trait, due to hemizygous pathogenic variant in *FANCB*
- **Feingold syndrome** (MIM 164280)
  - Autosomal dominant trait, caused by mutation in *MYCN*
  - Clinical features: esophageal, duodenal, or other GI atresia, hypoplastic thumbs; clinodactyly, toe syndactyly
- **Holt–Oram syndrome** (MIM 142900)
  - Autosomal dominant disorder, due to pathogenic variant in *TBX5*
    - Often familial with an affected parent
  - Clinical features: typically secundum type ASD or VSD; triphalangeal thumb, upper limb anomalies may be severe
- **Mandibulofacial dysostosis with microcephaly—Guion–Almeida type** (MIM 610536)
  - Autosomal dominant syndrome, caused by pathogenic variant in *EFTUD2*
  - Clinical features: thumb anomalies, esophageal atresia
    - Features atypical for VATER: microcephaly, ear anomalies, ID (Figure 12.4)
- **Thrombocytopenia absent radius syndrome** (TAR, MIM 274000)
  - Deletion at 1q21 (includes *RBM8A*) on one allele, and an unusual SNP in *RBM8A* on the other
  - Clinical features: bilateral radial defects; thumbs present
    - Cardiac and renal malformations
    - Features atypical for VATER: thrombocytopenia
- **Townes–Brocks syndrome** (MIM 107480)
  - Autosomal dominant disorder, caused by pathogenic variant in or deletion of *SALL1*
  - Clinical features: imperforate anus, thumb, renal, and cardiac malformations
    - Features atypical for VATER: abnormal ears, hearing deficit (Figure 24.2)
- **VACTERL anomalies with cryptorchidism and without limb anomalies**
  - Heterozygous pathogenic variant in *FGF8*
- **X-linked visceral heterotaxy-1** (VACTERL association with or without hydrocephalus, MIM 306955)
  - X-linked disorder, caused by hemizygous pathogenic variant in *ZIC3*
  - Clinical features: heterotaxy, VATER anomalies
    - Features atypical for VATER: hydrocephalus, cleft palate, ear anomalies, hypertelorism
  - VACTERL-H (hydrocephalus) can be autosomal recessive (MIM 276950).

## Evaluation and Management

- Pregnancy history: ART, teratogens, maternal diabetes mellitus
- Family history: other affected individuals, X-linked inheritance

*Pearl*: Consider diabetic embryopathy in every infant with VATER/VACTERL spectrum anomalies.

- Identify other congenital anomalies.
  - Head US, spine radiographs, abdominal US, echocardiogram
  - VCUG: when there are structural renal anomalies
- Chromosome testing
  - Chromosomal microarray: ~2% yield
  - Chromosome breakage study (DEB) for Fanconi anemia, especially with microcephaly or thumb anomalies
- Clinical features should guide further gene testing.
  - *ZIC3*: X-linked family history of cardiac defects
  - Methylation test for maternal UPD16 when microarray is normal
  - Consider exome sequencing trio, when microarray and DEB tests are negative *and* features are atypical (low BW, dysmorphic, microcephalic) *or* family history is positive.
- Expect normal growth and development; re-evaluate if they are not.

## Further Reading

Alter BP, Giri N. (2016) Thinking of VACTERL-H? Rule out Fanconi anemia according to PHENOS. Am J Med Genet A. 170:1520–4. PMID 27028275

Beauregard-Lacroix E, Tardif J, Lemyre E, et al. (2017) Genetic testing in a cohort of complex esophageal atresia. Mol Syndromol. 8(5):236–43. PMID 28878607

Brosens E, Ploeg M, van Bever Y, et al. (2014) Clinical and etiological heterogeneity in patients with tracheo-esophageal malformations and associated anomalies. Eur J Med Genet. 57:440–52. PMID 24931924

Chung B, Shaffer LG, Keating S, et al. (2011) From VACTERL-H to heterotaxy: Variable expressivity of ZIC3-related heterotaxy disorders. Am J Med Genet Part A. 155A:1123–8. PMID 21465648

Shaw-Smith C. (2010) Genetic factors in esophageal atresia, tracheo-esophageal fistula and the VACTERL association: Roles for FOXF1 and the 16q24.1 FOX transcription factor gene cluster, and review of the literature. Eur J Med Genet. 53:6–13. PMID 19822228

Shi H, Enriquez A, Rapadas M, et al. (2017) NAD deficiency, congenital malformations, and niacin supplementation. N Engl J Med. 377:544–552. PMID 28792876

van den Hondel D, Wijers CH, van Bever Y, et al. (2016) Patients with anorectal malformation and upper limb anomalies: Genetic evaluation is warranted. Eur J Pediatr. 175:489–97. PMID 26498647

Zhang R, Marsch F, Kause F et al. (2017) Array-based molecular karyotyping in 115 VATER/VACTERL and VATER/VACTERL-like patients identifies disease-causing copy number variations. Birth Defects Res. 109:1063–9. PMID 28605140

# 19S

## Williams Syndrome

## Definition

- Williams syndrome (Williams–Beuren syndrome, WS, MIM 194050) is an autosomal dominant contiguous gene deletion disorder caused by a 1.55 Mb (~95%) or a 1.84 Mb (5–10%) microdeletion at chromosome 7q11.23.
  - Encompasses 26–28 genes, including the elastin gene, *ELN*
  - Atypical chromosome 7q deletions account for 2%.
- 1 in 7,500 live births
- Usually sporadic and de novo; recurrence risk is low.
  - Rarely familial; MZ twins are concordant.
  - A parental inversion of chromosome 7 that includes the Williams syndrome critical region (WSCR) increases the risk for offspring with the syndrome.
    - 24% of unaffected parents, who transmitted the deleted chromosome 7 to their children with WS, have this inversion.
    - The risk for WS in subsequent offspring remains low, ~1/1,750.

## Diagnosis

- Clinical features: characteristic "elfin" face, puffy periorbital areas (Figure 19S.1), epicanthal folds, hypotelorism, depressed nasal bridge, short upturned nose, long philtrum, full lips, wide mouth, lax cheeks (Figure 19S.2), nail hypoplasia. Blue-eyed infants have a stellate iris pattern.
  - Cardiac: structural anomalies and/or symptomatic narrowing of the arteries in 80–90%, may not be detected prenatally
    - Most common cardiac anomalies: supravalvular aortic stenosis (SVAS) (75%), peripheral pulmonary artery stenosis (PPAS) (50%).
      - SVAS and PPAS generally improve with time.
      - Approximately one-third of patients have both lesions, raising risk for significant cardiac hypertrophy and adverse outcomes.
        - Bilateral outflow tract obstruction poses the highest risk for cardiovascular complications during anesthesia.

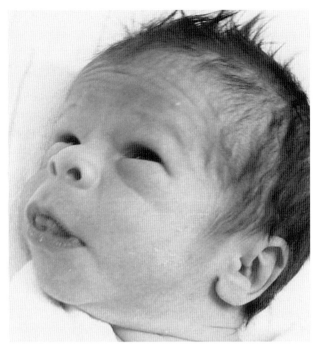

FIGURE 19S.1 The so-called elfin face of the newborn with Williams syndrome can be mildly coarse with periorbital fullness, infraorbital creases, short nose, long phitrum, and a wide mouth.

- Narrowing of systemic arteries: coronary, renal, aorta (coarctation, hypoplasia)
- Structural cardiac anomalies: VSD, bicuspid aortic valve, valvular aortic or valvular pulmonary stenosis, total

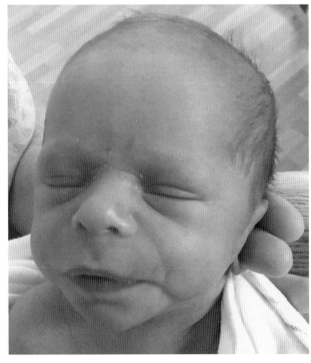

FIGURE 19S.2 This infant with Williams syndrome has a long phitrum, wide mouth, full lower lip, and lax cheeks.

anomalous pulmonary venous return, mitral and aortic valve prolapse or insufficiency
- QTc prolongation in 13%
- Hypertension: occasional in newborns; frequent in older children

*Pearl*: The risk of sudden death in WS is 25–100 times higher than expected for an age-matched population.

- Renal anomalies ~25%
- Musculoskeletal and connective tissues: scoliosis, kyphosis, radioulnar synostosis, joint laxity
- Growth: at least one growth parameter is <3rd percentile in 20%.
  - Poor weight gain in infancy 70%
- Endocrine
  - Hypercalcemia, hypercalcuria ~15%, resolves by 4 years
  - Elevated thyroid-stimulating hormone (TSH) 30%
- Feeding difficulties >80%: failure to thrive, colic, irritability, GE reflux, poor suck/swallow, constipation. G tube occasionally needed
- Neurodevelopment
  - Hypotonia in infancy
  - ID 75%, usually mild. Mean full-scale IQ 55–60 (range, 40–100). Anxiety is common. Autism in some
  - Cognitive profile: highly social, "cocktail party" personality. Verbal abilities exceed visual–spatial. Often musical. Hyperacusis
- Later: diabetes mellitus, celiac disease, precocious puberty 18%, short stature, widely spaced teeth
  - Frequent contractures and stiffness
  - Hypertension ≤50%
- Mean age at diagnosis: WS with a cardiac defect: ~5 years; WS without one: 10 years
  - Prenatal diagnosis is uncommon.
    - Occurs when prenatal microarray is ordered for IUGR
- Genetic testing
  - Chromosome microarray in all infants with SVAS.
  - FISH with *ELN* probe rapidly detects del 7q11.23.
  - Microarray delineates the size and extent of the deletion; preferred over conventional chromosome analysis or FISH.
  - Rarely, a parent is diagnosed with WS only after the birth of an affected child.

## Differential Diagnosis

- **Supravalvar aortic stenosis** (SVAS, MIM 185500)
  - Autosomal dominant trait, caused by pathogenic variant or intragenic deletion of *ELN*, which is located in the WSCR on chr 7

- Clinical features shared with WS: SVAS, cutis laxa, joint laxity
  - "SVAS plus": a smaller atypical deletion in WSCR that includes some genes adjacent to *ELN*, causes an overlapping phenotype
- **Noonan syndrome**\* (MIM 163950)
  - Autosomal dominant trait, caused by a heterozygous pathogenic variant in *PTPN11* or a related gene in the same pathway
  - Clinical features shared with WS: primarily right-sided cardiac lesions, puffy and coarse face in the newborn period
- **Smith–Magenis syndrome** (MIM 182290)
  - An interstitial deletion at chromosome 17p11.2
  - Clinical features shared with WS: short stature, cardiac anomalies, hypersensitivity to sound (Figure 1.3)
- *PPM1D*-**related syndrome** (MIM 617450)
  - Autosomal dominant trait, caused by pathogenic variant in *PPM1D*
  - Clinical features shared with WS: feeding and GI difficulties, short stature, ID, anxiety, ADHD, hypersensitivity to sound
- Other dysmorphic syndromes with cardiac anomalies
  - **Chromosome 22q11.2 deletion**\* (MIM 188400)
  - **Kabuki syndrome** (MIM 147920)

## Evaluation and Management

- Check calcium levels. Consult Pediatric Endocrinology for hypercalcemia.
  - Monitor calcium q 4–6 months in the first 2 years.
  - Assess dietary calcium intake. Utilize low-calcium formula if necessary.
  - Treat hypercalcemia with hydration.
    - Persistent symptomatic hypercalcemia may respond to bisphosphonate (Pamidronate) or oral steroids.
  - Check $T_4$, TSH.

*Pearl*: Avoid multivitamins in Williams syndrome: Absorption of calcium from the gut is increased in WS and vitamin D promotes $Ca^{2+}$ absorption.

- Consult Pediatric Cardiology during the newborn period.
  - Echocardiogram

- Repeat echocardiogram at regular intervals, even when initial study is normal.
  - SVAS and PPAS may develop over a short period of time.
- Measure blood pressure in all four limbs.
- ECG for long QTc
- Renal: US for structural anomalies; uric acid, BUN, creatinine
- Consult Anesthesiology prior to surgery or sedation: higher chance of cardiovascular complications, especially with bilateral outflow tract obstruction.
- Genetic testing
  - Microarray or rapid dx with FISH for *ELN* at 7q11.23 with reflex to microarray
- Genetic referral. Consider how to give the news to the family (Waxler et al., 2013).
- Refer for early infant intervention services
- Anticipate common medical problems: poor feeding, GE reflux, prolonged colic, chronic constipation, chronic otitis media, strabismus, rectal prolapse, abdominal or inguinal hernia, urinary tract infection, hypertension
- Follow AAP health supervision guidelines for WS.
  - Up-to-date summary with support group contact information is available at http://www.genereviews.com.
  - Use specific growth charts for Williams syndrome.

*Pearl*: Caring for infants with WS can be challenging in the early months due to irritability, colic, and failure to thrive. Provide parental support.

## Further Reading

Committee on Genetics of American Academy of Pediatrics. (2001) Health care supervision for children with Williams syndrome. Pediatrics, 107:1192–1204. PMID 11331709

Matisoff AJ, Olivieri L, Schwartz JM, et al. (2015) Risk assessment and anesthetic management of patients with Williams syndrome: A comprehensive review. Paediatr Anaesth. 25:1207–15. PMID 26456018

Morris CA. (2017) Williams syndrome. In: Pagon RA, Adam MP, Bird TD, et al. editors. GeneReviews [Internet]. Seattle, WA: University of Washington, Seattle; 1993–2018. PMID 20301427

Pober BR. (2010) Williams–Beuren syndrome. N Engl J Med. 362:239–52. PMID 20089974

Waxler JL, Cherniske EM, Dieter K, et al. (2013) Hearing from parents: The impact of receiving the diagnosis of Williams syndrome in their child. Am J Med Genet Part A. 161A:534–41. PMID 23401422

# Index